Principles
and Practice
of
Sleep Medicine
in the Child

DATE DUE FOR RETURN

This book may be recalled before the above date.

Principles and Practice of Sleep Medicine in the Child

RICHARD FERBER, MD

Assistant Professor of Neurology
Harvard Medical School
Boston, Massachusetts
Director, Center for Pediatric Sleep Disorders
Children's Hospital
Boston, Massachusetts

MEIR KRYGER, MD

Professor of Medicine
University of Manitoba
Director, Sleep Laboratory
St. Boniface General Hospital
Winnipeg, Manitoba

W.B. SAUNDERS COMPANY

An Imprint of Elsevier Science

W.B. SAUNDERS COMPANY

An Imprint of Elsevier Science

The Curtis Center
Independence Square West
Philadelphia, Pennsylvania 19106

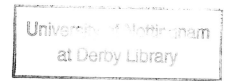
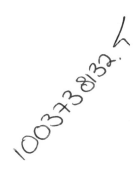
Library of Congress Cataloging-in-Publication Data

Principles and practice of sleep medicine in the child / [edited by] Richard Ferber, Meir Kryger.

p.   cm.

ISBN 0–7216–4761–8

1. Sleep disorders in children.   I. Ferber, Richard.   II. Kryger, Meir H.   [DNLM: 1. Sleep
   Disorders—in infancy & childhood.   2. Pediatrics.   WM 188 P9575 1995]

RJ506.S55P75 1995   618.92′8498—dc20

DNLM/DLC   94–37667

PRINCIPLES AND PRACTICE OF SLEEP MEDICINE IN THE CHILD   ISBN 0–7216–4761–8

Printed in the United States of America.

Last digit is the print number: 9   8   7   6   5

This book is dedicated to our families:

Geri, Matthias, and Thaddeus Ferber
Barbara, Shelley, Michael, and Steven Kryger

CONTRIBUTORS

Christine Acebo, Ph.D.
Associate Professor (Research), Sleep Research Laboratory, Department of Psychiatry and Human Behavior, E.P. Bradley Hospital/Brown University, East Providence, Rhode Island

Monitoring of Sleep in Neonates and Young Children

Thomas F. Anders, M.D.
Professor of Psychiatry, University of California Davis, Davis; Chief of Psychiatry, University of California Davis Medical Center, Sacramento, California

Normal Sleep in Neonates and Children

Viajya Appareddy, M.D.
Private Practice, Chattanooga, Tennessee

Normal Sleep in Neonates and Children

Ronald L. Ariagno, M.D.
Professor of Pediatrics, Stanford Medical Center, Stanford University, Stanford, California

Sleep and the Sudden Infant Death Syndrome

Michel Billiard, M.D.
Professor of Neurology, School of Medicine, Montpellier; Chef de Service, Neurology B, Gui de Chauliac Hospital, Montpellier, France

Narcolepsy, Kleine-Levin Syndrome, and Other Causes of Sleepiness in Children

Lawrence W. Brown, M.D.
Assistant Professor of Neurology and Pediatrics, University of Pennsylvania,
School of Medicine, Philadelphia; Department of Neurology, Children's Hospital of Philadelphia, Philadelphia, Pennsylvania

Narcolepsy, Kleine-Levin Syndrome, and Other Causes of Sleepiness in Children; Sleep in Children with Neurologic Problems

John L. Carroll, M.D.
Associate Professor of Pediatrics, The Johns Hopkins Children's Center; Director, The Johns Hopkins Pediatric Sleep and Breathing Disorders Center, Baltimore, Maryland

Primary Snoring in Children; Obstructive Sleep Apnea Syndrome in Infants and Children: Clinical Features and Pathophysiology; Obstructive Sleep Apnea Syndrome in Infants and Children: Diagnosis and Management; Sleep and Respiratory Disease in Children

Mary A. Carskadon, Ph.D.
Professor of Psychiatry and Human Behavior, Brown University, School of Medicine, Department of Psychiatry, East Providence; Director of Chronobiology, E.P. Bradley Hospital, Riverside, Rhode Island

Sleep and Its Disorders in Adolescence

Ronald E. Dahl, M.D.
Associate Professor of Psychiatry and Pediatrics, University of Pittsburgh, School of Medicine, Pittsburgh; Director, Child and Adolescent Sleep Laboratory, Western Psychiatric Institute and Clinic, Pittsburgh, Pennsylvania

Sleep and Its Disorders in Adolescence; Sleep in Behavioral and Emotional Disorders

Richard Ferber, M.D.

Assistant Professor of Neurology, Harvard Medical School, Boston; Director, Center for Pediatric Sleep Disorders, Children's Hospital, Boston, Massachusetts

Introduction: Pediatric Sleep Disorders Medicine; Assessment of Sleep Disorders in the Child; Sleeplessness in Children; Circadian Rhythm Sleep Disorders in Childhood; Sleepwalking, Confusional Arousals, and Sleep Terrors in the Child

Patrick C. Friman, Ph.D.

Associate Professor, Pediatrics and Otolaryngology, Creighton and University of Nebraska Schools of Medicine, Omaha; Director of Clinical Research, Father Flanagan's Boys Home, Boys Town, Nebraska

Nocturnal Enuresis in the Child

Steven F. Glotzbach, Ph.D.

Senior Research Scientist, Program in Human Biology, Stanford University, Stanford, California

Sleep and the Sudden Infant Death Syndrome

Christian Guilleminault, M.D.

Professor of Psychiatry, Stanford University, Sleep Disorders Clinic, Palo Alto, California

Sleep in Children with Neurologic Problems

Ronald M. Harper, Ph.D.

Professor of Anatomy, Brain Research Institute, University of California, School of Medicine, Los Angeles, California

Sleep and the Sudden Infant Death Syndrome

Gerald M. Loughlin, M.D.

Professor of Pediatrics, The Johns Hopkins Children's Center; Director, Eudowood Division of Pediatric Respiratory Sciences, Baltimore, Maryland

Primary Snoring in Children; Obstructive Sleep Apnea Syndrome in Infants and Children: Clinical Features and Pathophysiology; Obstructive Sleep Apnea Syndrome in Infants and Children: Diagnosis and Management; Sleep and Respiratory Disease in Children

Betsy Lozoff, M.D., M.S.

Professor of Pediatrics, University of Michigan, School of Medicine, Ann Arbor; Director, Center for Human Growth and Development, University of Michigan, Ann Arbor, Michigan

Culture and Family: Influences on Childhood Sleep Practices and Problems

Mark W. Mahowald, M.D.

Associate Professor in Neurology, University of Minnesota Medical School, Minneapolis; Director, Minnesota Regional Sleep Disorders Center, Department of Neurology, Hennepin County Medical Center, Minneapolis, Minnesota

Sleepwalking, Confusional Arousals, and Sleep Terrors in the Child; Nonarousal Parasomnias in the Child

Paul Maistros, M.D.

Fountain Valley Regional Medical Center, Sleep Disorders Laboratory, Fountain Valley, California

Sleep in Children with Neurologic Problems

Henrique Rigatto, M.D.

Professor of Pediatrics, University of Manitoba, Winnipeg; Director of Neonatal Research, Health Sciences Centre, Winnipeg, Manitoba

Control of Breathing During Sleep in the Fetus and Neonate

Gerald Rosen, M.D.

Assistant Professor, Department of Pediatrics, University of Minnesota Medical School, Minneapolis; Associate Physician, Department of Pediatrics, and Pediatrician, Minnesota Regional Sleep Disorders Center, Hennepin County Medical Center, Minneapolis, Minnesota

Sleepwalking, Confusional Arousals, and Sleep Terrors in the Child

Avi Sadeh, D.Sc.

Lecturer, Department of Psychology, Tel Aviv University, Tel Aviv, Israel

Normal Sleep in Neonates and Children

Evelyn B. Thoman, Ph.D.

Professor, Biobehavioral Sciences and Psychology, University of Connecticut, Storrs, Connecticut

Monitoring of Sleep in Neonates and Young Children

Michael J. Thorpy, M.D.

Associate Professor of Neurology, Albert Einstein College of Medicine, Albert Einstein School of Medicine, New York; Director, Sleep-Wake Disorders Center, Montefiore Medical Center, New York, New York

Nonarousal Parasomnias in the Child

Marc Weissbluth, M.D.

Associate Professor of Pediatrics, Northwestern University Medical School, Chicago; Attending Pediatrician, Children's Memorial Hospital, Chicago, Illinois

Colic

FOREWORD

In the very broad multidisciplinary area of sleep medicine, it is an entirely felicitous event that the diagnosis and treatment of sleep problems in infants and children will at last be represented and fostered by a comprehensive textbook. My first two sleep apnea patients were children, about 20 years ago.

A commonplace and often poignant tragedy in adults, the consequences of an unrecognized sleep disorder are often much more heartbreaking and far-reaching in children. To the extent that the burgeoning knowledge base about pediatric sleep disorders is widely scattered and difficult to encompass, it is now happily in one place.

Recently, I traveled to several medical centers that have organized and comprehensive programs dealing with sleep disorders in the child. I have been struck by the fact that these disorders are not widely known and, as with many other problems, require a uniquely pediatric approach. By now, those of us who have practiced sleep medicine for the two decades of its existence are able to feel an enormous satisfaction for lives resurrected and families uplifted. Nowhere is this more satisfying to contemplate than when it happens to infants, children, and their families. The only frustration has been the urgent desire for the practice of pediatric sleep medicine to increase 100-fold. This magnificent textbook will assure and foster progress.

WILLIAM C. DEMENT, M.D., PH.D.

Lowell W. and Josephine Q. Berry
Professor of Psychiatry and Behavioral Sciences
Director, Sleep Disorders Center
Stanford University School of Medicine
Stanford, California

ACKNOWLEDGMENTS

The editors wish to thank the staff at W.B. Saunders for their patience, perseverance, and help at every stage in the production of this volume. In particular, we wish to thank Judy Fletcher, Lorraine Kilmer, and Frank Polizzano. We also wish to credit the many secretaries, copy-editors, illustrators, and others without whose help such a volume could never have been completed.

The field of sleep medicine in the child would not have been possible without the scientific foundations laid by Nathaniel Kleitman, Arthur Parmelee, Jr., and Heinz FR Prechtl. We are also grateful to our colleagues and to the American Sleep Disorders Association who supported the field of pediatric sleep disorders medicine from the outset.

Finally, we wish to thank our wives, children, and other family members for their patience, support, and understanding.

PREFACE

This book is for any professional who sees children (or parents of children) with sleep problems including pediatricians, primary care physicians, nurses, mental health workers, pulmonologists, neurologists, and specialists in sleep medicine. This volume deals exclusively with sleep disorders in the child and is a companion to *Principles and Practice of Sleep Medicine,* 2nd edition, which focuses on similar issues in the adult and also reviews the biology of sleep in detail.

Although sleep disorders in children are very common, until recently the body of knowledge in pediatric sleep medicine was too limited to warrant a textbook devoted to this topic. In recent years, however, a robust scientifically based body of knowledge has emerged, and the tools to diagnose and effectively treat children with sleep disorders are now available. The first part of this book primarily reviews normal sleep patterns and clinical assessment techniques in the child. The second part deals with specific problems related to the sleep period, problems that may be developmental, neurologic, psychologic/psychiatric, or medical in origin.

Children with sleep problems are not merely small adults with sleep problems. Although nominally many of the same sleep disorders are seen in both children and adults (for example, sleeplessness and sleep-associated breathing abnormalities), the presentations, diagnoses, and treatments are quite different in the two groups. Cultural and parental factors turn out to be of great importance in children, and in many cases, changes in parental behavior or expectations turn out to be at least as important as changes made directly in the child.

Only by understanding the interactions among normal sleep patterns, parental desires, patient needs, and pathologic states can a rational approach to the evaluation and treatment of sleep disorders in children become feasible.

RICHARD FERBER
Boston

MEIR KRYGER
Winnipeg

CONTENTS

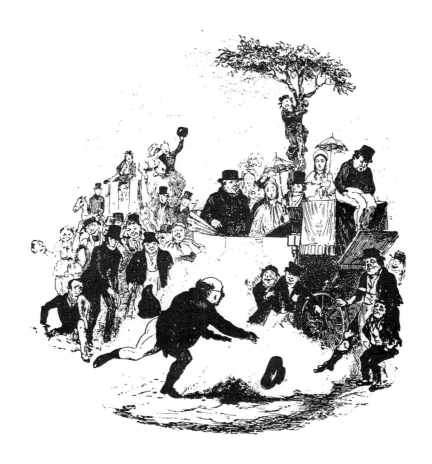

"...and on the box sat a fat and red-faced boy, in the state of somnolency."

Charles Dickens introduces us to Joe (in the upper right of the drawing). Dickens described many of the features of sleep apnea 120 years before this syndrome was identified by medical science.

Dickens, C.: The Posthumous Papers of the Pickwick Club, London, Chapman & Hall, Published in Serial Form 1836–1837.

Introduction: Pediatric Sleep Disorders Medicine

RICHARD FERBER

The general physiologic patterns of rapid eye movement (REM) and (at least after the early months) non-rapid eye movement (NREM) sleep are practically the same in children as in adults, and for the most part, the general physiologic patterns seen as part of the various sleep disorders are similar. Nevertheless, there are important differences. Some are physiologic in nature, and many reflect aspects of behavior, psychology, and development.

Important areas and questions to be considered are: physiology; behavior; psychology; parent–child interactions; disorders specific to childhood; age-related differences in presentation, evaluation, and management; normal vs abnormal; presentation: whose complaints are being evaluated, whose desires are being treated, and is a true sleep disorder present or just a variation of normal; and age-dependent responses to treatment.

Physiology

In the developing fetus and newborn, NREM or quiet sleep is slower to evolve than REM or active sleep.[1–3] In the newborn, the electroencephalogram during NREM shows predominantly a tracé alternant rhythm with bursts of large-amplitude slow waves separated by 4 to 8 seconds of attenuated activity of mixed frequencies (see Chapters 2 and 6).[1] This pattern disappears within a few weeks and is replaced by one of more continuous slow activity. Spindles appear by 6 weeks and are most prominent at 4 to 6 months.[4, 5] Early spontaneous K-complexes are always present by 6 months, sometimes as early as 4 months.[4, 6] Certainly by the second half-year NREM becomes classifiable into substages, although the deeper stages predominate. Thereafter, the electrical patterns of REM and NREM progressively resemble those seen in the adult. Starting between 1 to 3 months there is progressive consolidation of sleep into sustained periods and progressive concentration of these periods into the night, while daytime sleep becomes organized into regularly recurring naps. The patterns of sleep stage cycling and sleep-wake alternation become increasingly mature and by 3 months there is a switch from sleep-onset REM to sleep-onset NREM (see Chapter 2).[7, 8] However, even after 1 year of age, stage 4 sleep in the child may be distinguished from that seen in the adult because there is much more delta activity (approaching 100% of the record) of much higher voltage (often 300 μV or more).

The length of the ultradian REM-NREM cycle slowly increases across childhood from about 50 minutes in infancy to the adult value of 90 minutes by adolescence.[9] On the other hand, the circadian clock is probably functional at birth at the adult rate and becomes clearly linked to the sleep-wake rhythms by 6 to 8 weeks, if not before (see Chapter 10).[10, 11] Even as sleep consolidates into the night, napping continues and only gradually diminishes to 3 naps per day between 3 to 6 months, 2 naps per day from 6 to 12 months, 1 nap soon after reaching age 1, and no naps starting around age 3. Then, as the child reaches middle childhood (after the toddler years but before adolescence), he enters a phase of maximal daytime wakefulness. He sleeps well at night and is so wide awake during the day that napping under most situations is rare. This wakefulness may be so marked that it may overcome any need for napping that might be expected from causes such as sleep loss, sleep apnea, or narcolepsy (factors that may still lead to increased sleep at night). Increased daytime sleepiness returns with puberty (see Chapter 3).[12, 13]

In very early infancy, sleep may be fragile and easily broken, and the youngster may have difficulty smoothly negotiating transitions from waking to sleep and between REM and NREM. Within several months, sleep usually becomes quite stable. Even though parents may complain that their child has "poor sleep" or "many wakings," periods of very deep NREM sleep do occur that are well maintained and from which it actually may be difficult for a child to be wakened. This naturally deep sleep predisposes a child to the various "disorders of arousal" seen commonly in early childhood (see Chapter 11).[14] The strong drive into stage 4 sleep, its stability, and the improved respiratory control seen in that state also mean that this sleep stage is rarely reduced even in children with severe sleep apnea—a fact that may partially explain the usual absence of severe sleepiness in children with this disorder (see Chapters 18 and 19).

Across childhood there is progressive movement to more fully adult patterns (including shorter sleep time, less napping, less deep sleep with decreased delta activity, and longer sleep cycles). By the end of adolescence, adult patterns are seen.

Behavior

Habits and various learned behavior patterns associated with sleep transitions are present at all ages after the earliest weeks; but the specifics are quite different at different ages. Infants may be held, rocked, walked about, nursed, or given a pacifier. Toddlers hopefully have long since learned "self-soothing" techniques that will get them through the night,[13] although bedtime rituals of reading stories and "tucking in" remain appropriate. Transitional objects are commonly used and ease the nighttime separations (see Chapter 7). Older children may begin to take on the bedtime routines more independently (read to themselves, listen to the radio), but parental contact remains important. Adolescents may be "independent" to the point of not wanting any parental participation at night; however,

they still may be so immature as to choose inappropriate nighttime behaviors (phone conversations or rock music into the early morning hours) and increasingly irregular schedules (see Chapter 3).

Psychology

Here perhaps most strikingly do the features seen across childhood differ from those seen in the adult. During the newborn's initial adjustment to the outside world, all care and nurturance come from others. Gradually, the infant comes to recognize and need his parents and miss them when they are not present. By the second half-year these separation issues may become quite prominent. As the youngster grows, he must learn to deal with siblings, share, control his impulses, and obey rules and limits. Language develops and with it the ability to make requests and demands. Frustrations and disappointments are no longer limited to whether one is fed, cuddled, properly cared for, and loved. There is toilet training, the start of daycare and school, and learning to deal with peers. Academic pressures gradually grow. Middle childhood is usually a time of relative calm preceding the complicated course of adolescence with its attendant physical changes and drives, school and peer pressures, and increasing independence.

A youngster's age, stage, and particular psychologic stresses must be taken into account when trying to understand the sleep difficulties that may also be occurring (see Chapter 6). Children at any age can be anxious, frightened, angry, or needy, but the causes are usually different from those seen in the adult. Learning difficulties, crowded classrooms, unempathetic teachers, frightening movies or television, scary stories, or parental fights, drunkenness, illness, separation, or death may tip the balance from control to chaos. Although fear of sleeping alone is common, its significance is certainly not the same at ages 2, 12, and 17. Major psychiatric disturbances (depression, mania, psychosis) and associated sleep disturbances may also appear during childhood, but they present differently, have different significance, and demand different treatment than in the adult (see Chapter 16).[15–17]

Parent–Child Interactions

Particularly in the early years, a child's life is centered around the home. Most of the interactions, the most intense and the most important, take place between parent and child. Ideally this should be a rewarding experience for both. But not all parents are able to provide a warm, loving, consistently nurturing environment, and not all children are easy to manage or even fun to be with. If these interactions do not go well, there may be tension, stress, and anger. A child who is needy emotionally may not be able to handle the immense challenges that take place at night: separation, darkness, fantasy. If his nighttime difficulties are met by lack of empathy, even anger, threats, and punishment, the youngster should be expected to have even more nighttime problems not less. On the other hand, if the parents' attempts to "nurture" are too zealous, then the child sees an absence of limits, a true lack of proper caretaking, and another source of anxiety.

These patterns of parent–child interactions may reflect aspects of the parents' own upbringing. Thus, the child cannot be evaluated in isolation; the family must be evaluated as a unit. The parents' desires, needs, and problems must be taken into consideration as well as those of the child (see Chapters 6 and 7).

Disorders Specific to Childhood

Although many disorders occur in both children and adults and are phenomenologically the same in both groups (even if they have different significance), some disorders are unique to childhood. The main problems confined to the infant are the sudden infant death syndrome (SIDS), apnea of infancy, and colic (see Chapters 8, 18, 19, 21). In toddlers and older children certain problems may be fairly unique, especially those reflecting inappropriate sleep schedules. These may occur because children do not set their own bed- and naptimes; their parents do. The parents may set these times based more on convenience, habit, desire, wishful thinking, or even punishment than on physiologic need (see Chapter 10). Other problems fairly unique to childhood reflect the habitual patterns established when parents become intimately associated with the sleep transition process (see Chapter 9).

Age-Related Differences in Presentation, Evaluation, and Management

Certain sleep disorders seen in children and adults may be phenomenologically the same

but still have differences in presentation, significance, cause, and required treatment. This is particularly true of obstructive sleep apnea (OSA) (see Chapters 18 and 19). In normal children respiratory obstructions are very rare, and an arbitrary value for apnea index is not very helpful in deciding on the need for intervention. Similarly, setting a 10-second criterion for significance of an apnea has little meaning in children with respiratory rates faster than adults. Different criteria for determining the need for treatment are necessary. Daytime sleepiness is often mild, subtle, or seemingly absent. The occurrence of ventricular arrhythmias and hence the risk of hypoxia-triggered cardiac deaths are much less, and except for obesity, the causes of the obstruction are generally different and so is the treatment (uvulopalatopharyngoplasty is only occasionally useful, adenotonsillectomy often is, and continuous positive airway pressure [CPAP] is generally not necessary).

A sleepwalking toddler may be difficult to distinguish from a toddler who remains very sleepy after fully waking at night. Confusional arousals, seen commonly in early childhood, are relatively rare in adults; whereas, full-blown sleep terrors are usually not seen in the early years. Partial arousals in young children may be developmental in nature and need little evaluation or treatment; whereas, in older children and adults, they may imply an underlying medical or psychologic disorder and must be handled differently (see Chapter 11).

Anxiety is seen at most ages, but obviously the causes, significance, and proper management in young children must be determined relative to the child's level of psychologic development.

Although a sleepless toddler and an insomniac adult may both be awake at night, they have little else in common. Although there may be some overlap of possible causes (pain, anxiety), the etiologies of this problem in young children (generally more behavioral and interactional) and hence the usual treatments are quite different.

Excessive daytime sleepiness in an adult usually is evident because of unwanted napping, but both sleepy and normally alert 2-year-olds take naps and in both the naps may be unavoidable, coming on in almost any situation. On the other hand, a pathologically sleepy preteen may nap only rarely but have unusually long nocturnal sleep. Milder sleepiness in the young child may be evident more by overactivity, inattentiveness, whining, and difficult behavior than by the appearance of sleep itself. A narcoleptic child rarely shows cataplexy and other associated features are probably absent (or, if present, are very difficult to ascertain by history) (see Chapter 14).

Normal vs Abnormal

When does normal become abnormal and when does abnormal become normal? The same event or occurrence in a child and an adult may be considered normal in one and abnormal in the other. The most obvious examples of this are napping and enuresis. Both are normal early on but become relatively uncommon after 3 to 5 years of age. At some point they are considered abnormal; but given the gradual decrease in both napping and sleep-associated micturition with increasing age, it seems unrealistic to say that these become "abnormal" at the fifth birthday. Similarly, if a 1-year-old child sleeps only 8 hours a night and does not nap, this would be considered "abnormal"; but if the same pattern is continued through adolescence, it becomes "normal." Sleepwalking is usually considered to be a sleep disorder in adults, but it is often considered a normal developmental feature in toddlers. Similarly, it is abnormal for an unmedicated adult to be almost unarousable from sleep, but this is normal behavior in toddlers. Finally, REM onsets are ordinarily normal only during the first 3 months of life.

The answers to these questions of normality are, therefore, not always clearcut. When a child with an apparent sleep disorder is evaluated, one must first try to decide if a disorder is even present. Adult criteria certainly do not apply.

Presentation: Whose Complaints Are Being Evaluated, Whose Desires Are Being Treated, and Is a True Sleep Disorder Present or Just a Variation of Normal?

Most often adult sleep disorder patients present with their own complaint. They feel something is wrong with their sleep and they want it improved. Even when a spouse is making the complaint, it is usually out of concern for the patient (except perhaps for snoring). Infants and young children never complain about their sleep. In fact, they may even be happy about the current state of affairs or at least they may want something different than the parents do. It is the parents who complain. Although they may be truly concerned about their child's health ("he's not getting enough sleep"), usually it is they who will be happier if the sleep pattern is changed. This is particularly true for bedtime difficulties or struggles, frequent wakings, nighttime feedings, early wakings, difficulty napping, refusal to sleep alone, enuresis, sleepwalking, sleep terrors, confusional arousals, and headbanging. The child may be getting sufficient sleep and be functioning quite well. The parents may not be. Two brief wakings at night cannot be considered abnormal, but if a parent must quickly cover the child each time and if the parent cannot return to sleep quickly, the parent has a complaint. In childhood, many sleep patterns are possible (early bedtime and early waking, late bedtime and late waking, long naps and short night sleep, short naps and long night sleep, one long nap, several short naps) and these may all be variations of normal. The problem may come when the particular patterns occurring are ones that conflict with the desires of the parents.

Older children may start to voice concerns about insomnia, bedwetting, nighttime fears, and occasionally daytime sleepiness. Now it is their own complaints that must be evaluated. Still, the parents' desires must be taken into consideration. A 10-year-old having difficulty falling asleep may not be allowed to read in bed as an adult might do. His parents complain that he does not fall asleep early enough, but the child might be quite happy (and healthy) with a later bedtime.

All of these considerations present a dilemma to the practitioner who should see himor herself as an advocate of the child. But since variations of sleep-wake patterns are common despite normal underlying physiology and psychology, parents may describe a "problem" when there is no real "abnormality." Parents may say they are worried that their child "does not get enough sleep," when they really mean that their child does not give them enough time for themselves. One should not want to "fix" a problem that is not there, such as with the inappropriate use of medication, but it is usually possible to adjust the child's sleep patterns (and the parents' expectations) to allow a satisfactory match. By so doing, much may have been done to settle the issue of the child's sleep within the family structure, although little may have been done for the child's sleep per se. In such circumstances, parental anger toward the child may decrease, the child may learn that he was not misbehaving or "bad," and the quality of life for that child within the family may improve. Thus, it is the child's sleep pattern relative to the entire family that must be faced. This is no small task; but the rewards for the child, and for the family, are enormous.

Age-Dependent Responses to Treatment

Young children with partial arousals may respond well to schedule adjustment, assurance of sufficient sleep, and parental instruction, but they may respond poorly to medication. Adolescents and adults with somnambulism or sleep terrors may respond only to medication and perhaps psychotherapy or self-hypnosis (see Chapter 11). Four-year-old children who wet the bed are difficult to treat and probably should not be treated. Eight-year-old children are relatively easy to treat (see Chapter 12). Adolescents and adults with enuresis may respond poorly to usual therapy. Insomniac adults certainly may be treated, but they are often very fixed in their ways and change usually comes slowly, over weeks or months. Children are much more adaptive. Sleepless children, even with a very chronic history, usually can be treated extremely rapidly with normal sleep patterns appearing within a few days to a week or so.

Conclusion

Pediatric sleep disorders medicine has as many differences from adult sleep disorders medicine as does the specialty of pediatrics from internal medicine. The organs are all the same and their functions are similar, but the organisms as a whole are quite different. This brings special challenges and special benefits, which justify the writing of this book devoted to sleep disorders medicine in the child.

References

1. Parmelee AH, Jr, Schulte FJ, Akiyama Y, et al: Maturation of EEG activity during sleep in premature infants. Electroencephalogr Clin Neurophysiol 24:319, 1968.
2. Dreyfus-Brisac C: The electroencephalogram of the premature infant and full-term newborn. *In* Kellaway P, Petersen I (eds): Neurological and Electroencephalographic Correlative Studies in Infancy. New York, Grune & Stratton, 1964, pp 186–207.
3. Parmelee AH, Stern E: Development of states in infants. *In* Clemente C, Purpura D, Mayer F (eds): Maturation of Brain Mechanisms Related to Sleep Behavior. New York, Academic Press, 1972, pp 199–228.
4. Samson-Dollfus D, Forthomme J, Capron E: EEG of the human infant during sleep and wakefulness during the first year of life. *In* Kellaway P, Petersen I (eds): Neurological and Electroencephalographic Correlative Studies in Infancy. New York, Grune & Stratton, 1964, pp 208–229.
5. Tanguay PE, Ornitz EM, Kaplan A, et al: Evolution of sleep spindles in childhood. Electroencephalogr Clin Neurophysiol 38:175, 1975.
6. Metcalf DR, Mondale J, Butler FK: Ontogenesis of spontaneous K-complexes. Psychophysiology 8:340, 1971.
7. Hoppenbrouwers T: Sleep in infants. *In* Guilleminault C (ed): Sleep and Its Disorders in Children. New York, Raven Press, 1987, pp 1–15.
8. Coons S: Development of sleep and wakefulness during the first 6 months of life. *In* Guilleminault C (ed): Sleep and Its Disorders in Children. New York, Raven Press, 1987, pp 17–27.
9. Roffwarg HP, Muzio JN, Dement WC: Ontogenetic development of the human sleep-dream cycle. Science 152:604, 1966.
10. Kleitman N, Engelmann TG: Sleep characteristics in infants. J Appl Physiol 6:269, 1953.
11. Ferber R, Boyle MP: Persistance of a free-running sleep-wake rhythm in a one-year-old girl. Sleep Res 12:364, 1983.
12. Carskadon MA, Harvey K, Duke P, et al: Pubertal changes in daytime sleepiness. Sleep 3:453, 1980.
13. Anders TF, Carskadon MA, Dement WC: Sleep and sleepiness in children and adolescents. Pediatr Clin North Am 27:29, 1980.
14. Broughton R: Sleep disorders: disorders of arousal? Science 159:1070, 1968.
15. Puig-Antich J, Weston B: The diagnosis and treatment of major depressive disorder in childhood. Ann Rev Med 24:231, 1983.
16. Puig-Antich J: Affective disorders in childhood: a review and perspective. Psychiatr Clin North Am 3:403, 1980.
17. Demyer MK: The psychoses of childhood. *In* Noshpitz JD (ed): Basic Handbook of Child Psychiatry, Vol 5. New York, Basic Books, Inc, 1987, pp 362–374.

Normal Sleep in Neonates and Children

THOMAS F. ANDERS, AVI SADEH, and VIAJYA APPAREDDY

This chapter describes the characteristics of sleep-wake states during early development from their origins in fetal rest-activity cycles, to neurophysiologic patterns of inhibition and activation in premature infants and full-term neonates, to organized sleep-wake states in older infants and children. The development of common behaviors associated with the regulation of sleep and waking is also described. For the purposes of this chapter, a distinction is made between architectural and temporal organization of sleep. The former refers to the coordination of independent neurophysiologic systems into functional states; the latter refers to the establishment of two interdependent rhythms, an ultradian rapid eye movement–non-rapid eye movement (REM-NREM) sleep rhythm and a circadian sleep-wake rhythm.

Developmental Perspective

Although REMs in sleeping newborns had been described previously,[1, 2] credit for applying a developmental perspective to the study of sleep in humans belongs to Roffwarg, Muzio, and Dement, who published their classic description of sleep state ontogenesis in *Science* in 1966.[3] As a psychiatrist, Roffwarg was interested in the origins of dreaming and the relationship between dream mentation and REM sleep physiology. Contrary to his original speculation that newborns would not manifest REM sleep because, presumably, they did not dream, Roffwarg and associates[3] instead reported that newborns spent more time in REM sleep than did the young college students,

who had been the subjects of Dement and Kleitman's original description.[4]

Roffwarg and associates[3] presented a theoretical formulation that remains seminal about the significance of REM sleep in the immature nervous system. They speculated that the heightened activation of central and autonomic nervous systems processes during REM sleep was particularly important in newborns because of the neonate's relative inability to process information during wakefulness. REM sleep served to functionally stimulate immature neurons and synapses "internally" at an age when infants were in a partial state of waking sensory deprivation. They noted that visual pathways, in particular from the retina to the lateral geniculate body and the visual cortex, were activated during periods of REM sleep, and they surmised that a process of intense information processing from within was stimulating the visual system. Their ontogenetic hypothesis provided an explanation and rationale for the differences in the sleep of infants compared with the sleep of adults: the increased proportion of REM sleep, the occurrence of REM sleep onsets, the shorter REM-NREM sleep cycle lengths, and the increased amount of total sleep time in 24 hours. This hypothesis remains salient despite accumulated research, which reports that newborns are more responsive to their environment than was previously believed.[3] In addition, the infant's visual system is more mature at birth than are any of the other sensorimotor systems.[5] Its function supports dyadic gaze behavior, one of the critical modalities for mother–infant interaction, which is associated with the emergence of social and emotional competence and the establishment of the infant–caregiver attachment system.[6]

Since Roffwarg's report,[3] a number of studies have traced the developmental course of REM-NREM architectural and temporal organization of sleep states and sleep-wake state regulation in more detail. All of them continue to provide general confirmation of the descriptions reported in 1966. Denenberg and Thoman[7] have also provided indirect experimental evidence and an animal model that further supports the ontogenetic hypothesis.

Ethologic Perspective

The ethologic perspective, like the developmental perspective, has increased our understanding of infant sleep-wake regulation. Ethologists observe animal behavior in natural settings. Studies of the ecologic niche in which human newborns sleep and the parental tasks of regulating sleep and waking have focused attention on parent–infant interaction and primary relationships as contexts in which environmental stresses affect sleep.[6]

Sander and coworkers[8] first demonstrated differences in sleep-wake organization between newborns reared in the neonatal nursery during their first 10 days and newborns who roomed in with a single caretaker and fed on demand. The latter group began a shift from polyphasic sleep to daytime wakefulness and nighttime sleep earlier than the former group, who showed no evidence for this shift. Keffe[9] reported that newborns who slept in the same room with their mothers spent more time in quiet sleep and less time crying and in indeterminate sleep than newborns who slept in the nursery.

An important cross-cultural and evolutionary view has been expressed by James McKenna,[10] who suggests that only in very recent times, in an evolutionary sense, and only in a small part of the Western developed world, in a cross-cultural sense, do infants sleep alone in their own beds and in their own rooms. He speculates that in contrast to these modern practices mother–infant co-sleeping has had a long historical tradition and is a natural extension of prenatal mother–fetus physiologic regulation. McKenna proposes that maternal contact during sleep has significant effects on regulating the infant's breathing, temperature, and level of arousal. He further speculates that the sudden infant death syndrome (SIDS) may sometimes be related to the altered regulation of these processes in predisposed, vulnerable infants who sleep alone.[11]

To support these speculations, McKenna and associates[12] recorded sleep simultaneously in 3-month-old infants and their mothers with the infants alternately sleeping with their mothers and in separate beds. Compared with the separate bed condition, arousals in the co-sleeping condition were reported to be more frequent and more synchronized, and more time was spent in light stages of sleep or awake and less time in the deeper stages of sleep. Figure 2–1 portrays a sleep-wake histogram based on the video recording of a 3-month-old child co-sleeping. The middle-of-the-night awakening is evident.

Combining developmental and ethologic perspectives provides an opportunity to examine the effects of environmental perturbations on sleep-wake state organization at different ages. In general, studies have demonstrated that newborns, older children, and adults respond similarly in sleep to a variety of acute stresses.[13–15] They exhibit decreased amounts of REM sleep, increased amounts of wakefulness, and fragmentation of sleep continuity. Infants sleeping in neonatal nurseries compared with infants rooming-in demonstrate comparable shifts, and frequent handling in the nursery is associated with more frequent awakenings.[9]

Finally, attempts to selectively and totally deprive infants of sleep lead to rebound responses similar to those of adults. REM sleep deprivation leads to REM rebound responses; total sleep deprivation leads to NREM rebound responses followed by REM rebound responses.[16] Curiously, in situations of more chronic or persistent stress (ligature circumcision versus excisional circumcision),[17] infants may spend more time in quiet sleep, perhaps to reduce painful stimulation, which is akin to the conservation-withdrawal defense described by Engle.[18]

Sleep Architecture

Sleep-Wake Recording in Infants

Infant sleep can be studied using a polygraph in the sleep laboratory. However, after discharge from the hospital nursery, many parents are reluctant to return with their infants to a laboratory for even one night away from home. Thus, studies of normal infants and toddlers using adequate sample sizes and re-

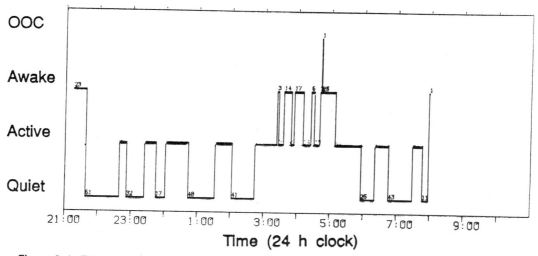

Figure 2–1. This all-night time-lapse histogram portrays the disrupted middle-of-the-night sleep of a co-sleeping 3-month-old child. Sleep state proportions are normal for age. OOC = Out of Crib.

peated nights of contiguous recording in the laboratory are few. In fact, much of our polygraphic information is derived from daytime naps or a single night of sleep. As a result, several other techniques have been developed that can record sleep in the home without instrumentation. Direct behavioral observation,[19] time-lapse video recording,[20] movement sensors in the crib mattress,[8, 19] and, most recently, actigraphic recording from a watch-sized wrist sensor[21] have been used from infancy through 5 years of age. These methods rely heavily on observed behaviors and movement patterns to establish algorithms that attempt to differentiate active (REM) sleep, quiet (NREM) sleep, and wakefulness. Some of these methods also provide information about parent–infant nighttime interaction around sleep-wake regulation.

In infants, as in adults (see Kryger MH, et al: Principles and Practice of Sleep Medicine, 2nd ed, Chap. 89), REM sleep is defined by a low-voltage, fast, desynchronized electroencephalogram (EEG) pattern; bilaterally synchronous REMs under closed lids; rapid and irregular heart rate and respiratory patterns; and muscle atonia. The eye movement bursts, peripheral small muscle twitches, and body jerks "break through" the muscle inhibition of REM sleep more in infants than in older children. Phasic breakthrough diminishes over the first few years of life. Until 6 months of age, NREM sleep cannot be subdivided into four EEG stages; rather it is characterized by a single high-voltage, slow-wave pattern, slowed

regular cardiac and respiratory rates, and resting levels of muscle tone. These patterns are illustrated in Figures 2–2 and 2–3.

In early development, the patterns of alternating activity and quiescence of each of the various physiologic parameters that characterize REM and NREM sleep have their own course of maturation. The studies that have examined the earliest development of these patterns have been carried out on premature infants while in the hospital nursery. For the most part, "normal" premature infants have been assessed, but in these populations it is especially difficult to be certain that samples are well defined and that conclusions can be generalized. Nevertheless, important developmental changes in each of these neurophysiologic systems are evident. Since the early nursery experience of premature infants is

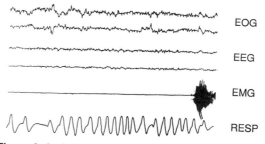

Figure 2–2. A 30-second epoch of REM sleep recorded polygraphically from a sleeping newborn infant. Single REMs in the electro-oculogram (EOG), tonically inhibited muscle tone in the electromyogram (EMG), and irregular, rapid respirations characterize the epoch.

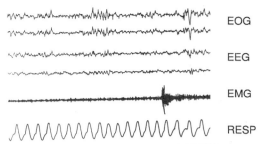

Figure 2–3. A 30-second epoch of NREM sleep recorded polygraphically from a sleeping newborn infant. The high-voltage, slow-wave activity in the EOG is reflected frontal EEG waves, not REMs. Muscle tone is present, and respirations are slow and regular.

significantly different from the more natural in utero experience of comparably aged fetuses, studies after 40 weeks gestational age that compare differences between premature and term infants, matched for conceptional age, contribute to our understanding of the relative effects of environmental stimulation and biologic maturation.

Although there may well be subtle differences in the way sleep states are organized, the way sleep-wake cycles develop, and the way parents interact with their infants around bedtime and during the night between premature and term infants of comparable conceptional ages, by and large there are no gross differences that are attributable to premature birth. That is, prematurity per se is not a risk factor for disordered or disorganized sleep. In fact, some of the subtle differences reported suggest more mature organization in premature infants; for example, there are slightly longer sustained periods of sleep, self-soothing seems more common, and quiet sleep may predominate earlier.[22–26]

Maturation of Individual Neurophysiologic Systems

The earliest tracings of EEG activity in humans have been obtained from in utero fetuses recorded transabdominally at a conceptional age of 3 months. Continuous low-voltage, irregular, brain activity patterns were noted.[27] The recordings could not distinguish alternating patterns of activity, so that sleep and waking states could not be defined. Maturational trends are apparent as early as 24 weeks of conceptional age, beginning with discontinuous activity, interhemispheric asynchrony, and absence of electrocortical reaction to stimuli and progressing to polymorphic, irregular electrical activity by 24 to 26 weeks. By 28 weeks, fast rhythms are superimposed on slow waves in both temporal and occipital regions.

Dreyfus-Brisac,[28, 29] Parmelee and colleagues,[30] and others have described the evolution of EEG patterns in premature infants. Between 24 and 27 weeks gestation, the EEG generally shows bursts of high-voltage, occipitally predominant, slow-wave pleomorphic activity alternating with long periods of very depressed activity (tracé discontinu). A tracé alternant pattern, which consists of 2- to 6-second bursts of high-amplitude slow waves separated by 4 to 8 seconds of low-voltage mixed activity, appears in an early form by 28 weeks, becomes associated with quiet sleep by 32 weeks, and appears in its mature form at about 36 weeks. Shortly thereafter, the high-voltage slow and low-voltage fast patterns typical of the neonate become evident.

Parmelee and colleagues[30] described a catalog of EEG frequency and amplitude findings that are characteristic of sleeping premature infants at different conceptional ages. Using this catalog, the authors were able to predict conceptional age within 2 weeks in 85% of infants scored blindly. Power spectra analysis of the patterns corresponding to the age-related EEG codes confirmed the validity of the visual impressions.[31]

Other studies have traced the appearance of specific wave forms in the EEG. Sleep spindles begin to appear at 4 weeks of age, develop rapidly through 8 weeks of age, and clearly characterize NREM sleep by 3 months of age.[32] Lenard[33] measured the numbers of spindles and interspindle intervals from age 2 months to 2.5 years. He noted a progressive lengthening of the interspindle interval with maturation. Metcalf and associates[34] noted that K-complexes appear first around 6 months of age and are fully developed by 2 years of age.

Petre-Quadens and colleagues[35] suggested that REM patterns could be divided into single, isolated REMs and REM burst patterns. Only the high-density burst patterns with interburst intervals of less than 1 second changed with age. Parmelee and colleagues[36] reported burst patterns as early as 28 weeks of conceptional age. Petre-Quadens and colleagues[35] describe bursts present in 33- to 36-week-old premature infants. The interburst interval length is decreased significantly by term and continues to change over the first year of life.[37] Dreyfus-Brisac[29] noted that eye movement burst patterns became associated with one specific EEG pattern by 37 weeks of conceptional age. Prechtl and Lenard demonstrated similar organization in full-term neonates.[38]

Parmelee[39] reported that four types of respiratory patterns could be defined: regular, irregular, periodic, and apneic. Little regular respiration, characterized by equal breath-to-breath intervals, occurs before 36 weeks of conceptional age; rather, periodic breathing and apneic patterns predominate during sleep. After 36 weeks of conceptional age, both of these patterns drop off dramatically as the amount of regular respiration increases.

The maturation of body movement patterns has also been studied. Dreyfus-Brisac[28] reported that movements of the upper limbs change little during sleep from 32 weeks of conceptional age to 41 weeks. Lower limb movements, prominent in the younger preterm infants, decrease with maturation; whereas facial movements increase. Periods of body quiescence become prominent after 30 weeks of conceptional age. The inhibition of chin muscle tone during REM sleep is irregular before 37 weeks of conceptional age. Even at term it remains variable and is the least dependable parameter for scoring state.

In summary, for any physiologic measure to be considered a criterion of state, some alternation of its active and inhibited pattern must be evident. Parmelee[39] has established a developmental guide related to conceptional age, indicating the effectiveness of each measure for scoring sleep: body movements at 28 weeks, eye movements at 30 weeks, respiration at 34 weeks, EEG at 36 weeks, and chin electromyogram (EMG) after 40 weeks.

Organization of Sleep States

Another outcome of development that characterizes mature sleep state architecture is the progressive coordination of the activated and inhibited neurophysiologic patterns into synchronous, functional sleep states. In healthy adults, the NREM and REM sleep states are well coordinated. In young infants, when epochs of active and quiet sleep are disorganized, *indeterminate sleep* (or "transitional" sleep) is coded. An underlying assumption of this concept is that as development proceeds the amount of poorly organized indeterminate sleep will diminish, at least in normally developing infants. Scoring manuals for sleep-wake

states in neonates[40] and infants[41] have been published. Parmelee[36] reported that the amount of indeterminate sleep drops from 67% in the 30-week premature infant to 38% when the preemie reaches 40 weeks of conceptional age and 29% at 3 months past term. Dreyfus-Brisac[26] suggested that the sleep of premature infants at 40 weeks of conceptional age is not as well organized architecturally as the sleep of full-term infants of the same age. A discrepant report[22] suggested that premature infants and full-term infants matched for conceptional age do not differ in the proportions of their indeterminate sleep, although this study used videosomnography instead of polysomnography for state identification.

Table 2–1 summarizes some of the maturational changes that distinguish sleep state organization in neonates from adults. During the first 3 months of life, infants spend 50% of their sleep time in REM, or active sleep, and 50% in NREM, or quiet sleep. When the young infant falls asleep, the initial sleep episode is typically a sleep onset REM period. By 3 months of age, the proportion of REM sleep begins to diminish and sleep onset REM periods begin to be replaced by sleep onset NREM periods. The intensity of body motility during REM sleep decreases with increased peripheral muscle atonia and the proportion of indeterminate sleep decreases as sleep states become better organized (Fig. 2–4).[42]

Temporal Organization of Sleep

There are two biorhythmic processes that define the temporal organization of sleep: a circadian sleep-wake rhythm and an ultradian REM-NREM rhythm. Both of these systems change with age as internal biologic "clocks" become coordinated with regularly recurring environmental zeitgebers such as the light-dark cycle, ambient temperature/noise changes, and regularly scheduled periods of social interaction, and with internal body signals such as hunger, pain, core temperature, and hormone secretion.

Diurnal Organization: The Sleep-Wake Cycle

At birth, normal full-term newborns spend 16 to 18 of 24 hours asleep. At this age, sleep is polyphasic so that sleep-wake states alternate in 3- to 4-hour cycles. There is as much wake-

Table 2–1. THE DEVELOPMENTAL CHANGES IN SLEEP AND SLEEP CYCLE ORGANIZATION FROM THE NEONATAL PERIOD TO ADULTHOOD

	Infant	Adult
Sleep state proportions (%) REM/NREM	50/50	20/80
Periodicity of sleep states	50–60 min	90–100 min
Sleep onset state	REM sleep onset	NREM sleep onset
Temporal organization of sleep states	REM-NREM cycles equally throughout sleep period	NREM stages 3–4 predominant in first third of night **** REM state predominant in last third of night
Maturation of EEG patterns	LVF pattern HVS pattern 1 NREM EEG stage	K-complexes Delta waves 4 NREM EEG stages
Concordance of sleep measures (organization of sleep states)	Poor	Good

fulness at night as there is sleep during the day.[42] Within the first month following birth, sleep-wake state organization begins to adapt to the light-dark cycle and to regularly recurring associated social cues.

By 6 months of age, the longest continuous sleep period has lengthened to 6 hours. Two long sleep periods make up the night, interrupted by a brief awakening for a nighttime feeding. The wakeful periods similarly consolidate, lengthen, and shift to the daytime, while still being interrupted by brief periods of sleep. By the end of the first year, the number of sleeping and waking hours have changed relatively little. The infant still sleeps 14 to 15 hours per day; yet, except for 1 to 2 daytime naps, sleep periods have shifted to the nighttime and waking periods to the day.[43]

During the second year of life, infants sleep 50% of the time. During this year, one of the daytime naps disappears and sleep becomes restricted to two times: one long episode during the night and one brief nap during the afternoon. In the preschool years, depending on social expectations, many children give up the remaining daytime nap and sleep becomes truly monophasic, although a tendency for an afternoon nap remains throughout adulthood (see Kryger MH, et al: Principles and Practice of Sleep Medicine, 2nd ed, p 44). Failures in the process of nighttime sleep consolidation, manifested by prolonged and repeated periods of night waking, constitute a significant developmental problem for infants and their parents.

Sleep-wake Consolidation and Night Waking

Studies of sleep-wake consolidation in infants have relied largely on data derived from parental reports, which describe difficulties in "settling" or sleeping through the night. Recently, more objective time-lapse video recordings and actigraphic monitoring have demonstrated that nighttime awakenings in infancy are more prevalent than reported by parents.[21, 44] These methods indicate that in-

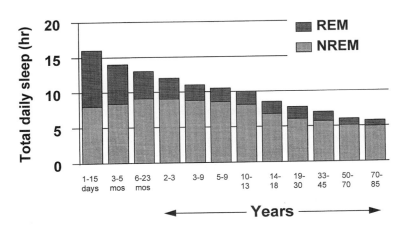

Figure 2–4. The changes in total daily sleep, REM sleep, and NREM sleep with age. Notice the large amount of REM sleep in the neonate and infant. (Based on data from Roffwarg HP, Munzio JN, Dement WC: Ontogenetic Development of the Human Sleep-Dream Cycle. Science 152:604, 1966.)

fants usually arouse one or more times for 1 to 5 minutes each night. Parents, however, are often unaware of these awakenings because the child does not cry. Infants who can put themselves back to sleep without arousing their parents have been described as "self-soothers"; infants who cry have been described as "signalers."[44, 45]

During the first few months of life, 95% of infants cry (signal) after a nighttime awakening and require a parental response before returning to sleep. By 1 year of age, 60 to 70% of infants are able to self-soothe and return to sleep on their own.[45] A study using an activity monitor has reported that infants from 9 to 24 months woke up twice nightly on average. Most of these infants were able to soothe themselves and return to sleep without signaling.[21] Using the actigraph, it was also demonstrated that sleep-disturbed infants could become self-soothers and consolidate their sleep following a behavioral intervention.[46] Thus, the problem of night waking is more appropriately redefined as a problem with the infant's response to the awakening rather than the awakening per se.

Ultradian Organization: The REM-NREM Cycle

Sterman[47] recorded fetal activity in utero from strain gauges taped to the mother's abdomen while she slept. He was able to differentiate clearcut periods of fetal rest and activity that coincided with maternal REM and NREM sleep cycles by 8 months of conceptional age. Thus, it appears that, although EEG activity can be recorded early in post-conceptional development,[27] organization of sleep states into alternating cycles of activity and rest (REM and NREM) does not appear until the last trimester of gestation.

In the neonatal period, active (REM) and quiet (NREM) sleep periods alternate in 50 to 60 minute sleep cycles. In each sleep cycle during the sleep period there is as much REM sleep as NREM sleep.[42, 43] After 3 months of age, although REM periods continue to recur with a periodicity of 50 to 60 minutes, the amount of REM sleep in each cycle begins to shift. REM sleep predominates in the later sleep cycles of the night and NREM (eventually stage 4) sleep predominates during the earlier cycles. The longer adult sleep cycle periodicity of 90 minutes is not observed until adolescence.

Sleep Patterns in Children 2 to 6 Years of Age

Relatively little laboratory research has been carried out with preschool and school-age children. In the early toddler period, mothers are reluctant to have their children sleep away from home. In addition, the children may experience instrumentation and the unfamiliar laboratory procedures as stressful. Also, since they still nap at this age, it is necessary to record daytime and nighttime sleep to understand changes in proportional relationships between sleep states that occur as a result of maturation.

Roffwarg and associates[3] described the longer REM latency of 5-year-olds compared with 2-year-olds and suggested that 5-year-olds were more fatigued as a result of having given up their daytime naps. Webb and Agnew[48] and Maron and associates[49] demonstrated that significant amounts of stage 3–4 NREM sleep occurred in afternoon naps (19–25% of nap time) and that the amounts were greater in naps taken later in the day compared with morning naps.

Kahn and associates[50] hypothesized that lesser amounts of stage 4 NREM sleep at night at young ages might be explained by more stage 4 NREM sleep during the afternoon nap. They studied daytime naps and nighttime sleep in 2-year-olds and nighttime sleep in 5-year-olds who no longer napped. The amount of stage 4 NREM sleep of 5-year-olds at night was significantly greater than that of 2-year-olds; however, when the naps of the 2-year-olds were included, the amount of stage 4 NREM sleep for both groups was similar. Total REM time in the 2-year-olds tended to be greater and the number of REM periods per 24 hours was significantly greater, possibly related in part to a longer total sleep time of 2-year-olds. The longest individual REM period of the night was equal for both groups, and successive REM episode durations were not significantly different. However, the REM-NREM cycle lengths of 2-year-olds were shorter than corresponding cycles in 5-year-olds. The mean length for the first three cycles was 75 minutes and 84 minutes, respectively.

Comparing nighttime sleep only, 2-year-olds had higher percentages of REM sleep, perhaps related to the predominance of NREM sleep during the afternoon nap. The 5-year-olds had the longest sustained stage 3–4 NREM periods. There was a gradual decrease in the number and nature of body movements and position shifts during sleep. Older children tended to sleep on their sides and younger infants on their stomachs or backs. Other reports have confirmed these developmental trends.[3, 51–53]

Williams and associates[54] compared sleep in 3- to 5-year-old and 6- to 9-year-old boys and girls. At each age, boys slept longer and spent more time in stage 2 NREM sleep. There were other subtle gender differences at each age suggesting that sleep characteristics, like many other physical, cognitive, and social attributes, develop earlier in girls than boys.

Several investigators have attempted to examine the correlation between the lengths of daytime and nighttime total sleep.[52, 54] That is, are long nappers also long nighttime sleepers and vice-versa? There is some suggestion that during infancy long nappers also have long nighttime sleep periods. After 2 years of age, the relationship between the lengths of the daytime sleep period and nighttime sleep is more controversial.

Sleep Patterns From 6 to 12 Years of Age

There are few studies on sleep patterns in this age group. Coble and associates[55] compared computer-based, automated REM and delta scoring techniques with standard visual scoring methods. Children were divided into three age groups: 6- to 7-year-olds, 8- to 9-year-olds, and 10- to 11-year-olds. The results suggested that first night effects (such as increased sleep latency and decreased stage 4 and REM sleep) were more extreme in the 6- to 7-year-old group, but they showed adaptation by the second and third nights. As a group, the children spent 8 to 9.5 hours in bed and were asleep approximately 95% of the time. After the first night, they fell asleep in 20 to 25 minutes and subsequently had on average only 1 to 3 brief awakenings. Stage 4 NREM sleep decreased from 18% in 6- to 7-year-olds to 14% in 11-year-olds. The decline in stage 4 NREM sleep was associated with an increase in the proportional amount of stage 2 NREM sleep. Other NREM sleep stage percentages remained the same. The proportion of REM sleep was constant across ages, but the REM latency decreased from 140 minutes in 6- to 7-year-olds to 124 minutes in 10- to 11-year-olds. The number of REM periods and the amount of activity during REM periods also decreased with increasing age. These developmental changes have been corroborated.[52, 54]

Origins and Significance of Sleep-Wake Relevant Behaviors

Since some sleep-related behaviors are considered normal at early ages but symptoms of a sleep disorder at later ages, it is important to describe their occurrence in normal development.

Repetitive Motor Activity

Repetitive rhythmic behaviors during the transition to sleep are common sleep-related behaviors of infants. They include bodyrocking, headturning, and headbanging (see Chapter 13). Behaviors such as sucking (thumb, pacifier, or bottle) and playing with transitional objects are considered separately. It is important to note that rhythmic stimulation is an ubiquitous experience in early life. Caregivers often spontaneously, or in response to an infant's distress, rock, pat, or use strollers and car rides to soothe their children. The mechanisms whereby rhythmic stimulation produces quieting and sleep are not understood fully, but its effectiveness seems well recognized cross-culturally. The prevalence of repetitive motor behavior seems to peak during the latter part of the first year of life and gradually disappears during the second year, although in some children it persists. Klackenberg[56] reported that 58% of infants at 9 months of age exhibited at least one of these repetitive behaviors. The prevalence decreased to 33% by 18 months of age and to 22% by 2 years of age.

Even premature infants seek rhythmic stimulation. In fact, such experiences may facilitate neurobehavioral organization. Premature infants in the intensive care nursery given an opportunity to spend time with a "breathing" bear spent more time in contact with the rhythmic bear than with a "nonbreathing" bear. Following discharge from the nursery, they showed more quiet sleep, which persisted over several months.[57] Other studies have reported that rhythmic stimulation results in reduction of sleep apnea and bradycardia in preterm infants.[58]

Sucking

Thumb-sucking is a self-soothing rhythmic behavior that can be observed in utero and in neonates. A recent survey reported that more than 20% of children between 6 months and 4 years of age in an urban metropolitan area sucked their thumbs.[59] The prevalence of thumb-sucking varies among cultures. In a survey conducted in Israel, only 8.4% of the infants reportedly fell asleep sucking their thumb. Nevertheless, more than 80% of the group used other sucking behaviors (pacifier or a bottle) during the transition to sleep.[60] Woodson and associates[61] demonstrated decreased restlessness in both full-term and preterm babies following periods of sucking. Infants who suck their thumbs are also more likely to be attached to a "transitional" object such as a piece of cloth, blanket, or teddy bear at a later age. Breast-fed infants are more likely to suck their thumbs than bottle-fed infants.[59]

In addition to the general self-soothing effects of repetitive sucking during wakefulness, studies have shown that thumb- and pacifier-sucking become linked to the process of falling asleep. Infants who suck their thumbs are more likely to be left by their parents to fall asleep on their own.[59, 60, 62] Because these studies have been correlated, the findings can be interpreted in two ways: infants who are born with or who acquire an early propensity for sucking as a self-soothing behavior do not need the help of a caregiver to fall asleep, and infants who are left alone to fall asleep tend to develop self-soothing sucking in order to induce sleep. Further longitudinal research is needed to unravel the interaction of sucking and sleep onset during early infancy.

Self-soothing behavior after a nighttime awakening is significantly correlated with falling asleep at bedtime. Those infants who are put into their cribs at the beginning of the night already asleep are likely to signal in the middle of the night. In contrast, those infants who are put into their cribs awake at the beginning of the night are more likely to return to sleep on their own after a nighttime awakening.[46, 63, 64] The pattern of returning to sleep following a nighttime awakening resembles the pattern of falling asleep at bedtime. The relationship between feeding and night waking remains controversial. In the first 3 months of life, nighttime awakenings have been associated with hunger and physical discomfort.[65] Some studies[66, 67] report a relationship between breast-feeding and prolongation

of night awakenings, while others have failed to find such a relationship.[68, 69] Kahn and associates[70, 71] identified cow's milk allergy in a group of infants with persistent night waking who did not benefit from behavioral interventions. However, the sleep-wake patterns of 4-week-old and 4-month-old infants who were fed an enriched diet did not differ from those of infants on a regular diet.[72] Feeding styles (demand vs schedule) were not found to be related to nighttime awakenings,[66] although inconsistent and unsatisfying feedings were. It is possible that consistency in feeding, rather than nutritional factors, may influence the consolidation of sleep-wake patterns.

Temperament

Infant temperament may influence night waking and self-soothing. Carey[73] found, in a pediatric clinic sample, that infants with night waking had lower sensory thresholds (a component of temperament) than infants without night waking. In support of this hypothesis, Weissbluth and associates[74] found that children with "difficult" temperaments slept less than children with "easy" temperaments, and Schaefer[75] found a higher than expected incidence of "difficult" temperament in young children referred for night awakenings. Inconsistent feedings, difficult temperament, and disrupted sleep have been reported for infants with colic.[76] Finally, parental stress, maternal personality, and attachment classification have been identified as contributing factors to infant nighttime awakening.[77–80] In a conflicting report, Keener and associates,[81] in a sample of non-referred, normal infants, did not find difficult temperament to be associated with differences in sleep-wake patterns. Sleep-wake patterns and crying were scored from time-lapse video tapes (not from maternal reports) and temperament was scored from maternal ratings. No relationship could be demonstrated between these independent measures.

Transitional Objects

The transitional object is a term used by Winnicott[82] to describe inanimate objects, such as a piece of cloth or diaper, a blanket, a teddy bear, or even a bottle or pacifier, that older infants use at times of stress to provide comfort and security in the absence of the mother. A transitional object serves as a maternal substitute or psychologic representation of the mother. Characteristically, transitional objects are chosen by the infant and lead to distress if absent. Even changes, such as washing, cause disruption. Since going to bed and falling asleep each night are regularly recurring experiences of separation and since separation from parents is considered to be stressful for some infants at certain ages, transitional objects are especially useful when falling asleep. Developmentally, transitional objects assume their salience from 9 months of age to 3 years of age, the period when infants begin to move progressively from attachment and dependency to some physical independence and psychologic autonomy.

In a sample of 212 Swedish children, Klackenberg[56] noted that only 7% of the children never used a transitional object. There was a progressive decrease in regular use at sleep onset from 45% at the age of 4 years to 7% at the age of 14 years. Klackenberg found no significant relationships between sleep disruption and the use of transitional objects. Wolf and Lozoff[59] reported that 44% of American children under 4 years of age regularly used a transitional object at bedtime. The use of transitional objects was more prevalent in children who fell asleep alone (57%) compared with children who fell asleep in the presence of a caregiver (30%). Older children were more likely than younger children to use transitional objects.

There is controversy about the psychologic significance of transitional objects and about whether insecure or secure infants use them more. There is little disagreement, however, that many infants use such objects as ''sleep aids'' to assist them in falling asleep, both at the beginning of the night and after a middle-of-the-night awakening.

Conclusions

The development of sleep-wake states has been reviewed from several perspectives: maturation of neurophysiologic systems, state architecture, environmental influences, and the appearance of behaviors that may become problematic at older ages. Two models, the developmental model and the ethologic model, are particularly suited for the study of sleep in young infants and children. The knowledge generated from these studies has improved our ability to understand sleep-wake state organization in young subjects, especially as it relates to normal and disordered functioning and to treatment of sleep perturbations and problems.

References

1. Denisova M, Figurin N: Periodic phenomena in the sleep of children. Nov Refl Fiziol Nerv System 2:338, 1926.
2. Aserinsky E, Kleitman N: A motility cycle in sleeping infants as manifested by ocular and gross bodily activity. J Appl Physiol 8:11, 1955.
3. Roffwarg H, Muzio J, Dement W: Ontogenetic development of the human sleep-dream cycle. Science 152:604, 1966.
4. Dement W, Kleitman N: Cyclic variations in EEG during sleep and their relationships to eye movements, body motility and dreaming. Electroencephalogr Clin Neurophysiol 9:673, 1957.
5. Stern D: The goal structure of mother-infant play. J Am Acad Child Adolesc Psychiatry 13:402, 1974.
6. Sroufe A: Relationships, self and individual adaptation. *In* Sameroff AJ, Emde R (eds): Relationship Disturbances in Early Childhood: A Developmental Approach. New York, Basic Books Inc, 1989, pp 70–94.
7. Denenberg V, Thoman E: Evidence for a functional role for active (REM) sleep in infancy. Sleep 4:185, 1981.
8. Sander L, Stechler G, Julia H, et al: Mother-infant interaction and 24-hour patterns of activity and sleep. J Am Acad Child Adolesc Psychiatry 9:103, 1970.
9. Keffe M: Comparison of neonatal nighttime sleep-wake patterns in nursery versus rooming-in environments. Nursery Res 36:140, 1987.
10. McKenna J: Evolution and sudden infant death syndrome (SIDS): infant reseponsivity to parental contact. Human Nat 1:145, 1990.
11. McKenna J, Thoman E, Anders T, et al: Infant-parent co-sleeping in an evolutionary perspective: implications for understanding infant sleep development and the sudden death syndrome. Sleep 16:263, 1993.
12. McKenna J, Mosko S, Dungy C, et al: Sleep and arousal patterns of co-sleeping human mother/infant pairs: A preliminary physiological study with implication for the study of Sudden Infant Death Syndrome (SIDS). Am J Phys Anthropol 83:331, 1990.
13. Anders T, Sostek A: The use of time lapse video recording of sleep-wake behavior in human infants. Psychophysiology 13:155, 1976.
14. Anders T, Chalemian R: The effects of circumcision on neonatal sleep. Psychosom Med 36:174, 1974.
15. Freudigman K, Thoman E: Newborn sleep: effects of age, sex and mode of delivery. Sleep Research 20:103 (abstract), 1991.
16. Anders T, Roffwarg H: The effects of selective interruption and total sleep deprivation in the human newborn. Dev Psychobiol 6:79, 1973.
17. Emde R, Harmon R, Metcalf D, et al: Stress and neonatal sleep. Psychosom Med 33:491, 1971.
18. Engle G: Anxiety and depression-withdrawal: the primary effects of unpleasure. Int J Psychoanal 43:89, 1971.
19. Thoman E: Sleeping and waking states in infants: a functional perspective. Neurosci Biobehav Rev 14:93, 1990.
20. Anders T: Home recorded sleep in two- and nine-month-old infants. J Am Acad Child Adolesc Psychiatr 17:421, 1978.

21. Sadeh A, Lavie P, Scher A, et al: Actigraphic home monitoring of sleep-disturbed and control infants and young children: a new method for pediatric assessment of sleep-wake patterns. Pediatrics 87:494, 1991.
22. Anders T, Keener M: Developmental course of nighttime sleep-wake patterns in full-term and pre-term infants during the first year of life. Sleep 8:173, 1985.
23. Parmelee A, Akiyama Y, Monod N, et al: EEG patterns in sleep of full-term and premature newborn infants. Electroencephalogr Clin Neurophysiol 17:445, 1969.
24. Ungerer J, Sigman M, Beckwith L, et al: Sleep behavior of preterm children at three years of age. Dev Med Child Neurol 25:297, 1983.
25. Booth C, Leonard H, Thoman E: Sleep states and behavior patterns in preterm and fullterm infants. Neuropediatrics 11:354, 1980.
26. Dreyfus-Brisac C, Monod N: Sleep of premature and full-term neonates: a polygraphic study. Proc R Soc Med 58:6, 1965.
27. Okamoto Y, Kirikae T: Electroencephalographic studies on brain of fetus, children of prebirth and newborn, together with a note on reactions of fetus brain upon drugs. Folia Psychiatr Neurol Jap 5:135, 1951.
28. Dreyfus-Brisac C: Ontogenesis of sleep in human prematures after 32 weeks of conceptional age. Dev Psychobiol 3:91, 1971.
29. Dreyfus-Brisac C: Sleep ontogenesis in early human prematurity from 24–27 weeks of conceptual age. Dev Psychobiol 2(3):162, 1968.
30. Parmelee A, Shulte F, Akiyama Y, et al: Maturation of EEG activity during sleep in premature infants. Electroencephalogr Clin Neurophysiol 24:319, 1968.
31. Parmelee A, Akiyama Y, Shultz M, et al: Analysis of electroencephalograms of sleeping infants. Activ Nerv Suppl 11:111, 1969.
32. Tanguay P, Ornitz E, Kaplan A, et al: Evolution of sleep spindles in childhood. Electroencephalogr Clin Neurophysiol 38:175, 1975.
33. Lenard H: The development of sleep spindles in the EEG during the first two years of life. Neuropediatrie 1:264, 1970.
34. Metcalf D, Mondale J, Butler F: Ontogenesis of spontaneous k-complexes. Psychophysiology 8:340, 1971.
35. Petre-Quadens O, deLee C, Remy M: Eye movement density during sleep and brain maturation. Brain Res 26:49, 1971.
36. Parmelee A, Wenner W, Akiyama Y, et al: Sleep states in premature infants. Dev Med Child Neurol 9:70, 1967.
37. Ktonas P, Bes F, Rigoard M, et al: Developmental changes in the clustering pattern of sleep rapid eye movement activity during the first year of life: A Markov-process approach. Electroencephalogr Clin Neurophysiol 75:136, 1990.
38. Prechtl H, Lenard H: A study of eye movements in sleeping newborn infants. Brain Res 5:477, 1967.
39. Parmelee A: The ontogeny of sleep patterns and associated periodicities in infants. In Falkner F, Kretchmer N, Rossi E (eds): Modern Problems in Pediatrics. Vol 13, Prenatal and Postnatal Development of the Human Brain. Basel, S. Karger, AG, 1974, pp 298–311.
40. Anders T. Emde R, Parmelee A (eds): A Manual of Standardized Terminology, Techniques and Criteria for the Scoring of States of Sleep and Wakefulness in Newborn Infants. Los Angeles, UCLA Brain Information Services, 1971.
41. Guilleminault C, Souquet M: Sleep states and related pathology. In Korobkin R, Guilleminault C (eds): Advances in Perinatal Neurology. New York, Spectrum, 1979, pp 225–247.
42. Coons S, Guilleminault C: Development of sleep-wake patterns and non-rapid eye movement sleep stages during the first six months of life in normal infants. Pediatrics 69:793, 1982.
43. Thoman E, Whitney M: Sleep states of infants monitored in the home: individual differences, developmental trends, and origins of diurnal cyclicity. Infant Behav Dev 12:59, 1989.
44. Anders T: Night waking in infants during the first year of life. Pediatrics 63:860, 1979.
45. Anders T, Halpern L, Hua J: Sleeping through the night: origins in early infancy. Pediatrics 90:554, 1992.
46. Sadeh A: Actigraphic home-monitoring of sleep-disturbed infants: comparison to controls and assessment of intervention. In Horne J (ed): Sleep '90. Bochum, Pontenagal Press, 1990, pp 469–470.
47. Sterman B: The relationship of intrauterine fetal activity to maternal sleep stage. Exp Neurol 19:98, 1967.
48. Webb W, Agnew H: Sleep cycling within 24-hour periods. J Exp Psychol 74:158, 1967.
49. Maron L, Rechtschaffen A. Wolpert E: Sleep cycle during napping. Arch Gen Psychiatry 11:503, 1964.
50. Kahn E, Fisher C, Edwards A: Twenty-four hour sleep patterns: comparison between 2- to 3-year-old and 4- to 6-year-old children. Arch Gen Psychiatry 29:380, 1973.
51. Kohler W, Coddington R, Agnew H: Sleep patterns in 2-year-old children. J Pediatr 72:228, 1968.
52. Feinberg I: Effects of age on human sleep patterns. In Kales A (ed): Sleep, Physiology and Pathology: A Symposium. Philadelphia, JB Lippincott, 1969, pp 39–52.
53. Basler K, Largo R, Molinari I: Die entwicklung des schlafverhaltens in den ersten funf lebensjahren. Helv Pediatr Acta 35:211, 1980.
54. Williams R, Karacan I, Hursch C: EEG of Human Sleep. New York, J Wiley & Sons, 1974, pp 26–68.
55. Coble P, Kupfer D, Reynolds C: EEG sleep of healthy children 6 to 12 years of age. In Guilleminault C (ed): Sleep and Its Disorders in Children. New York, Raven Press, 1987 pp 29–41.
56. Klackenberg G: Incidence of parasomnias in children in a general population. In Guilleminault C (ed): Sleep and Its Disorders in Children. New York, Raven Press, 1987, pp 99–113.
57. Thoman E, Ingersoll E, Acebo C: Premature infants seek rhythmic stimulation and the experience facilitates neurobehavioral development. J Dev Behav Pediatr 12:11, 1990.
58. Korner A, Guilleminault C, Hoed V, et al: Reduction of sleep apnea and bradycardia in pre-term infants on an oscillating waterbed: a controlled polygraphic study. Pediatrics 61:528, 1978.
59. Wolf A, Lozoff B: Object attachment, thumb-sucking and the passage to sleep. J Am Acad Child Adolesc Psychiatry 28:287, 1989.
60. Scher A, Tirosh E, Jaffe M, et al: Survey of sleep patterns of Israeli infants and young children. Sleep Res 16:209 (abstract), 1987.
61. Woodson R, Drinkwin J, Hamilton C: Effects of non-nutritive sucking on state and activity: term-preterm comparisons. Inf Behav Develop 8:435, 1985.
62. Ozturk M, Ozturk O: Thumbsucking and falling asleep. Br J Med Psychol 50:95, 1977.
63. Adair R, Bauchner H, Phillip B, et al: Night waking during infancy: the role of parental presence at bedtime. Pediatrics 87:500, 1991.
64. Johnson C: Infant and toddler sleep: a telephone survey of parents in one community. J Dev Behav Pediatr 12:108, 1991.

65. Moore T, Ucko L: Night waking in early infancy. Arch Dis Child 32:333, 1957.
66. Wright P, Macleod H, Cooper M: Waking at night: the effect of early feeding experience. Child Care Health Dev 9:309, 1983.
67. Eaton-Evans J, Dugdale A: Sleep patterns of infants in the first year of life. Arch Dis Child 63:647, 1988.
68. Beal V: Termination of night feeding in infancy. J Pediatr 75:690, 1969.
69. Jones B, Ferreira M, Brown M, et al: The association between perinatal factors and nightwaking. Dev Med Child Neurol 20:427, 1978.
70. Kahn A, Mozin M, Rebuffat E, et al: Milk intolerance in children with persistent sleeplessness: a prospective double-blind crossover evaluation. Pediatrics 84:595, 1989.
71. Kahn A, Rebuffat E, Sottiaux M, et al: Arousals induced by proximal esophageal reflux in infants. Sleep 14:39, 1991.
72. Macknin M, Medendorp S, Maier M: Infant sleep and bedtime cereal. Am J Dis Child 143:1066, 1991.
73. Carey W: Night waking and temperament in infancy. J Pediatr 84:756, 1974.
74. Weissbluth M, Davis A, Poucher J: Night waking in 4- to 8-month-old infants. J Pediatr 104:477, 1984.
75. Schaefer C: Night waking and temperament in early childhood. Psychol Rep 67:192, 1990.
76. Weissbluth M: Sleep Well: Peaceful Nights For Your Child and You. London, Unwin Hyman Limited, 1987.
77. Scott G, Richards M: Night waking in infants: effects of providing advice and support for parents. J Child Psychol Psychiatry 31:551, 1990.
78. Coutrona C, Troutman B: Social support, infant temperament and parenting self-efficacy: a mediational model of post-partum depression. Child Dev 57:1507, 1986.
79. Richman N: A community survey of characteristics of one to two year olds with sleep disruptions. J Am Acad Child Adolesc Psychiatry 20:281–291, 1981.
80. Benoit D, Zeanah C, Boucher C, et al: Sleep disorders in early childhood: association with insecure maternal attachment. Am Acad Child Adolesc Psychiatry 131:86, 1992.
81. Keener M, Zeanah C, Anders T: Infant temperament, sleep organization, and nighttime parental interventions. Pediatrics 81:762, 1988.
82. Winnicott D: Transitional objects and transitional phenomena. Int J Psychoanal 34:89, 1953.

Acknowledgment

The authors gratefully acknowledge the helpful suggestions and careful editing of Christine Acebo, PhD.

Sleep and its Disorders in Adolescence

RONALD E. DAHL and MARY A. CARSKADON

Adolescence encompasses the awkward years spanning early sexual maturation (puberty) until through attainment of adult status in society. This developmental interval has expanded significantly in recent human history as improved nutrition and physical health have contributed to earlier pubertal onset, while adult roles have required lengthier preparation and training. A wide range of physical changes, emotional and psychologic alterations, and social transitions accompany this developmental phase, and many adolescents experience a tumultuous barrage of stresses, challenges, and adaptations. Near the center of this maelstrom of changes lies the regulation of sleep and arousal. Several factors highlight the intimate relation between adolescent development and sleep-wake regulation: major developmental changes in the control of sleep and circadian systems occur during adolescence; emotional turmoil and stress affect the sleep system directly, while sleep deprivation may cause or exacerbate emotional difficulties; adolescents in modern western culture often follow erratic late-night schedules resulting in sleep deprivation; and experimentation with drugs, alcohol, and other substances can further interfere with sleep. For these reasons, adolescence likely represents a relatively vulnerable period with respect to sleep regulation. Because adolescence is a critical period to establish health and life habits and to begin career pursuits, this time of life provides an important opportunity for health-related interventions, such as treatment of sleep-related disorders and establishment of good sleep habits into adulthood.

Normal Sleep Related Changes in Adolescence

Prepubertal children are remarkably efficient sleepers, showing excellent alertness during the daytime and highly efficient, very deep sleep at night with abundant slow wave stages 3 and 4 (delta) sleep. A decrease in the amount of delta sleep accompanies adolescence, with approximately a 40% decrement between the ages of 10 and 20.[1] One hypothesis suggests that this age-related decline in delta sleep parallels the loss of cortical synaptic density ("cortical pruning") that occurs during adolescence.[2] Adolescents also show reduced REM latency and some increase in stages 1, 2, and awake during the night compared with preadolescents.

Changes in the *amount* of sleep are difficult to characterize during adolescence. Laboratory data compiled by Carskadon and associates[3] indicate that, if anything, adolescents require *more* sleep. On the other hand, field studies show that they frequently *obtain* much less.[4] The most parsimonious explanation for these observations is that adolescents get less sleep because of social schedules and late night activities combined with early school schedules, even though their physiologic sleep requirements do not appear to decrease. One outcome of these observations is significant daytime sleepiness among many adolescents.[5]

A third but related set of changes associated with adolescent sleep patterns is an apparent tendency for a delay of circadian phase; that is, adolescents tend to stay up later and to sleep in later than preadolescents. This developmental pattern has conventionally been attributed to study and work schedules, social activities, and striving for independence. Recent data, however, point to the possibility of a biologic component that may involve an alteration of the biologic timing mechanism in association with puberty.[6] One hypothesis consistent with these observations is that the period of the intrinsic circadian oscillator ("tau") may lengthen in association with pubertal maturation. This tendency for an adolescent delay of sleep phase has also been reported by Brazilian and Japanese investigators.[7, 8]

Assessment/Interview of Adolescent Sleep Symptoms

The clinical assessment of adolescents with sleep complaints requires a thorough interview of the patient and relevant family members to obtain a wide range of information about sleep and related habits, including usual sleep/wake habits, bedtime routines, descriptions of middle-of-the-night behaviors, wake-up times, morning routines, and symptoms of daytime sleepiness or irritability. The interview should assess the duration, frequency, and patterns of symptoms, including timing, changes with weekends and vacations, and changes with stressors and special events. Past medical history, medications (especially stimulants, asthma medications, antiseizure drugs, and sedatives), and family history of sleep problems are also important. A 2-week *prospective* sleep log or diary is often critical to obtaining detailed and accurate information because parents and adolescents will frequently describe a "usual schedule" that may bear little resemblance to more carefully documented details of bedtime and wake-up time. In the prospective log, the adolescent should record bedtime, estimated time to fall asleep, wake-up times, and details of sleep-related symptoms. If there is any doubt, the parent should initial each page of the form to verify accuracy. A continuous measure of activity may also be helpful in documenting waking and sleeping schedules.

The Sleepy Adolescent

Excessive sleepiness is a frequent complaint among adolescents. A thorough detailed history is clearly the first step in evaluating these complaints. This history must characterize the nature of the sleepiness (i.e., difficulty staying awake vs fatigue or decreased interest in activities), the frequency and duration of symptoms, and whether the symptoms occur at any particular time(s) of the day or only in certain situations.

The differential diagnosis of the sleepy adolescent includes four categories of problems: (1) insufficient amounts of sleep; (2) disturbed nocturnal sleep; (3) increased sleep requirements despite adequate nighttime sleep; and (4) circadian schedule disorders (Table 3–1). The history and evaluation should be directed at characterizing the problem with respect to these categories.

Insufficient Sleep

The most common cause of sleepiness in adolescence is an inadequate number of hours in bed. The combination of late night social schedules and activities with early morning school requirements can significantly compress the hours available to sleep. Part-time jobs, sports activities, clubs, hobbies, and active social lives can further exacerbate the problem. Further, as described previously, a biologic component may augment the tendency toward late night schedules in adolescents. Nonetheless, high school students frequently must begin their days very early on school days in order to catch buses, make schedules, and so forth. The emergence of such a problem and resultant daytime sleepiness may coincide

Table 3–1. SOURCES OF SLEEPINESS IN THE ADOLESCENT

Inadequate amounts of sleep
    Late night and erratic schedules
    Difficulty falling asleep
    Early morning awakening

Disturbed nocturnal sleep
    Obstructive sleep apnea syndrome
    Frequent nocturnal arousals
    Medical problems disturbing sleep
    Use of drugs and/or alcohol
    Withdrawal from drugs/alcohol

Circadian and scheduling disorders
    Delayed sleep phase syndrome

Increased sleep requirements
    Narcolepsy
    Idiopathic CNS hypersomnolence
    Some cases of depression
    Kleine-Levin syndrome

with the transition to a new school schedule (Fig. 3–1).

A typical pattern of sleep-related problems and daytime sleepiness often ensues when catch-up sleep on weekends and holidays promotes an even later circadian schedule, leading to a very erratic sleep/wake schedule. Such erratic patterns contribute to fragmented night sleep or the inability to fall asleep early on school nights, thus creating a repeating cycle of poor and inadequate sleep (see scheduling disorders). In other adolescents, the sleep deficit on school nights is exacerbated by the inability to obtain any catch-up sleep

on weekends owing to activities on weekend mornings or parental reluctance to foster catch-up sleep.

When insufficient sleep is identified, recommending that the adolescent "go to bed earlier" is rarely an effective remedy. The primary role of the clinician is often to help the entire family understand and acknowledge the consequences resulting from inadequate sleep and the relationship of insufficient sleep to specific behaviors. Sleep deprivation frequently contributes to many factors that the family does identify as major problems, including falling asleep in school, oversleeping in

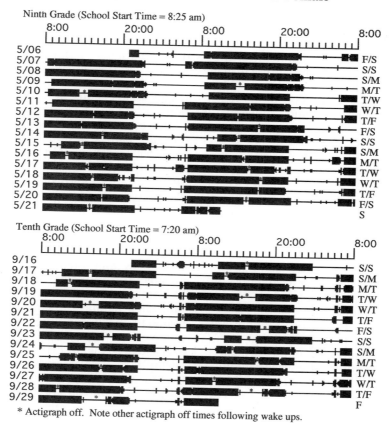

Figure 3–1. This diagram illustrates activity and rest patterns in an adolescent girl participating in a research project over the transition from ninth to tenth grade. The data are displayed as a double plot, wherein two consecutive days are placed side by side and then placed over consecutive days vertically. The dark areas illustrate portions of the day in which activity levels were high; light areas indicate sleep or, as designated by an asterisk, times when the activity monitor was not worn. In addition, many of the wake-up times are followed by a brief interval of actigraph off, particularly evident in the bottom graph. In the top graph, this girl was in ninth grade attending a junior high school that started at 8:25 AM. In the bottom graph, the girl was in tenth grade attending a school that started at 7:20 AM. The average school-night sleep time in the ninth grade was 491 minutes. In tenth grade, the average school-night sleep time was 385 minutes. The difference principally resulted from an earlier rising time in tenth versus ninth grade (approximately 5:30 AM vs approximately 7:30 AM).

the morning, fatigue, irritability, and mood lability. As with many areas of health, strategies to prevent poor habits and to promote and maintain healthy habits make great common sense but have little salience in the decision making process of many adolescents until problems become severe. If the adolescent's school or social functioning is significantly impaired by the sleep problem, a strict behavioral contract agreed on by the family can be an essential component of the intervention. The contract should specify hours in bed (with only small deviations on the weekends) and target the specific behaviors contributing to bad sleep habits, such as particular late night activities, erratic napping, and oversleeping for school. The choice of rewards for successes and negative consequences for failures as well as an accurate method of assessing compliance are essential components of the contract. The clinician should be sensitive in making recommendations for the gradual attainment of the new schedule—abrupt advancing of nocturnal bedtime by several hours may not be possible. For each adolescent, construction of a schedule to maximize sleep may require individualized strategies.

Disturbed Nocturnal Sleep

When symptoms of sleepiness occur despite an adequate sleep schedule, disruptions of sleep should be considered. Disturbances within sleep can be more difficult to assess by history alone than insufficient sleeping time. Although some families may describe that the child or adolescent is waking frequently, in other cases the family may be unaware of subtle sleep disruptions that lead to daytime sleepiness. Drug or alcohol use is an important consideration in these cases. In addition to the obvious effects of late night stimulants, such as cocaine, more complex drug/sleep interactions also can occur. For example alcohol can facilitate sleep onset but subsequently leads to decreased delta and REM sleep along with sleep fragmentation. Further, withdrawal from stimulants, alcohol, and marijuana can produce transient but severe sleep disruptions. Caffeine is also commonly used by adolescents in the form of caffeinated sodas, coffee, and tea and may produced sleep fragmentation particularly when used late in the day. Although it may seem a paradoxical approach to the treatment of excessive sleepiness, elimination of caffeine can be an important step in treating symptoms when daytime sleepiness is associated with disrupted nocturnal sleep. Prescription medications such as beta-adrenergic agonists for asthma or stimulants for attention deficit disorder (ADD) can also result in significant sleep disruptions.

Another cause of disturbed nocturnal sleep and consequent excessive daytime sleepiness is obstructive sleep apnea (OSA). This syndrome is uncommon in adolescents, usually associated with an obvious physical malformation (retrognathia, micrognathia), hypertrophied tonsils and/or adenoids, or a significant degree of obesity. This disorder is discussed in Chapters 18 and 19.

Circadian and Scheduling Disorders

The most common circadian problem relevant to adolescents is delayed sleep phase syndrome (DSPS).[9, 10] DSPS often begins with a tendency to stay up late, sleep in, and/or take a late afternoon nap. This process typically begins on weekends, holidays, or summer vacations. Problems become apparent when the adolescent and parent experience morning wake-up battles and difficulties getting the teenager to school. Often these adolescents cope through catch-up sleep (sleeping well into the afternoon) on the weekends. Although some of these behaviors occur in many normal adolescents, the circadian system in extreme or highly susceptible youngsters can become entrained at a phase position that places sleep at such a late time that even exceptionally motivated adolescents find it impossible to shift their sleep to an earlier time. In some instances, attempts by adolescents (and their families) to correct the problem by trying to make adjustments that exceed the range of entrainment of the intrinsic circadian oscillator goes against circadian principles. For example, an adolescent who has been going to bed at 3:00 AM and getting up at noon during vacation will abruptly try to go to bed at 10:00 PM on the night before the first day back at school. He or she will experience an exceedingly long delay in falling asleep, and for a few days may manage to get up for school by a strenuous effort to awaken at the wrong phase of his or her cycle. Then, the adolescent will take long naps after school to replace missed sleep, which only further retards sleep onset at night. Thus, despite numerous nights of trying to go to bed at 10:00 PM, he or she remains unable to achieve a stable entrainment of the circadian system to an earlier phase.

The treatment of DSPS consists of three parts: *stabilize* the schedule, then proceed with a *gradual realignment* to the desired schedule, and finally *maintain* the new alignment. After stabilizing on a schedule at a time when the adolescent usually goes to sleep without difficulty, the process of alignment requires small, *consistent* advances in bedtime and wake-up time (about 15 minutes earlier each day). During this process naps must be avoided and the realignment procedures must be consistent on weekends and holidays. In severe cases, adolescents on very late schedules may respond more favorably to going around the clock with successive delays in bedtime. This process has been described as phase delay "chronotherapy."[11] Since the intrinsic period of the biologic clock is generally longer than 24 hours, phase delays may be accommodated more easily than phase advances.[12] Delay schedule changes, therefore, can proceed with longer (2–3 hour) adjustments each day. Although the change can be accomplished quicker in the phase delay direction, the chief difficulty with this approach is that extremely unusual bedtimes and rising times occur along the course of the realignment, and such changes may require a great deal of assistance to ensure that the teenager keeps the appropriate schedule (e.g., staying awake from midnight until 6:00 PM on day 4).

This example of phase delay chronotherapy starts with an adolescent who has been falling asleep at 3:00 AM and getting up at noon. After stabilizing on this schedule, chronotherapy on day 1 calls for bedtime at 6:00 AM and risetime at 3:00 PM, with enforced awakening at that time and no sleep permitted until the next scheduled bedtime. On day 2, bedtime is 9:00 AM and wake-up is 6:00 PM; on day 3, noon until 9:00 PM; day 4, 3:00 PM until midnight; day 5, 6:00 PM until 3:00 AM; day 6, 9:00 PM until 6:00 AM; and on day 7, 10:00 PM until 7:00 AM. This last sleep schedule (or similar schedule adequate for the adolescent's needs) is then strictly maintained. During the course of chronotherapy, the adolescent must avoid napping and when possible should have physical activity and bright light exposure (such as walking outside) on waking up in each cycle.

Although many adolescents do very well with this type of phase delay chronotherapy or with a more gradual phase advance, the first weekend or vacation of returning to old habits can undo a lot of hard work. During the first 2 to 3 weeks following chronotherapy, rigid requirements should be set about wake-up time *seven days a week.* Later, if the adolescent wants to stay up late on an occasional weekend night, he may be able to do so but should not be permitted to sleep in more than 1 or 2 hours later than his usual wake-up time for school. Strict behavioral contracts (worked out with the parents) involving specific rewards for success and serious consequences for failures are essential in this type of intervention.

Some clinicians have advocated the use of melatonin for the treatment of DSPS on the basis of one encouraging study in adults.[11a] One approach is to use a physiological dose orally approximately 1.5 to 2 hours before bedtime (Lavie, et al personal communication, 1995). There are, however, no controlled clinical trials with any age group, and no long-term outcome data to support the effectiveness of this treatment over time. Although melatonin is widely available at health food stores in many countries (including the United States), it is also important to point out that currently this use of melatonin is not approved by the FDA. Further, there are theoretic concerns about using melatonin before or during puberty, since in many animal species melatonin has been shown to have an important function in reproductive physiology. Finally, it is worth re-emphasizing the clinical experience with this population, which suggests that addressing issues of motivation, mood, sleep hygiene and habits, and other behavioral issues discussed above are likely to be critical to long-term success in many adolescent patients.

At least two other disorders can mimic a DSPS. One disorder involves the adolescent who has trouble following an early schedule but does not find the pattern particularly distressing. Such youngsters are not motivated to correct the problem, are not particularly concerned about their recurrent experiences of being late for or missing school, and express little motivation to change their late night habits.[9] These adolescents are essentially *choosing* a late night schedule—some as a way of avoiding school, some because of situations in the home that foster late schedules, and some for possible secondary gain from a family situation. Unless the clinician is able to alter the larger realm of priorities and motivators, these adolescents are very unlikely to respond to any treatment of a sleep/schedule problem. The second disorder involves adolescents who initially appear to have DSPS but reveal a history of experiencing very long periods of time to fall asleep no matter how late they go to bed and yet are able to wake for school with little difficulty. In these adolescents, insomnia rather than the sleep schedule is the principal component of the problem.

Clinicians occasionally encounter a child or adolescent who appears to have a totally chaotic sleep schedule. Sleep appears to be scattered across night and day in a random fashion with no clear pattern. One of the most helpful assessment tools for such a problem is a well-documented sleep diary or sleep chart. Details of individual sleep bouts collected prospectively can then be plotted on a chart, which can indicate patterns not evident by history taking alone. An example of one such child is shown in Figure 3–2 displayed as a "double plot." Sleep is shown in black, awake in white, with 48 hours of data on each line. A completely erratic sleep schedule was reported. He was described as staying up all day

and all night followed by long sleep episodes, then short naps, and so forth. The sleep chart, however, shows that between 8/19 and 9/07, his sleep was following a periodicity of 25.6 hours—despite going to school from 8 AM to 3 PM. This child had a free-running circadian system with his sleep following the internal cycle rather than entraining to environmental cues. This boy had several features of autism, and his free-running rhythm may have been related to his limited capacity for spontaneous social interactions. As shown in the diagram, however, an intervention that included a structured behavioral program to eliminate naps and enforcement of a strict sleep and social schedule resulted in a sleep pattern in synchrony with a 24-hour rhythm. Of interest was that following this intervention, he no longer showed evidence of inadequate sleep and the family reported significant improvement in his irritability and other behavioral problems. Although this case is somewhat unusual, it highlights the value of obtaining specific sleep schedule information in a way that permits visual evaluation of the sleep pattern.

Increased Sleep Requirements

Narcolepsy

Adolescence has been reported as the peak age of onset for narcolepsy,[13] which is typically the second most prevalent cause of hypersomnolence in adolescent patients presenting at sleep disorder centers.[14] The full-blown narcolepsy syndrome is characterized by a tetrad of symptoms including sleep attacks (excessive intrusive daytime sleepiness), cataplexy (characterized by brief episodes of muscle weakness, often associated with an emotional precipitant such as laughter), sleep paralysis (an atonic condition occurring at the onset or offset of sleep), and hypnagogic hallucinations (vivid dream-like visual/auditory hallucinations at sleep onset).

Rarely, however, does a teenager with narcolepsy show all of these symptoms.[15-17] In a recent review of 16 consecutive cases of early-onset narcolepsy, only one case experienced the full tetrad.[18] Excessive sleepiness was the prominent symptom in all 16 cases, although only three showed the classic pattern of uncontrollable "sleep attacks." In several cases, the only manifestation of sleepiness was an increase in the total sleep time per 24 hours. In some cases, where the patient was able to ob-

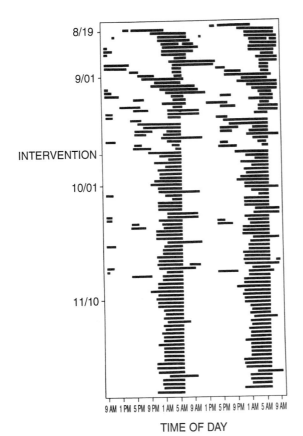

Figure 3–2. Double plot of sleep in a boy with free-running rhythm. Black bars indicate sleep with 48 hours of data on each line.

tain 12 or more hours of sleep per night, daytime sleepiness was minimal; while in other patients, no matter how much nightime sleep was obtained, severe daytime sleepiness was a major problem. In the majority of cases, daytime sleepiness was significantly exacerbated (or began) near the onset of physical pubertal changes. We emphasize that all of these patients demonstrated *true sleepiness* while following a good sleep/wake schedule with adequate hours in bed. By true sleepiness we are distinguishing "tiredness" or fatigue (the decreased motivation and difficulty initiating activities as is often seen in depressed adolescents) from repeated episodes of falling asleep during the day despite adequate night sleep, as is usually seen in narcoleptic adolescents.

Cataplectic episodes were dramatic in two cases, and cataplexy was mild or subtle in seven others. In patients with definite cataplexy, the symptoms were missed by experienced clinicians who mistook the behaviors for willful unresponsiveness or convergence symptoms. In the 16 cases, hypnagogic hallucinations were dramatic and disturbing in three, mild or subtle in six, and absent in seven. In three subjects, the hypnagogic hallucinations were so frightening that they significantly interfered with sleep. Sleep paralysis was present in only one of the 16 adolescents.

Other observations included very high rates of emotional and behavioral disturbances (12 of 16 cases). Four of the patients had been misdiagnosed with a psychiatric disorder before narcolepsy was recognized. These diagnoses included major depressive disorder, major depressive disorder with psychotic features, and ADD. Obesity was an unexpected association in the case series, with 11 of the 16 narcoleptic patients overweight at the time of diagnosis. Relationships among emotional regulation, appetite regulation, and sleep regulation in these narcoleptic patients were not disentangled.[18] These results are consistent with previous studies of early onset narcolepsy.[15–17, 19] Taken together, these studies indicate that narcolepsy is often missed in children and adolescents and that behavioral and emotional problems are often prominent features of adolescent narcolepsy.

The multiple sleep latency test (MSLT) is useful in the diagnosis of adolescent narcolepsy.[20] Importantly, sleepiness can antedate by years the manifestation of REM onset episodes in the MSLT. Clinical follow-up and repeat studies are often necessary to make a definitive diagnosis.[16, 18] Care must be taken, however, to ensure adequate nocturnal sleep prior to the MSLT testing and appropriate timing of the MSLT naps, as both insufficient sleep and naps at the trough of the circadian cycle may be associated with sleep onset REM episodes in nonnarcoleptic adolescents. With respect to treating adolescent narcolepsy, few data are available to indicate any potential differences from treatment of adult narcolepsy. One critical issue, however, is the necessity for young patients to follow a good sleep/wake schedule and to maintain good sleep hygiene. Although these concerns are crucial among adolescent narcoleptics, these youngsters are vulnerable to the same tendencies and social pressures as other adolescents making education, counseling, support, and psychosocial issues equally or more important to treatment than medications when working with young narcoleptics.

Another diagnosis to be considered in the sleepy adolescent is idiopathic hypersomnia, where there is often a familial history of excessive sleep need and the individual shows clear objective sleepiness during nap studies despite well-documented adequacy of night time sleep. This disorder is frequently treated with stimulant medication when the diagnosis is definitively established and daytime functioning is impaired.

Kleine-Levin syndrome, characterized by symptoms of excessive somnolence, hypersexuality, impulsive overeating, was first described by Kleine in 1925 and Levin in 1929 (see Chapter 14). Mental disturbances including irritability, confusion, and occasional auditory/visual hallucinations have frequently been reported in association with this disorder. The syndrome appears to occur more frequently in males, begins during adolescence, and in about half the cases has an onset following flu-like illness or injury with loss of consciousness. An episodic recurrence of symptoms is frequently observed with cycles lasting anywhere from 1 to 30 days. The syndrome usually disappears spontaneously during late adolescence or early adulthood; however, cases have been described with chronic changes.[21]

Depression

Adolescents with depressive disorders frequently complain of excessive sleepiness. One study demonstrated that depressed adolescents were capable of greater oversleeping in the morning than control adolescents.[22] Other studies have found no objective evidence of increased sleep in depressed adolescents, despite subjective complaints of excessive sleepiness among depressed adolescents.[23] This finding suggests that fatigue and a subjective sense of tiredness may play a more prominent role than true sleepiness in these depressed teens. Nevertheless, the diagnosis of major depressive disorder should be considered in the differential of adolescents complaining of excessive sleepiness (see Chapter 16).

Insomnia

Clinical experience with sleep disorders among adolescents suggests that the most frequent cause of the complaint of insomnia stems from sleep/wake schedule problems. As previously discussed, adolescents can follow a phase delayed schedule during the summer and holidays and experience extraordinary difficulty adjusting to the early demands of a school schedule. Their optimal bedtime on school nights may coincide with the so-called "forbidden zone" of the circadian system making it quite impossible to fall asleep. This pattern can also lead to a conditioned psychophysiologic insomnia, where the adolescent experiences performance anxiety about getting sufficient sleep for school and begins to associate bedtime and the bedroom with stress and anxiety.

Other common sources of insomnia in adolescents are anxiety and depressive disorders and/or traumatic or stressful events. These issues are addressed in Chapter 16. Childhood-onset insomnia, or "idiopathic insomnia," can also present during adolescence. The etiology of this disorder is unknown; however, an imbalance between arousal and sleep systems has been suggested.[24] This type of insomnia may indicate a hyperarousal or a hyposomnolence and is likely to be related to neurophysiologic alterations in sleep/wake systems. The seriousness of idiopathic insomnia cannot be explained by other psychologic or medical problems. Typically, the adolescent with idiopathic insomnia complains of poor concentration, impaired vigilance and attention, low energy, bad mood, and increased fatigue. These adolescents also may have some neurologic signs, which can appear as dyslexia or hyperactivity, and may show subtle EEG abnormalities. Idiopathic insomnia is believed to be a very rare clinical disorder, distinguished by the following diagnostic criteria: a complaint of insom-

nia that is longstanding, typically beginning in very early childhood; the insomnia is unceasing and persists equally through intervals of relatively good or poor emotional functioning; and no medical or psychiatric cause can be associated with the onset of symptoms. Prognosis for this disorder is poor unless the patient is particularly responsive to hypnotic medication.

Psychophysiologic Insomnia

As with adults, psychophysiologic insomnia can present in adolescence. As previously described, adolescents can have acute periods of stress or hyperarousal that interfere with sleep onset and can develop performance anxiety and negative associations with bedtime. This chronic difficulty with sleep onset is very similar to that described in adults. Behavioral regimens, including stimulus control, sleep restriction, and biofeedback, have shown some efficacy in adults with psychophysiologic insomnia. No controlled studies of such treatments specifically for adolescents have been done.

Summary

Adolescent sleep patterns in many western cultures show several common features that lead to inadequate sleep. These include a marked tendency to delay the timing of preferred sleeping hours, which often conflicts with the time that school begins in the morning—the "zero hour" as it is termed in Israel. Furthermore, teenagers require at least as much sleep as preteens. As a consequence of these factors, many teens have a chronic sleep deficit or develop wildly erratic sleeping patterns. For some, these pressures may lead to serious consequences in terms of excessive daytime sleepiness, reactive mood and behavior disruptions, and family conflict; for others, serious sleep pathology develops, such as DSPS or chronic insomnia.

Although adolescence clearly poses unique risks for the development of sleep disorders, few clinical reports have described diagnosis and treatment specifically for this age group. Most of our appreciation of adolescent sleep disorders is based on experiences with childhood and adult sleep problems, for which there is a far richer literature. Consequently, clinicians may attempt to apply techniques for treating adolescents that are successful with younger children or adults. However, in developing treatment strategies for adolescents, one must remember the teenager's psychosocial milieu. The adolescent is capable of independent action and self-management, yet remains dependent on parents. The motivating factors, the daily stressors, the psychosocial pressures will differ in teenagers versus preteens and adults. These factors can either interfere with or be recruited to assist in treatment. The successful approach requires a careful balance that involves the adolescent and parents in a program taking into account the particular life circumstances of the adolescent and the family.

References

1. Carskadon MA: The second decade. *In* Guilleminault C (ed): Sleeping and Waking Disorders: Indications and Techniques. Menlo Park, Addison-Wesley, 1982.
2. Feinberg I: Schizophrenia: caused by a fault in programmed synaptic elimination during adolescence? J Psychiatr Res 17(4):319, 1982–83.
3. Carskadon MA, Harvey K, Duke P, et al: Pubertal changes in daytime sleepiness. Sleep 2:453, 460, 1980.
4. Carskadon MA: Patterns of sleep and sleepiness in adolescents. Pediatrician 17:5, 1990.
5. Carskadon MA, Dement WC: Sleepiness in the normal adolescent. *In* Guilleminault C (ed): Sleep and Its Disorders in Children. New York, Raven Press, 1987, pp 53–66.
6. Carskadon MA, Vieira C, Acebo C: Association between puberty and delayed phase preference. Sleep 16(3):258, 1993.
7. Andrade MMM, Benedito-Silva EE, Domenice S, et al: Sleep characteristics of adolescents: a longitudinal study. J Adolesc Health 14:401, 1993.
8. Ishihara K, Honma Y, Miyake S: Investigation of the children's version of the morningness-eveningness questionnaire with primary and junior high school pupils in Japan. Percept Motor Skills 71:1353, 1990.
9. Ferber R, Boyle PM: Delayed sleep phase syndrome versus motivated sleep phase delay in adolescents. Sleep Res 12:239, 1983.
10. Thorpy MJ, Korman E, Spielman AJ, et al: Delayed sleep phase syndrome in adolescents. J Adolesc Health 9:22, 1988.
11. Czeisler CA, Richardson GS, Coleman RM, et al: Chronotherapy: resetting the circadian clocks of patients with delayed sleep phase insomnia. Sleep 4:1, 1981.
11a. Dahlitz M, Alvarez B, Vignau J, et al: Delayed sleep phase syndrome response to melatonin. Lancet 337(8750):1121, 1991.
12. Weitzman ED, Czeisler CA, Coleman RM, et al: Delayed sleep phase syndrome. Arch Gen Psychiatry 38:737, 1981.
13. Aldrich MS: Narcolepsy. Neurology 42(suppl 6):34, 1992.
14. Guilleminault C: Narcolepsy and its differential diagnosis. In Guilleminault C (ed): Sleep and Its Disorders in Children. New York, Raven Press, 1987, pp 181–194.
15. Young D, Zorick F, Wittig R, et al: Narcolepsy in a pediatric population. Am J Dis Child 142:210, 1988.
16. Kotagal S, Hartse KM, Walsh IK: Characteristics of narcolepsy in preteenaged children. Pediatrics 85:205, 1990.
17. Navelet Y, Anders T, Guilleminault C: Narcolepsy in children. *In* Guilleminault C, Dement W, Passouant P (eds): Narcolepsy. New York, Spectrum, 1976, pp 171–177.
18. Dahl RE, Holttum J, Trubnick L: A clinical picture of child and adolescent narcolepsy. J Am Acad Child Adolesc Psychiatry 6:834, 1994.
19. Allsopp MR, Zaiwall Z: Narcolepsy. Arch Dis Child 67:302, 1992.
20. Carskadon MA and Dement WC: MSLT—what does it measure. Sleep 5:S67, 1982.
21. Critchley M: Periodic hypersomnia and megaphagia in adolescent males. Brain 85:627, 1962.
22. Hawkins DR, Taub JM, Van de Castle RL: Extended sleep (hypersomnia) in young depressed patients. Am J Psychiatry 142:905, 1985.
23. Dahl RE, Puig-Antich J, Ryan ND, et al: EEG sleep in adolescents with major depression: the role of sucidality and inpatient status. J Affect Disord 19:63, 1990.
24. Hauri P, Olmstead E: Childhood-onset insomnia. Sleep 3(1):59, 1980.

Control of Breathing During Sleep in the Fetus and Neonate

HENRIQUE RIGATTO

The control of breathing has been extensively studied over the years, yet the effect of sleep on this control has not. There are two basic reasons for this. First, the notion that sleep profoundly alters breathing became clear only recently.[1, 2] Second, to study the effect of sleep on breathing, it is essential to work with the intact subject and this became available only during the last three decades.[3] It is still not known how breathing may relate to carotid body discharges, since there are no accurate methods to record evoked potentials chronically from the carotid sinus nerve. As some of these technical problems are solved, we may understand better the role of sleep on specific mechanisms regulating breathing.

A major difference in behavior between the newborn infant and the adult subject is that the newborn sleeps about three-quarters of the time while the adult sleeps only about one-third (see also Chapter 2).[2] The fetus, on the other hand, sleeps all or almost all of the time.[4-6] This behavioral difference has methodologic implications: many of the previous studies on the control of breathing have compared ventilatory variables in the sleeping neonate with those in the awake adult, which is inappropriate and leads to erroneous conclusions.[2, 7-10] In order for comparisons to be meaningful, it is essential that they be made during similar sleep states.

Sleep has important effects on the modulation of breathing. In 1972, Rigatto and Brady stated "periodic breathing occurs physiologically in the state of sleep associated with rapid eye movements in infants[2] and adults.[11, 12] This type of sleep is ontogenetically primitive and related to immaturity of the reticular formation in the medulla.[13] Because sleep is 90% primitive (REM) at 30 to 31 weeks of gestation in contrast to 50% at term and 20% in adult life,[14] and because it depresses ventilation and shifts the CO_2 response curve to the right with a small decrease in slope,[12, 15] it may be an important factor in producing periodic breathing in the preterm infant."[2] Indeed, subsequent studies have confirmed that sleep state is a very important factor in the control of respiration. In addition to powerfully modulating resting breathing, sleep state may also be important in the establishment of extrauterine breathing[5, 6, 16, 17] and may be a vital physiologic factor in triggering the irreversible apnea leading to sudden infant death syndrome (SIDS).[18, 19]

In this chapter the important effects of sleep on breathing in the fetus and neonate are reviewed. Much of our knowledge of fetal breathing stems from work in experimental animals.

History

Study of the specific effects of sleep on breathing dates back to the nineteenth century. It was not until 1944, however, that a systematic work was published by Magnussen showing that ventilation decreases during sleep in healthy adults and that alveolar carbon dioxide tension ($PaCO_2$) increases.[20] The next major study was in 1963 when Bulow described the effect of sleep on breathing in adult subjects.[12] His study was essentially only on the effects of NREM (quiet) sleep, although, in the preceding decade, Aserinsky and Kleitman[21] and Dement and Kleitman[22] had published their important discovery of REM sleep. The first description of the effect of sleep on breathing in the neonate was probably that of Aserinsky in 1965, who reported periodic breathing in conjunction with eye movements during sleep.[11] Although the effect of sleep on breathing was obviously important, there was a long delay before a systematic analysis of its effect on respiration began. This occurred in the 1970s and was in great part stimulated by studies done on sleeping newborn infants.[2, 23–25] In 1972, Dawes and coworkers published a classic paper showing that the fetus normally breathes in utero during periods of REMs associated with low-voltage electrocortical activity (LVECoG) but not during periods of high-voltage electrocortical activity (HVECoG, quiet sleep).[3] This discovery generated a great deal of interest about the influence of "fetal state" on control of breathing. This interest remains strong today and much of the information derived from studies on the effect of sleep on breathing may well be crucial to our improved understanding of the central control of breathing.[13]

The Fetus

Breathing Pattern at Rest

The history of the concept of fetal breathing really began in 1972 with the Oxford discovery of fetal breathing during REM sleep in sheep.[3] The investigators showed that deflections in tracheal pressure episodically occurring during periods of LVECoG could only reflect breathing activity by the fetus. However, in the preceding decade in Paris, Merlet and associates published findings of deflections in esophageal pressure which could only be explained on the basis of fetal breathing.[26] As occurs with most new ideas and discoveries, it took time for the concept of fetal breathing in utero to be universally accepted. Most subsequent studies, however, confirmed the initial observations (Fig. 4–1).[27–33] Some of these later studies showed electrical activity of the diaphragm occurring simultaneously with changes in tracheal pressure, clearly defining a central respiratory output.[5, 31, 34–36]

Fetal breathing occurs primarily during periods of LVECoG which accounts for 40% of the fetal life during the last trimester of gestation in sheep.[3, 5] In the human fetus, this percentage is similar or somewhat higher (see Chapter 2).[33, 37, 38] During HVECoG, there is no established breathing present, but occasional breaths may surface after episodic, generalized, tonic muscular discharges associated with body movements (Fig. 4–1).[5] During LVECoG, breathing is irregular and diaphragmatic electromyogram (EMG) is characterized by abrupt beginning and ending. Less frequently, there is a progressive increase in envelope amplitude, comparable to the inspiratory slope observed in the anesthetized newborn lamb (Fig. 4–2). A gradual decrease in diaphragmatic EMG at the end of a breath, reflecting postinspiratory activity, as observed in the newborn infant, is rarely seen in the fetus.[5, 6, 36, 39–41] This irregular diaphragmatic activity generates a negative tracheal pressure of about 2 to 5 mmHg. The corresponding changes in tracheal flow are less than seen postnatally, likely because of the higher viscosity of lung fluid in the system. The irregular breathing activity observed during this period probably reflects the influence of the reticular formation on breathing so characteristic of REM sleep. The average breath has an inspiratory time of 0.45 second, expiratory time of 0.74 second, and a total duration of 1.12 seconds.[39] These measurements are similar to those obtained in the newborn lamb. The breathing activity in the fetus serves no gas exchange function, which is performed by the placenta, and therefore its purpose has been the object of considerable debate. Geoffrey Dawes postulated that its purpose is to train the respiratory apparatus for extrauterine activity.[42] The physiologic mechanism responsible for the occurrence of fetal breathing only in LVECoG is unknown.

Fetal State

The occurrence of fetal breathing in LVECoG has led some investigators to believe that the fetus might be awake during part of this period.[43, 44] In fact, using electrophysiologic criteria, it was postulated that the fetus was awake in about 5% of the time during the last part of gestation in sheep.[16, 17, 44, 45] It was further postulated that a number of chemical and pharmacologic agents could alter fetal breathing by "arousing" the fetus.[16, 17, 44, 45] In

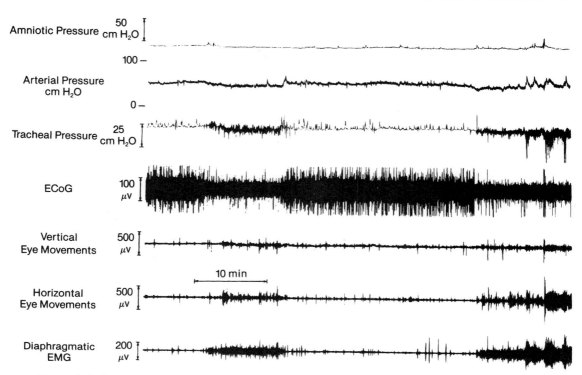

Figure 4–1. Breathing in a fetal lamb at 134 days of gestation. Note that the deflections in tracheal pressure and diaphragmatic activity occur during periods of rapid eye movement (REM) in low-voltage electrocortical activity (LVECoG) only. In high-voltage electrocortical activity (HVECoG, quiet sleep) breathing is absent. (From Rigatto H: Control of breathing during sleep in the fetus and neonate. *In* Kryger MH, Roth T, Dement WC: Principles and Practice of Sleep Medicine. Philadelphia, WB Saunders, 1989.)

the late 1970s Rigatto and associates became interested in determining whether the fetus, at times, was awake at rest in utero and whether arousal could be induced by chemical or pharmacologic agents. They reported the polysynaptic reflexes obtained from the hindlimbs in the chronic fetal sheep preparation to be unusually intense during transition from LVECoG to HVECoG.[36] They further speculated that this might represent fetal wake-fulness and subsequently implanted a window on the left flank of the ewe to directly observe the fetus in utero (Fig. 4–3).[6] The technique proved to be powerful and has generated substantial new information. Wakefulness, defined by open eyes and purposeful movement of the head, was never observed in the fetus under resting conditions. Analysis of videotapes now amounting to more then 2000 hours of observation over 5 years has shown clearly that the

Figure 4–2. Tracheal pressure and diaphragmatic activity in a fetal lamb at 129 days' gestation. Note the abrupt beginning and ending of diaphragmatic activity in some of the breaths and the progressive increase in activity in others. A gradual decrease in diaphragmatic activity, reflecting postinspiratory activity, as seen in the newborn infant, is rarely seen in the fetus. (From Rigatto H: Control of breathing during sleep in the fetus and neonate. *In* Kryger MH, Roth T, Dement WC: Principles and Practice of Sleep Medicine. Philadelphia, WB Saunders, 1989.)

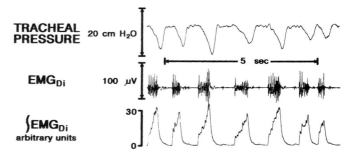

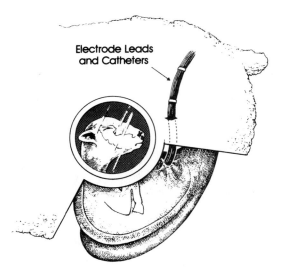

Electrode Leads and Catheters

Figure 4–3. View of the head of the fetus as it appears after surgery is completed. Note that the bundle with catheters and electrical leads cross the abdominal and uterine walls at some distance from the window. (From Rigatto H: Control of breathing during sleep in the fetus and neonate. *In* Kryger MH, Roth T, Dement WC: Principles and Practice of Sleep Medicine. Philadelphia, WB Saunders, 1989.)

fetal lamb alternates between two basic behavioral states, REM (LVECoG) sleep and quiet (HVECoG) sleep.[5] Activities such as movement, swallowing, licking, breathing occur during REM sleep (Fig. 4–4). During quiet sleep the fetus is still and occasionally shows generalized ample movements associated with tonic discharges. The enhancement of the polysynaptic reflexes observed previously was associated with generalized tonic discharges and rotation of the body and head during the transition from LVECoG to HVECoG. It was not associated with wakefulness.[5] This generalized discharge is typical of the transition from LVECoG to HVECoG. We speculate that understanding the neurophysiologic basis for this intense discharge may provide the explanation of how the change from low to high voltage occurs.

Besides the normal irregularity of the respiratory pattern seen in REM sleep, licking and swallowing clearly disturb breathing activity.[5, 40] Breathing becomes slower and irregular, and the diaphragmatic activity becomes interrupted by clusters of esophageal electromyographic activity. This digestive activity occurs primarily during REM sleep and is translated behaviorally and electrophysiologically as a general increase in EMG activity, blood pressure, and heart rate.

Modulation of Fetal Breathing by CO_2, Hypoxia, Pulmonary Reflexes, and Pharmacologic Agents

Initially, fetal breathing was thought by some investigators to depend on behavioral influences since it was observed only during REM sleep and seemed somewhat refractory to chemical stimuli.[46] Subsequent studies, however, clearly showed that the fetal breathing apparatus is capable of responding well to chemical stimuli and other agents known to modify breathing postnatally. Thus it became clear that the fetus responds to an increase in $Paco_2$ with an increase in breathing.[6, 27, 28, 39, 45, 47] This increase is associated with increases in tracheal pressure, integrated diaphragmatic activity, and frequency (Fig. 4–5). Both inspiratory and expiratory times decrease as would be expected from postnatal studies.[6, 39, 47] The increased breathing activity continues into the period of transitional HVECoG, but it does not continue into the period of established HVECoG despite suggestions to the contrary.[16, 17, 45, 47] Rigatto and associates specifically investigated whether they could raise arterial Pco_2 during rebreathing or during direct administration of CO_2 to the fetus via an endotracheal tube.[47] Breathing activity was always abolished during periods of HVECoG except when $Paco_2$ was unphysiologically high (>100 mmHg) and pH low (< 7.0). In this situation low pH could be the primary stimulus, as acidosis has been shown to induce continuous breathing.[48] This increased breathing activity was not associated with wakefulness.[5] Administration of low oxygen to the fetus, by having the ewe breathe hypoxic mixtures, abolished fetal breathing and was associated with a decrease in body movements and in the amplitude of the ECoG.[49] Conversely, the administration of 100% O_2 to the fetus via an endotracheal tube induced continuous fetal breathing with clear manifestations of arousal. Together the findings appear to suggest a strong link between oxygen tension, fetal breathing, and sleep with low oxygen inhibiting and sedating the fetus and high oxygen facilitating fetal breathing and arousal.

Pharmacologic agents such as indomethacin, pilocarpine, 5-hydroxytryptophan (5-HTP), and morphine induced continuous breathing in the fetus for a variable duration.[6, 50–53] This continuous breathing classically crosses the ECoG barrier; that is, it occurs in LVECoG and HVECoG (Fig. 4–6). As the response starts to fade, the HVECoG breaks in, inhibiting

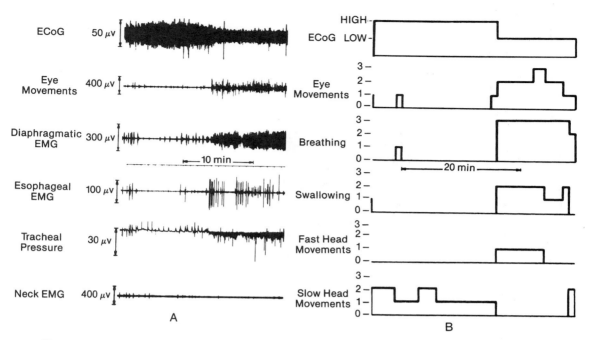

Figure 4–4. A comparative representation of observations made *(A)* on polygraph and *(B)* through double-wall Plexiglas window. Fetal breathing, eye movements, and swallowing are predominantly present in LVECoG. 0, absent; 1, low activity; 2, medium; 3, high. (From Rigatto H: Control of breathing during sleep in the fetus and neonate. *In* Kryger MH, Roth T, Dement WC: Principles and Practice of Sleep Medicine. Philadelphia, WB Saunders, 1989.)

breathing and restricting the still intense breathing to periods of LVECoG. Once the pharmacologic effects subside and breathing becomes normal again, the intensity of breathing activity decreases. Two interesting facts about this prolonged breathing response to pharmacologic agents are that the fetus in general does not tend to wake except in the case of morphine stimulus and prolonged breathing tends to cross the HVECoG barrier. In response to morphine given during a breathing interval, the fetus becomes apneic and simultaneously switches from LVECoG (REM sleep) into HVECoG (quiet sleep); this is fol-

lowed by a prolonged run of continuous breathing, lasting an average of about 2 hours in which the fetus switches back into LVECoG (REM sleep).[51, 54] During the period of maximal breathing, the fetus may open his eyes, increase body movements, and have some swallowing activity, a behavior suggesting arousal.[51] This is transient and accounts for only part of the breathing response to morphine. During administration of pilocarpine, a fetus was once noticed opening his eyes, but behaviorally he seemed to be in REM sleep.[6] All these pharmacologic agents produce an increase in tracheal pressure and an increase in diaphragmatic

Figure 4–5. Fetal breathing during control and during CO_2 rebreathing. Note the increase in tracheal pressure and diaphragmatic activity during CO_2 rebreathing. Fetal breathing was prolonged into the transitional low- to high-voltage ECoG, but stopped in established high-voltage ECoG. (From Rigatto H: Control of breathing during sleep in the fetus and neonate. *In* Kryger MH, Roth T, Dement WC: Principles and Practice of Sleep Medicine. Philadelphia, WB Saunders, 1989.)

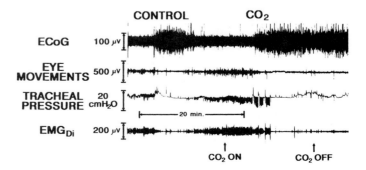

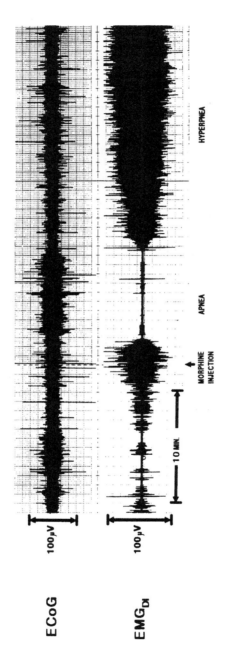

Figure 4-6. The fetal response to intravenous injection of morphine. Administration of morphine induced apnea followed by prolonged and intense continuous breathing. Apnea coincided with a change in ECoG from low to high voltage, and conversely, hyperpnea was associated with a change in ECoG from high to low voltage. During hyperpnea, at times, the fetus showed signs of arousal, such as open eyes, squirming, and licking. (From Rigatto H: Control of breathing during sleep in the fetus and neonate. *In* Kryger MH, Roth T, Dement WC: Principles and Practice of Sleep Medicine. Philadelphia, WB Saunders, 1989.)

EMG, but only indomethacin, pilocarpine, and morphine increase respiratory frequency. With 5-HTP, breathing was deep and slow.[6] As endogenous opiates have been hypothesized to inhibit fetal breathing, some investigators reported that naloxone given to the fetus produced continuous breathing, decreased the threshold for CO_2 stimulation of breathing, and possibly wakened the fetus.[45] Rigatto was unable to corroborate these findings in experiments using the window technique.[6] Indeed, in dosages of naloxone equivalent to those used by Moss and Scarpelli,[45] intense and prolonged convulsions were produced in the fetus, followed by limited periods of continuous breathing. Thus, the action of naloxone is likely agonist depending on its stimulant effects, not on its inhibitory action on endogenous opiates.

There are numerous pieces of experimental evidence suggesting that the action of CO_2 and pharmacologic agents occurs centrally. The mechanism by which hypoxia affects respiration in the fetus is poorly understood but is probably central also. The peripheral chemoreceptors were thought to be inactive in utero, but the idea that they are completely silent was probably derived from incorrect experimental evidence.[55] Blanco and associates have clearly documented activity of the peripheral chemoreceptors in the fetal lamb showing that they are reset at the time of delivery.[56] Resection of the carotid bodies did not alter fetal breathing or fetal state substantially and apparently did not alter the establishment of breathing at birth.[34] The exact relevance of peripheral chemoreceptors to intrauterine breathing remains undetermined. Finally, it seems that pulmonary reflexes are present in fetal life. Lung distention with saline infusion produced decreased frequency of breathing.[30] Section of the vagi, however, did not alter breathing pattern and the relevance of the pulmonary reflexes to fetal breathing is still not clear.[3, 57]

The Neonate

Breathing Pattern at Rest

The neonate, and particularly the premature infant, breathes irregularly. There is great breath-to-breath variability and long stretches of periodic breathing in which breathing and apnea alternate.[2, 9, 10, 58] Haldane's statement that "the surprising fact is not that we breathe regularly but that we do not breathe periodi-

cally most of the time" applies more at this age than at any other.[59] The resting breathing pattern of the neonate is not sleep state dependent, although sleep greatly modulates it. Neonates spend 90% of their time in REM sleep at 30 weeks of gestation and 50% at term as compared to 20% in adult subjects.[2] Quiet sleep becomes definable only after 32 weeks of gestation, and wakefulness occurs only 6 to 8 hours a day in the newborn (see also Chapter 2).[37] Periodic breathing with alternation between regular breathing periods and 5 to 10 seconds of apnea is commonly seen in premature infants. It occurs in the three states, wakefulness, REM, and quiet sleep, but is most common in REM sleep.[60] It is frequently stated that in quiet sleep, in analogy with criteria used for adult subjects, infant breathing is regular. Prechtl and others, however, have clearly shown that periodic breathing is common in quiet sleep.[58, 61, 62] The difference is that periodic breathing in quiet sleep is regular, that is, the breathing and apneic intervals are of the same duration, and very irregular in REM sleep. The most well-defined periodic breathing observable in small babies is in quiet sleep during tracé alternans (Fig. 4–7). The cause of this periodic breathing is not known but most investigators believe that it depends on oscillations in blood gases.[63] The overall minute ventilation is increased in REM sleep as compared to quiet sleep, and this is due to a primary increase in respiratory frequency with little change in tidal volume.[23, 58, 60]

Chemical Regulation

Inhalation of CO_2 increases ventilation during REM and quiet sleep in newborn infants. The response to steady-state inhalation of CO_2 is the same in these two sleep states, but the response during rebreathing of CO_2 is less in REM than in quiet sleep (Fig. 4–8).[15, 23, 60, 61] Moriette and associates postulated that the differences in response using these two techniques are due to the fact that with rebreathing, it is only possible to measure the response in "phasic" REM, whereas with the steady-state technique the response is measured in both "phasic" and "tonic" REM sleep.[61] Since the CO_2 response in "tonic" REM is the same as in quiet sleep, the results obtained using the steady-state method resembled those seen in quiet sleep.[54, 64] The breathing pattern in response to CO_2 may change in two different ways. If inhaled CO_2 is low, less than 2%, dur-

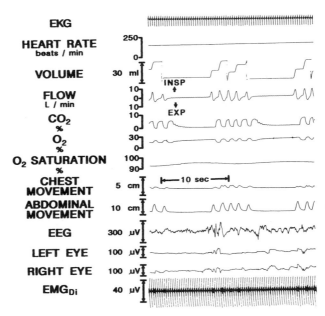

Figure 4–7. Periodic breathing during quiet sleep in an 8-day-old preterm infant born at 32 weeks. Note the regular periodicity of breathing, with both apneic and breathing intervals keeping a constant length. Note also the classic tracé alternans pattern on EEG. (From Rigatto H: Control of breathing during sleep in the fetus and neonate. *In* Kryger MH, Roth T, Dement WC: Principles and Practice of Sleep Medicine. Philadelphia, WB Saunders, 1989.)

ing steady state inhalation, the response consists primarily of an increase in tidal volume.[58] If inhaled CO_2 is high, more than 2%, the response in both sleep states consists of an increase in respiratory frequency and in tidal volume.[2, 61] Periodic breathing is abolished with a small increase in inhaled CO_2 of about 1 to 2%.[2] This response has been attributed to the increased central drive and increased stores of CO_2 with better buffering capacity for the oscillations in Pa_{CO_2}.

Inhalation of low oxygen produces an immediate increase in ventilation (1 min) followed by a later decrease (5 min).[10, 65] The response is similar in wakefulness, REM and quiet sleep, although hyperventilation seems more sustained during late hypoxia in quiet sleep (Fig. 4–9).[60] The more sustained hyperventilation in these infants during quiet sleep reflects the increase in autonomic control that occurs during this sleep state and which makes the system more responsive to chemical stimuli.[1, 64] The immediate increase in ventilation reflects peripheral chemoreceptor stimulation and is associated with an increase in frequency and in tidal volume. The late response is primarily mediated through a decrease in respiratory frequency.[2, 10] The mechanism responsible for this response is still unclear, but recent experi-

ments in kittens and newborn monkeys suggest that the late decrease in ventilation is a mechanical effect rather than a depression of the central respiratory neurons.[66–68] In these experiments, diaphragmatic activity and frequency remained elevated during hypoxia, but tidal volume decreased below control values during late hypoxia (Fig. 4–10). These experiments were carried out during quiet sleep. Because the response to low oxygen in the fetus and in the premature infant is clearly related to some degree of central inhibition, these findings may have to be viewed cautiously: they may reflect a difference between species with a predominant peripheral mechanism in animals and a central mechanism in humans. The peculiar response of the neonate to low inhaled oxygen is of great clinical significance. Infants who are borderline hypoxic tend to breathe periodically or develop apneic spells. Hypoxia can induce periodic breathing in these infants, as shown previously.[10] The relief of these apneic spells, which are frequently associated with bradycardias, can be obtained by increasing the inspired oxygen concentration.[2]

Administration of high oxygen, on the other hand, produces an immediate decrease in ventilation followed by hyperventilation, a re-

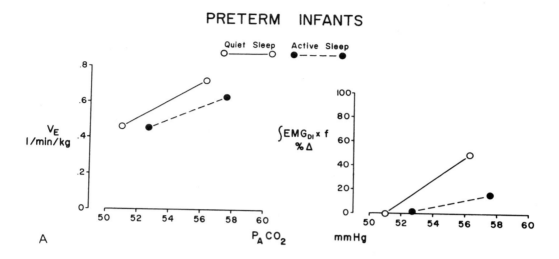

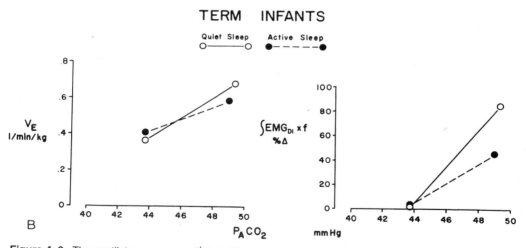

Figure 4–8. The ventilatory response ($\dot{V}E$) to CO_2 rebreathing in neonates. Note that *(A)* preterm and *(B)* term infants showed a decreased response to CO_2 in "phasic" REM sleep as compared to quiet sleep. (From Rigatto H: Control of breathing during sleep in the fetus and neonate. *In* Kryger MH, Roth T, Dement WC: Principles and Practice of Sleep Medicine. Philadelphia, WB Saunders, 1989.)

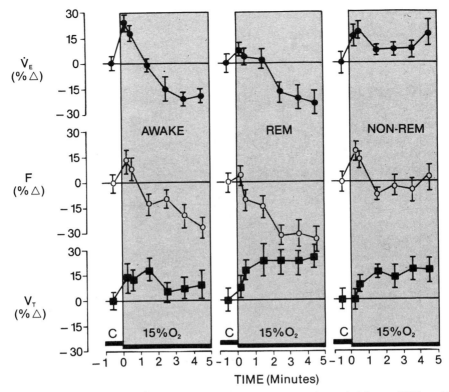

Figure 4–9. Ventilatory response ($\dot{V}_E$) to 15% O_2 in preterm infants during wakefulness, REM, and NREM sleep. With 15% O_2 there is an immediate increase followed by a decrease in ventilation in wakefulness and REM sleep; in NREM sleep or quiet sleep hyperventilation is more sustained. V_T, tidal volume; F, frequency. (From Rigatto H: Control of breathing during sleep in the fetus and neonate. *In* Kryger MH, Roth T, Dement WC: Principles and Practice of Sleep Medicine. Philadelphia, WB Saunders, 1989.)

sponse which is similar during wakefulness, REM sleep, and quiet sleep. These findings suggest a lack of major differences in the activity of the peripheral chemoreceptors during these sleep states.[60, 65] The immediate decrease in ventilation following the administration of 100% oxygen is related to a decrease in frequency—apnea being common in preterm infants—and a decrease in tidal volume. The late increase in ventilation with oxygen is likely related to cerebral vasoconstriction, but a mechanical change related to effects at the level of the airways cannot be ruled out.[69]

Pulmonary Reflexes

The effect of sleep state on pulmonary reflexes has been investigated less thoroughly than its effect on chemical control of breathing. The evidence suggests that pulmonary stretch receptors and irritant receptors are in-

active during REM sleep.[1, 25] Airway mechanisms responsible for clearing may be impaired during REM sleep.

Respiratory Muscles

Sleep has a profound effect on respiratory muscles, as tonic activity of most respiratory muscles is abolished during REM sleep.[25, 41, 70, 71] For instance, disappearance of tone in the intercostal muscles is likely responsible for the increase in chest distortion seen in these infants during REM sleep. Lack of tone leads to chest wall collapse during inspiration, and the caudal displacement of the diaphragm has to be twice as long to produce the same lung volume displacement.[70, 72] Because of chest wall collapse, functional residual capacity is decreased in these infants during REM sleep.[70] Luz and associates also found that distorted and nondistorted breaths produce the same

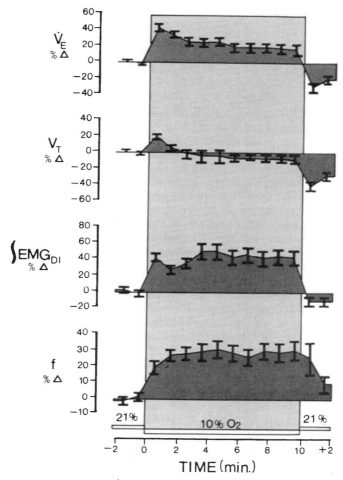

Figure 4–10. The ventilatory response ($\dot{V}E$) to hypoxia in newborn kittens. Note the immediate increase in ventilation followed by a decrease during inhalation of low O_2. The late decrease was primarily related to a decrease in tidal volume (VT), diaphragmatic activity (EMGDI), and frequency (f) remaining elevated during hypoxia. This suggested that the late decrease in ventilation during hypoxia was not primarily central but peripheral, possibly related to bronchoconstriction and increased pulmonary impedance or uncoupling of diaphragm and lungs. (From Rigatto H: Control of breathing during sleep in the fetus and neonate. *In* Kryger MH, Roth T, Dement WC: Principles and Practice of Sleep Medicine. Philadelphia, WB Saunders, 1989.)

instantaneous ventilation as long as they are of the same duration, although the work of the diaphragm is 40% greater when the respiratory movements are out of phase (Fig. 4–11).[72] Another important influence of sleep on the respiratory muscles is on the postinspiratory activity of the diaphragm. This activity controls, in part, the duration of expiratory time.[73, 74] In neonates, Rigatto and associates observed that this activity was more pronounced in the lateral than in the crural part of the diaphragm, longer in quiet than in REM sleep, and more prolonged in preterm than in term infants (Fig. 4–12).[75] The length and

variability of this activity in preterm infants suggest that because of their highly compliant chest wall, these infants use the postinspiratory diaphragmatic activity as a breaking mechanism whose role in maintaining lung volume and controlling expiratory time is much more important than in older children and adults. Similarly, sleep state profoundly affects the muscular control of upper airway resistance. Studies by Harding and associates in fetal and neonatal lambs suggest that the abductor muscles of the larynx—the posterior cricoarytenoid and cricothyroid—have inspiratory activities in parallel with that of the diaphragm,

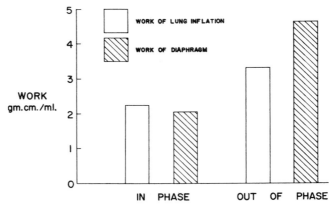

Figure 4–11. Work of lung inflation and of diaphragm when breathing is in-phase or out-of-phase. The work of lung inflation is not significantly different when the breath is in phase or out of phase. However the work of the diaphragm is approximately 40% greater when the breath is out of phase as opposed to in phase. (From Rigatto H: Control of breathing during sleep in the fetus and neonate. *In* Kryger MH, Roth T, Dement WC: Principles and Practice of Sleep Medicine. Philadelphia, WB Saunders, 1989.)

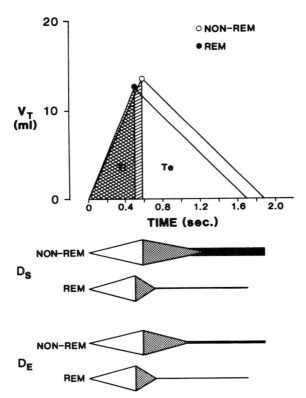

Figure 4–12. Diagrammatic changes in tidal volume (VT), "timing," and diaphragmatic EMG in NREM (quiet) and REM (active) sleep. Note that total phasic activity diminishes from NREM to REM sleep. Also, in both sleep states, it is shorter in esophageal (DE) than in surface EMG (DS). Expiratory phase activity as a proportion of total phasic activity decreases significantly from NREM to REM sleep. (From Rigatto H: Control of breathing during sleep in the fetus and neonate. *In* Kryger MH, Roth T, Dement WC: Principles and Practice of Sleep Medicine. Philadelphia, WB Saunders, 1989.)

during both quiet and REM sleep. On the other hand, the adductor muscles of the larynx—the thyroarytenoid, lateral cricoarytenoid, and intra-arytenoid—have a phasic expiratory activity only during quiet sleep. This activity is lost during REM sleep in the fetus and in the newborn lamb (Fig. 4–13).[41] In conjunction with decreased intercostal and postinspiratory diaphragmatic activity during REM sleep, a reduction in adductor activity of the larynx may be partly responsible for the decrease in lung volume observed during this sleep state. Thus, these studies indicate that sleep profoundly affects upper airway resistance and findings fit with general observations that obstructive apneas occur more frequently in REM sleep than in quiet sleep.

Summary

Sleep is an important modulator of breathing. Conversely, consciousness represents "the forgotten stimulus to breathe."[1] The effects of sleep on the fetus and neonate are profound: fetal breathing only surfaces during REM sleep and there is no tonic respiratory muscular activity during REM sleep in neonates. Although sleep seems to have more of a modulatory than causal effect on breathing at the time of delivery, in many situations, such as during apneas, it may represent the difference between death and survival, if arousal is impaired.[1, 18] Clarification of the precise mechanisms of how sleep interacts with breathing is likely to provide substantial information on how breathing is controlled centrally.

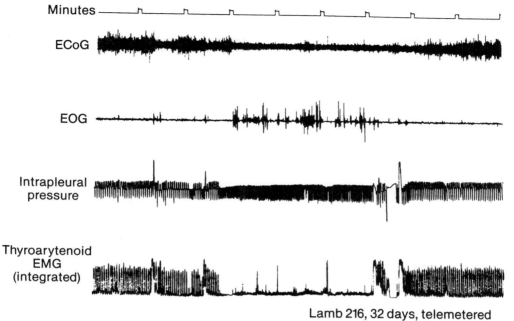

Figure 4–13. The influence of sleep state on thyroarytenoid (TA) activity. The recording shows a short period of REM sleep preceded by and followed by quiet sleep. TA activity and simultaneous positive overshoot of intrapleural pressure were absent in REM sleep. (From Rigatto H: Control of breathing during sleep in the fetus and neonate. *In* Kryger MH, Roth T, Dement WC: Principles and Practice of Sleep Medicine. Philadelphia, WB Saunders, 1989.)

References

1. Phillipson, EA: Control of breathing during sleep. Am Rev Respir Dis 118:909, 1978.
2. Rigatto H, Brady JP: Periodic breathing and apnea in preterm infants. I. Evidence for hypoventilation possibly due to central respiratory depression. Pediatrics 50:202, 1972.
3. Dawes GS, Fox HE, Leduc MB, et al: Respiratory movements and rapid eye movement sleep in the fetal lamb. J Physiol (Lond) 220:119, 1972.
4. Dreyfus-Brisae C: Sleep ontogenesis in early human prematurity from 24–27 weeks of conceptual age. Dev Psychobiol 2(3):162, 1968.
5. Rigatto H, Moore M, Cates D: Fetal breathing and behavior measured through a double-wall Plexiglas window in sheep. J Appl Physiol 61:160, 1986.
6. Rigatto H: A new window in the chronic fetal sheep model. *In* PW Nathanielsz (ed): Animal Models in Fetal Medicine. Ithaca, NY, Perinatology Press, 1984, pp 57–67.
7. Brady JP, Ceruti E: Chemoreceptor reflexes in the newborn infant. Effects of varying degrees of hypoxia on heart rate and ventilation in a warm environment. J Physiol (Lond) 184:631, 1966.
8. Brady JP, Cotton EC, Tooley WH: Chemoreflexes in the newborn infant: effects of 100% oxygen on heart rate and ventilation. J Physiol (Lond) 172:332, 1964.
9. Cross KW, Oppe TE: The effect of inhalation of high and low concentrations of oxygen on the respiration of the premature infant. J Physiol (Lond) 117:38, 1952.
10. Rigatto H, Brady JP: Periodic breathing and apnea in preterm infants. II. Hypoxia as a primary event. Pediatrics 55:604, 1975.
11. Aserinsky E: Periodic respiratory pattern occurring in conjunction with eye movement during sleep. Science 150:763, 1965.
12. Bulow K: Respiration and wakefulness in man. Acta Physiol Scand 59(Suppl 209):1, 1963.
13. Jouvet M: Neurophysiology of the states of sleep. Physiol Rev 47:117, 1967.
14. Parmelee AH, Wenner WH, Akiyama Y, et al: Sleep states in premature infants. Dev Med Child Neurol 9:70, 1967.
15. Reed DJ, Kellogg RH: Changes in respiratory response to CO_2 during natural sleep at sea level and at altitude. J Appl Physiol 13:325, 1958.
16. Ioffe S, Jansen AH, Russel BJ, et al: Respiratory response to somatic stimulation in fetal lambs during sleep and wakefulness. Pflugers Arch 388:143, 1980.
17. Ioffe S, Jansen AH, Russell BJ, et al: Sleep, wakefulness and the monosynaptic reflex in fetal and newborn lambs. Pflugers Arch 388:149, 1980.
18. Kelly DH, Shannon DC: Sudden infant death syndrome and near sudden infant death syndrome: a review of the literature 1964 to 1982. Pediatr Clin North Am 29:1241, 1982.
19. Rigatto H: Disorders of the control of breathing. *In* Pediatric Respiratory Diseases. Bethesda, MD, National Institutes of Health, Publication #86–2107, 1986, p 20.
20. Magnussen, G: Studies on the Respiration During Sleep. London, Lewis, 1944.
21. Aserinsky E, Kleitman N: Regularly occurring periods of eye motility, and concomitant phenomena, during sleep. Science 118:273, 1953.

22. Dement WC, Kleitman N: Cyclic variations in EEG during sleep and their relation to eye movements, body motility, and dreaming. Electroencephalogr Clin Neurophysiol 9:673, 1957.

23. Davi M, Sankaran S, MacCallum M, et al: Effect of sleep state on chest distortion and on the ventilatory response to CO_2 in neonates. Pediatr Res 13:982, 1979.

24. Gabriel M, Albani M, Schulte FJ: Apneic spells and sleep state in preterm infants. Pediatrics 57:142, 1976.

25. Hagan RAC, Bryan CA, Bryan MH, et al: The effect of sleep state on intercostal muscle activity and rib cage motion. Physiologist 19:214, 1972.

26. Merlet C, Hoerter J, Devilleneuve C, et al: Mise en evidence de mouvements respiratoires chez le foetus d'agneau. CR Acad Sci Ser D 270:2462, 1970.

27. Boddy K, Dawes GS: Fetal breathing. Br Med Bull 31:3, 1975.

28. Boddy K, Dawes GS, Fisher R, et al: Fetal respiratory movements, electrocortical and cardiovascular responses to hypoxaemia and hypercapnia in sheep. J Physiol (Lond) 243:599, 1974.

29. Maloney JE, Adamson TM, Brodecky V, et al: Diaphragmatic activity and lung liquid flow in the unanesthetized fetal sheep. J Appl Physiol 39:423, 1975.

30. Maloney JE, Adamson TM, Brodecky V, et al: Modification of respiratory center output in the unanesthetized fetal sheep "in utero." J Appl Physiol 39:552, 1975.

31. Maloney JE, Bowes G, Wilkinson M: "Fetal breathing" and the development of patterns of respiration before birth. Sleep 3:299, 1980.

32. Patrick J, Campbell K, Carmichael L, et al: A definition of human fetal apnea and the distribution of apneic intervals during the last ten weeks of pregnancy. Am J Obstet Gynecol 136:471, 1980.

33. Patrick J, Campbell K, Carmichael L, et al: Patterns of human fetal breathing during the last 10 weeks of pregnancy. Obstet Gynecol 56:24, 1980.

34. Jansen AH, Ioffe S, Russell BJ, et al: Effect of carotid chemoreceptor denervation on breathing in utero and after birth. J Appl Physiol 51:630, 1981.

35. Jansen AH, Ioffe S, Russell BJ, et al: Influence of sleep state on the response to hypercapnia in fetal lambs. Respir Physiol 48:125, 1982.

36. Rigatto H, Blanco CE, Walker DW: The response to stimulation of hindlimb nerves in fetal sheep, in utero, during the different phases of electrocortical activity. J Dev Physiol 4:175, 1982.

37. Dreyfus-Brisae C: Ontogenesis of sleep in human prematures after 32 weeks of conceptual age. Dev Psychobiol 3(2):91, 1970.

38. Perrin DG, Becker LE, Madapallimatum A, et al: Sudden infant death syndrome: increased carotid body dopamine and noradrenaline content. Lancet 2:535, 1984.

39. Dawes GS, Gardner WN, Johnston BM, et al: Effects of hypercapnia on tracheal pressure, diaphragm and intercostal electromyograms in unanesthetized fetal lambs. J Physiol (Lond) 326:461, 1982.

40. Harding R, Johnson P, McClelland ME, et al: Laryngeal function during breathing and swallowing in foetal and newborn lambs. J Physiol (Lond) 272:14P, 1977.

41. Harding R, Johnson P, McClelland ME: Respiratory function of the larynx in developing sleep and the influence of sleep state. Respir Physiol 40:165, 1980.

42. Dawes GS: Breathing before birth in animals and man. N Engl J Med 290:557, 1974.

43. Condorelli S, Scarpelli EM: Somatic-respiratory reflex and onset of regular breathing movements in the lamb fetus in utero. Pediatr Res 9:879, 1975.

44. Ruckebusch Y: Development of sleep and wakefulness in the foetal lamb. Electroencephalogr Clin Neurophysiol 32:119, 1972.

45. Moss IR, Scarpelli EM: Generation and regulation of breathing in utero: fetal CO_2 response test. J Appl Physiol 47:527, 1979.

46. Chernick V: Fetal breathing movements and the onset of breathing at birth. Clin Perinatol 5:257, 1978.

47. Rigatto H, Lee D, Davi M, et al: The effect of increased arterial CO_2 on fetal breathing and behavior in sheep. J Appl Physiol 64:982, 1988.

48. Molteni RA, Melmed MH, Sheldon RE, et al: Induction of fetal breathing by metabolic acidemia and its effect on blood flow to the respiratory muscles. Am J Obstet Gynecol 136:609, 1980.

49. Clewlow F, Dawes GS, Johnston BM, et al: The developing relationship between breathing, electrocortical, ocular and nuchal muscle activity in unanesthetized fetal lambs. J Physiol (Lond) 341:463, 1983.

50. Brown ER, Lawson EE, Jansen A, et al: Regular fetal breathing induced by pilocarpine infusion in the near-term fetal lamb. J Appl Physiol 50:1348, 1981.

51. Hasan SU, Lee DS, Gibson D, et al: Dose response of behavior and breathing to intravenous injection of morphine in the fetal sheep. J Appl Physiol 64:2058, 1988.

52. Kitterman JA, Liggins GC, Clements JA, et al: Stimulation of breathing movements in fetal sheep by inhibitors of prostaglandin synthesis. J Dev Physiol 1:453, 1979.

53. Quilligan EJ, Clewlow F, Johnston BM, et al: Effect of 5-hydroxytryptophan on electrocortical activity and breathing movements of fetal sheep. Am J Obstet Gynecol 141:271, 1981.

54. Olsen GD, Dawes GS: Morphine effects on fetal lambs. Fed Proc 42:1251, 1983.

55. Biscoe TJ, Purves MJ, Sampson SR: Types of nervous activity which may be recorded from the carotid sinus nerve in the sheep fetus. J Physiol (Lond) 190:443, 1967.

56. Blanco CE, Dawes GS, Hanson MA, et al: The response to hypoxia of arterial chemoreceptors in fetal sheep and newborn lambs. J Physiol (Lond) 351:25, 1984.

57. Condorelli S, Scarpelli EM: Fetal breathing. Induction in utero and effects of vagotomy and barbiturates. J Pediatr 88:94, 1976.

58. Kalapesi Z, Durand M, Leahy FN, et al: Effect of periodic or regular respiratory pattern on the ventilatory response to low inhaled CO_2 in preterm infants during sleep. Am Rev Respir Dis 123:8, 1981.

59. Douglas CG, Haldane JS: The causes of periodic or Cheyne-Stokes breathing. J Physiol (Lond) 38:401, 1908–1909.

60. Rigatto H, Kalapesi Z, Leahy FN, et al: Ventilatory response to 100% and 15% O_2 during wakefulness and sleep in preterm infants. Early Hum Dev 7:1–10, 1982.

61. Moriette G, Van Reempts P, Moore M, et al: The effect of rebreathing CO_2 on ventilation and diaphragmatic electromyography in newborn infants. Respir Physiol 62:387, 1985.

62. Prechtl H: The behavioural states of the newborn infant (a review). Brain Res 76:185, 1974.

63. Waggener TB, Stark AR, Cohlan BA, et al: Apnea duration is related to ventilatory oscillation characteristics in newborn infants. J Appl Physiol 57:536, 1984.

64. Phillipson EA, Kozar LF, Rebuck AS, et al: Ventilatory and waking responses to CO_2 in sleeping dogs. Am Rev Respir Dis 115:251, 1977.
65. Aizad T, Bodani J, Cates D, et al: Effect of a single breath of 100% oxygen on respiration in neonates during sleep. J Appl Physiol 57:1531, 1984.
66. LaFramboise WA, Guthrie RD, Standaert TA, et al: Pulmonary mechanics during the ventilatory response to hypoxemia in the newborn monkey. J Appl Physiol 55:1008, 1983.
67. LaFramboise WA, Woodrum DE: Elevated diaphragm electromyogram during neonatal hypoxic ventilatory depression. J Appl Physiol 59:1040, 1985.
68. Rigatto H, Wiebe C, Rigatto C, et al: The ventilatory response to hypoxia in the unanesthetized newborn kitten. J Appl Physiol 64:2544, 1988.
69. Davi M, Sankaran K, Rigatto H: Effect of inhaling 100% O_2 on ventilation and acid-base balance in cerebrospinal fluid in neonates. Biol Neonate 38:85, 1980.
70. Henderson-Smart DJ, Read DJC: Reduced lung volume during behavioral active sleep in the newborn. J Appl Physiol 46:1081, 1979.
71. Lopes J, Muller NL, Bryan MH, et al: Importance of inspiratory muscle tone in maintenance of FRC in the newborn. J Appl Physiol 51:830, 1981.
72. Luz J, Winter A, Cates D, et al: Effect of chest breathing and abdomen uncoupling on ventilation and work of breathing in the newborn during sleep. Pediatr Res 16:296A, 1982.
73. Remmers JE, Bartlett JR: Reflex control of expiratory airflow and duration. J Appl Physiol 42:80, 1977.
74. Remmers JE, DeGroot WJ, Sauerland EK, et al: Pathogenesis of upper airway occlusion during sleep. J Appl Physiol 44:931, 1978.
75. Rigatto H, Reis F, Cates D, et al: Effect of sleep on phasic and "tonic" diaphragmatic EMG in preterm infants. Fed Proc 41:1103, 1982.

5

Assessment of Sleep Disorders in the Child

RICHARD FERBER

It is now possible to approach the youngster with sleep-related symptoms in a systematic manner.[1-11] Although the assessment in children is similar to that in adults, including a history, physical examination, and laboratory study, there are important differences. Certain disorders are specific to childhood and others have different childhood presentations, manifestations, etiologies, and significance.

Until late childhood or adolescence (and often even then), the complaints usually come from the parents or caretakers, not from the child. Thus, the parents' perception of a disorder is what must be assessed. Often there is a problem but no true disorder. The child's sleep is technically normal but occurring at times or in patterns that cause a problem for the parents. Assessment is still important. It allows the current condition to be understood, the parents to be so informed, and the professional and the caretaker to work together to make the necessary changes. By so doing, the problem can be resolved by curing the disorder or "correcting" an undesirable variation of normal.[2, 4, 10, 12]

An initial assessment of a child should include: (1) a detailed sleep history, (2) a general medical history, (3) a complete social history, (4) psychologic/developmental screening, and (5) a physical examination. Based on these findings, a decision should be made as to the importance of more complete psychologic testing or psychiatric evaluation, general or specialized laboratory screenings, and sleep laboratory study.[9]

Largely because so many of the sleep problems seen in childhood are behavioral, interactive, or schedule related, a careful and extended history becomes particularly important. The physical examination in most of these circumstances adds relatively little information, but it remains very important for complaints or history suggestive of sleepiness, neurologic impairment, or respiratory abnormalities. Sleep laboratory studies are required less frequently than in the adult but are critical for the evaluation of certain complaints, notably excessive sleepiness, unusual sleep-associated motor behavior, suspected sleep-associated respiratory disorders, and unexplained sleeplessness.

Sleep History

Some factors may be primarily involved, directly and initially causing the sleep problems, such as enlarged tonsils causing sleep apnea and marital discord causing children's fears. Other factors may be secondarily involved. For example, a child's poor sleep, perhaps initially due to excessive nighttime feeding, may cause parental anger, sleep deprivation, arguments, tension, threats, and spankings, all of which may lead to anxiety in the child. This anxiety may then become a secondary cause of ongoing sleep problems. Many factors may be involved. Sorting through these factors is often time-consuming but necessary if proper intervention is to be assured.

The sleep history has many components, which are detailed in the following sections.

Presenting Complaint

Although a detailed history of the evolution and variability of a symptom over time is important, knowledge of the current sleep pattern is usually most important because many different paths can lead to the same symptom. Some parents want to begin with a description of their youngster's neonatal sleep pattern and proceed slowly from there, month-by-month. A better approach is to get a brief idea of the evolution, concentrate on the current pattern, and then go back and fill in the rest of the evolution as needed.

It is often useful to have the child, if old enough, describe the problem first. The parent/child differences in perception as to the nature, seriousness, specifics, and even existence of a problem are often quite revealing. Parents may complain that a child does not go to sleep "early enough," but the child may tell you that he is not at all sleepy. Time in bed may be unpleasant (typical adult insomnia with tossing and turning) or quite pleasant (the child enjoying the time to think, fantasize, review the day's activities, or listen to the radio). The child may be complaining of a problem and asking for help or may deny the existence of any problem and be brought to the doctor against his or her wishes. The older child and adolescent may be the only one who can report with any accuracy the time of sleep onset and the number and length of nighttime wakings. However, if there is no direct parental confirmation, the accuracy of these histories must still be viewed with suspicion. The child may only know about his problem second-hand, being told by his parents (perhaps about his sleepwalking). In this case, it is important to learn what he has been told. Also, the manner in which the child relates to the examiner during this phase provides a great deal of information as to the child's shyness, nervousness, independence, confidence, affect, and activity level.

Most often the history is obtained from the parents. In a two-parent family, it is best to have both present. Much can be learned about family dynamics and function by the way this history is presented. One parent may present everything, both parents may talk but constantly disagree, and one or both parents may show evidence of marked anger, frustration, or depression. The examiner must be empathetic and understanding, willing to listen to the parents, yet at the same time control the session and focus the history.

The facts should be ascertained as precisely as possible, which may be no small task. Statements such as "he *never* sleeps" or "she has *always* been a bad sleeper" provide little infor-

mation. Tired frustrated families often want to present worst case scenarios: "It can be as bad as . . ." or "He can wake as many as . . . times each night." Focusing on the *usual* rather than the extraordinary is generally helpful. Typical ranges are easier for some parents to describe than precise times or frequencies: "Although he has wakened as many as nine times a night, he usually wakes two to five times and most often three." If several scenarios are possible, it is helpful to have the parents describe each separately. They should try to assign a relative frequency to each, that is, the number of nights per week or the percentage of wakings that occur for each scenario. If the numbers don't add up, for example, they sum to 12 nights per week or 250%, then go over it again. It is easier to remember bad nights than good ones, so parents understandably may inflate their descriptions. But as a practitioner, *you cannot make a proper diagnosis or institute proper treatment if you do not know what is happening.* Such insistence on facts also helps the parents gain a better sense of reality.

Sometimes no amount of effort provides a reasonable history. The parents may insist that their child sleeps 1 hour at a time, wakes eight times a night, and each time he wakes he is up for 1 hour. Going through the night with them hour-by-hour does not seem to help. There may be several explanations for this. The sleep problem may be significantly overestimated, which may reflect the degree of trouble some parents have dealing with even mild problems. More significant psychosocial problems within the home may be involved including depression, marital problems, or alcoholism, which some parents cannot face directly and instead focus all their anger and frustration on their youngster and "his or her sleep problem." This may be the only way they can ask for help for themselves. Sometimes the parents or parent presenting the history has no first-hand knowledge of the problem because the other parent or a nanny gets up at night. Or, they may just be so disorganized that they cannot present a history in any orderly fashion.

Always ask about the onset, duration, character, frequency, and consistency of the sleep symptom, and the length of time it has existed in its "current" pattern. The onset may coincide with psychologic stress such as the birth of a sibling, a family illness, a fire, an accident, or the start of school. It may begin when controls are lost such as when a child is moved from crib to bed. It may be related to start of a medication or the occurrence of frequent ear or throat infections. Over the time that symptoms have existed, they may have been constant, waxed and waned, worsened, or improved, and the so-called "current pattern" may actually describe a relatively new symptom. A 3-year-old who has had the symptom of sleeplessness "from birth" may have had different causes over the years (colic at 3 months, separation anxiety at 1 year, an improper schedule at age 3). The current problem, lasting perhaps 3 months, may have little to do with what came before.

All treatments attempted by the parents or a physician, and the results, should be described. These might include warm milk at bedtime, elimination of naps, bringing the child into the parents' bed, threats and punishments, or "letting the child cry." Medications may have been prescribed for sleeplessness, sleepwalking, or enuresis. Enuresis alarm systems may have been used but perhaps at too early an age, inconsistently, incorrectly, with an improper device, and without proper supervision and follow-up. Again, it is important to know exactly what was done, for example, bringing a child into the parents' bed can mean once in a while, every night, only after waking in the middle of the night, only after periods of crying, or only when one parent agrees to move to a different room.

The occurrence of symptoms at naptime in addition to or instead of at night is of interest. Some children nap easily but fight at night; others do the reverse. Some only have sleep terrors from naps, whereas for most, this usually occurs at night.

Sleep in different settings or conditions is relevant. Some children may sleep fine at daycare or for sitters and only the parents have trouble. Other children panic whenever parents are not present.

For certain problems such as sleep terrors and sleepwalking, it is useful to find out if parents can predict at bedtime if these problems are likely to occur that night. Young children often are more likely to have arousal events when they go to bed overtired. Illness increases or decreases the likelihood of problems in some children. There may be a relationship to external events such as school exams or athletics. The events themselves need careful description (time of night, characteristics, or atypical behavior) to distinguish benign from ictal episodes. For example, there should be no clonus; the events should not be confined to the early morning hours; and if there

are multiple events, they should lessen in intensity across the night. (See Chapter 11.)

For enuresis, the frequency and, if possible, the time of wetting are important as is the distinction between primary (no previous dry periods) and secondary (an intervening period of several months without wetting). Other urinary tract symptoms should be reviewed, and it must be known if the incontinence is confined to sleep and to urine. One should know if the child cares or is teased about the wetting. The responses to previous treatments should be learned. (See Chapter 12.)

Sleep Associations, Current Sleep-Wake Schedule, and Sleep Rhythm

Sleep associations are those conditions that are present at the time of the transition from wakefulness to sleep. Since this often involves the parents in some capacity at bedtime and at times of waking, these conditions underlie many of the problems parents discuss.[2–4, 7, 8, 13–15] Thus, this is a critical part of the interview, and the clinician must be willing to spend whatever time is necessary to determine the facts with the greatest certainty. Sleep onset at bedtime and again after normal nighttime wakings may require rocking, backrubbing, a parent's shoulder, a bottle, or a pacifier.[2, 4, 10, 16, 17] (See Chapter 9.)

The *sleep-wake schedule* is the specific timing of bedtime and naptimes, the actual hours of sleeping and waking, and the pattern of meals and other daytime activities. The *sleep rhythm* represents the current pattern of circadian functioning, that is, the position of the nocturnal sleep phase, the timing of daytime dips (nap tendency), and the overall sleep requirement. No childhood sleep evaluation is complete without this.[4, 10, 18–20] Even if the problem is felt to be "purely" behavioral or medical, secondary alterations in the schedule and rhythm are likely and must be taken into account when trying to interpret and correct the original problem. (See Chapter 10.)

The schedule can be obtained from the history, but it is important to note day-to-day and weekday-weekend variations. The sleep rhythm can usually be sorted out as well but with more effort. The main items to consider are (1) the hour the child actually falls asleep (this is often fairly constant regardless of bedtime; hence, late nights should have less bedtime problems, very late nights may find the youngster asleep before arriving home); (2) the hour he wakes spontaneously (when allowed to do so); (3) the time of day in the morning he starts acting wide awake; (4) his naptimes, including catnaps in the car or stroller; and (5) the total hours of sleep, night and day (especially on days when allowed to wake spontaneously).

Information on sleep associations and circadian and other factors can usually be obtained during a single part of the interview. Rather than limiting oneself to questions focused on the symptom, this information can be obtained while establishing the pattern of the child's whole day. One might start at suppertime first asking, for example, when and where the child eats, who else is present, how much is eaten, and then taking a history in stepwise fashion of the remaining activities that occur during the evening. Typical evenings usually include play, bath, television, and bedtime routines. By following this procedure, one should gain a sense of the consistency, appropriateness, pattern of parent–child interaction, and tension throughout the evening. How is bedtime decided and who handles it? Is there a bedtime routine and what does it consist of (story, TV, nothing)? Get the facts, the answers are there.

The bedtime routines should be described in detail from the start of bedtime until the child is sound asleep.[2–4] This includes all the conditions present before sleep through the moment of sleep transition—the struggles, demands, enforcement or absence of limits, stories, rocking, pacifiers, transitional objects, night lights, bright lights, radios, lullaby tapes, white noise generators, and bed, crib, floor, or lap. Transfer from lap or breast to crib or bed may be easy or difficult. The parent may be able to leave while the child is still awake or only if he is very drowsy or sound asleep. There may be complaints of fear (sometimes convincing, sometimes not), tantrums, or refusal to stay in the room.

The pattern of behavior should be explored carefully throughout the night. When complaints are of nighttime wakings, it is not sufficient just to know that they take place. One needs to know when they occur, what the child does, what the parents do, and how the child goes back to sleep. It should be known if the child wakes gradually or suddenly and if he stays in the crib or bed (calling softly, crying, or screaming) or comes into the parent's bedroom (walking calmly or running hysterically).

If any form of rapid intervention—rocking, nursing, pacifier, or transfer to the parents' bed—can lead to quick return to sleep, then this suggests absence of an underlying disorder (medical or schedule) interfering with sleep; habitual associations are likely the cause. If there are nighttime feedings, then the number of ounces (or the mother's impression of nursings as minimal or substantial) should be specified. Substantial intake can lead to conditioned nighttime hunger.[4, 21] If no rapid intervention helps, the child may be in pain or may be wide awake because of an improper schedule and is not ready to return to sleep.[3, 4, 6, 19, 20]

Consistency should be ascertained. Are these wakings always handled in the same manner or does it depend on the time of night and which parent is intervening?

Prolonged wakings may be described for children who are not really awake. A youngster in the midst of a confusional arousal or calm sleepwalking may be considered by parents to have wakened.[22] Similarly, bodyrocking and headbanging may occur even though a child is asleep.[23] These distinctions are critical, because to assume that habitual factors underlie all of the problems would mean that many children would be treated inappropriately.

Even a child that seems frightened at night may not be all that anxious. If the child acts and seems truly frightened and if this upset persists despite a parent's willingness to stay with the child, true anxiety is probable and may imply a nightmare or a nondream-related arousal with fear secondary to ongoing daytime issues.[10, 24] But if certain interventions, such as taking the child into the parents' bed, provide immediate calming and rapid return to sleep, then the anxiety (if present at all) is likely less severe. However, other possibilities such as habits and manipulations must be considered. The manner in which the complaints of fear are made may help in this distinction. Some children making protestations of fear seem and act perfectly calm, and it is unlikely that any significant anxiety is present. Others demonstrate behavior convincing of real fright. Sleep problems reflecting major or minor anxiety, habits (accustomed to coming into the parents' bed), inappropriate schedules (in bed but wide awake), and limit-setting difficulties may all "present" as fear but need to be handled differently.

Patterns of waking in the morning should then be explored: when, spontaneous or not, easily or with difficulty. Next, the organization of daytime activities should be explored including breakfast, lunch, and snacks, daycare, walks, playground play, structured activities, and school and afterschool programs. It is important to know if there are organized activities in the child's day; if there is peer interaction and gross motor exercise; if the day is spent mostly alone by the television; if there is any separation from the parents; if the child is ever left with a sitter, or if the only attempted separation takes place at bedtime. It may help to know if the child ever plays in his or her room during the day or if the only associations with that location are negative ones (punishment, nighttime separation).

The timing and occurrence of naps are very important to clarify, as are the circumstances under which they take place (car, crib, stroller, living room floor, or in school; easily or with difficulty; held, rocked, or sleeping next to a parent) and whether or not they end spontaneously. Early naps, late naps, or too much napping can have major impacts on nocturnal sleep.[3, 4, 6, 19] (See Chapter 10.)

Sleep Environment

The environment in which the child sleeps, and the circumstances present during sleep, are important to ascertain. It may be in a one bedroom apartment or a three story house. The child may have his or her own room or share a room and perhaps a bed with siblings or parents. It may be quiet at night and in the morning, or the child may be kept awake or wakened in the morning by outside activity. There may be shades and curtains to darken the room or little protection from the bright morning sun. At night the room may be completely dark, lit by a night light (1.5–7.0 watts), by lights from the street or hallway, or from a room light (60–100 watts) kept on all night or until sleep onset. The door may be closed, left ajar, or wide open. From bed or crib the child may be able to see the parents in the living room or in their bedroom. The child may be several floors away from the parents or close enough to hear or observe arguments or sexual activity, both of which may be scary. The child may be attached to a blanket, teddy bear, or doll, using it as a transitional object, or only want to be held at his mother's breasts or twirl her hair. An intercom may be left on all night which although reassuring to some parents allows other parents to hear and respond to every nighttime sound.

Development of Sleep Patterns and Problems and Review of Sleep Symptoms

Remaining details regarding the development of the child's sleep patterns and problems can now be filled in, and one can also now screen for the existence of other problems. A 3-year-old may still nurse three times a night simply because he was always nursed to sleep and no decision was ever made as to weaning, or patterns that developed to help a colicky child sleep (such as rocking) just persisted after the colic resolved. Often one learns that the child did settle (start sleeping through the night) at one point even though it may have only lasted a few weeks or months, but the problems restarted in a new context, perhaps during an illness. Parents may have had the child sleep with them early on, but found that at age 3, 5, or 10 they were not able to switch the child to his own room.

An adolescent with full-blown sleep terrors may have had confusional arousals as a toddler that may have continued unabated over the years, although with somewhat changing characteristics, or the events might have disappeared at age 4 and returned at 16. In the latter case psychologic or medical factors might be suspected. In the former case, this would be less certain.

Similarly, a 9-year-old who starts wetting the bed after years of not doing so must be evaluated for organic and psychologic problems rather than assuming a diagnosis of functional enuresis.

The adolescent may have the sudden onset of definite symptoms of narcolepsy but careful history may reveal the existence of subtle symptoms (long sleep, napping until a late age, or "hyperactivity") early on.

The onset of loud snoring in a child may be traced to the early months when pharyngeal lymphoid tissue became hypertropic. The snoring may have disappeared for some months after a tonsillectomy/adenoidectomy but returned suggesting adenoidal regrowth.

Finally, a review of sleep symptoms is appropriate: difficulty in sleeping, sleep terrors, sleepwalking, confusional arousals, nightmares, snoring, headbanging or rocking, bruxism, or excessive sleepiness. Positive responses should be pursued.

Current Symptoms of Excessive Daytime Sleepiness

This complaint is made less often in children than in adults. Not only are the relevant disorders seen less often in young children, but especially in infants and pre-school children, the symptoms may be less obvious.[25] The children are less likely to complain, and the symptoms may be less noticeable to the observer. Long nighttime sleep and naps may be considered a blessing. Since naps may be occurring anyway (i.e., the child is still at an age where napping is considered normal), their length and frequency may not be recognized as abnormal. The main concern arises when the total amount of sleep is clearly excessive (e.g., 18 hours per day in a 3-year-old), when the amount of napping is clearly abnormal (two naps per day in a 5-year-old), or when the youngster frequently seems sleepy during periods of expected wakefulness.

Another problem is that sleepiness in young children does not always appear in a clear-cut manner. Rather than yawning and wanting to sleep, a sleepy toddler may show behavioral deterioration, tantrums, and increased activity. The distinction between behavioral problems per se and excessive sleepiness is not always easy to make.

By middle childhood and the start of school, a child should no longer be napping. Furthermore, he has entered the most wakeful time of his whole life, which continues until adolescence.[26] Any signs of sleepiness at these ages (an 8-year-old who falls asleep in school, a 10-year-old who naps after school, a 12-year-old who sleeps 14 hours each night) should be a serious concern. If there is napping, the timing, length, and ease of waking should be explored. The tendency of the naps to be refreshing should be questioned. However, short refreshing naps may not be reported in young narcoleptic patients; naps may be long or skipped altogether with only long nocturnal sleep described. A *sleepy* syndrome occurring at a very *wakeful* time of life may present differently from the expected.

Although marked sleepiness is less often a symptom of sleep apnea in children than it is in adults, respiratory symptoms should be ascertained. Snoring, particularly in children sleeping in other rooms, may be dismissed by parents as insignificant. It is helpful to know if there is snoring; if it is present every night, most nights, or just occasionally; and if it occurs all night or just intermittently. Parents may be able to distinguish loud irregular snoring with pauses, gasps, inspiratory struggles, and retractions from soft regular snoring without obviously increased effort. They may describe unusual sleep positions such as sitting or with head extended. They often know if snoring occurs only when the child is supine or has an upper respiratory infection and if the child always sleeps with his mouth open. They may be able to describe how loud the snoring is and whether it is audible in other rooms, downstairs, or with the door closed. In addition, a full otolaryngologic history (surgery, infections) is appropriate.

The possible existence of other symptoms of narcolepsy should be explored. This is very important in older children and adolescents. However, it is a very difficult history to obtain from young children. Parents are likely unaware of the existence of symptoms such as sleep paralysis and hypnagogic hallucinations, and the child may be unable to describe them accurately. Even cataplexy, which may be witnessed, is difficult to assess because most young children collapse to the ground when laughing very hard. It may help to ask if the child seemed frightened at these times, if the child continued laughing and rolling about in a silly but normal fashion, and if the child was able to get up immediately when he stopped laughing.

Family History of Sleep Problems

It is worth asking if other family members have had similar symptoms. A strong familial tendency is perhaps most clearly established for enuresis,[27] and genetic factors are known to exist in narcolepsy.[28, 29] Certain other disorders of excessive somnolence are likely familial as well. There are known familial tendencies in sleepwalking and sleep terrors, and it has been reported that headbanging, sudden infant death syndrome, or independent cataplexy has occurred in several generations of families.[30–32] However, in disorders such as early childhood sleeplessness and sleep apnea, familial tendencies are less clear.

Past History and Review of Systems

In most cases this can be obtained quickly by interview or questionnaire and follows the format generally used in pediatrics. This would include a description of the pregnancy, natal and neonatal courses, and history of recurrent or significant illnesses, medications, hospitalizations, surgery, and standard review of systems. This is not only important to help identify medical factors directly contributing to the patient's symptoms, but (if the child has had significant medical difficulties) this information may help to explain certain behavior patterns that may indirectly contribute to the problem (for example, a youngster with nocturnal asthma attacks may be too frightened to go bed or a parent of a youngster who recovered from leukemia may be hesitant to set limits).

Social History

Even if there are no psychosocial problems suggested by the history and by general observation and interaction, nothing should be taken for granted. The examiner should be prepared to ask probing questions of the parents and perhaps the child. It is important to learn the family structure, educational levels, occupations, history of marital problems—separation, divorce, or frequent arguments, financial status, drug or alcohol abuse, previous or current psychotherapy, depression or thought disorders, and medications. The medical and psychologic status of siblings should be ascertained. Significant illnesses or death of siblings may have major impact on the parent's interaction with the patient. Specific questions regarding the patient's activities, peer group, siblings, parent relationships, and school performance are appropriate. If the child is old enough, he should also be examined privately. At that time questions about school pressures, sexual and drug exposures, and his feelings about his parents can be further explored.

For clinicians not accustomed to such psychosocial probing, this part of the evaluation may prove somewhat difficult. However, since many of the sleep problems seen in childhood are at least partially dependent on such factors, not taking them into account may risk inadequate care.

Psychologic, Developmental, and Psychiatric Assessment

At the initial session one should generally evaluate the youngster's developmental/cognitive function, which may be accomplished by direct evaluation coupled with history. General screening tests for infants and toddlers may be used. Older children are capable of direct interview; younger ones have to be assessed through observation and play. It is important to evaluate children's thought processes, affective states, fears, worries, and concerns; manner of dealing with feelings of anger; and the manner of coping with issues of control, separation, and individualism.

Full psychiatric or psychologic evaluation usually is not necessary, but findings such as depression, truancy, learning disabilities, attentional deficit disorder, significant anxiety or fears, mania, thought disorders, or family dysfunctions would suggest such referrals.

Physical Examination

A general physical examination is worthwhile, but unless the history is suggestive, unsuspected findings with diagnostic implication are unlikely to be found. Certainly patients with snoring and suspected apnea should have careful examination of nose, mouth, and facial features; chest auscultation; sphygmomanometry; abdominal palpation; and neuromotor screening. A neurologic assessment should be conducted on all those with excessive sleepiness or possible seizures. Enuretic children should have inspection of the lower spine, urethral meatus, and perhaps of the sphincter tone, perineal sensation, and urinary flow. Infants and toddlers with poor sleep should have a general examination, including careful otoscopic examination of the ears.

Laboratory Studies, Polysomnography

No studies are mandatory for all children. Depending on the history and initial examination, laboratory studies may be indicated, including routine hemograms and screening chemistries, as they might with any child. Enuretic children should have a routine urinalysis and perhaps a urine culture. Full urologic testing is sometimes indicated because of urinary tract infections, daytime incontinence, secondary enuresis, age of patient, unusual symptoms, or specific physical findings. Patients with snoring and suspected or documented sleep apnea may require radiographic assessment of the upper airway and the bony structures of the head and face. Patients with unexplained sleepiness should have a hemogram, sedimentation rate, and a broad panel of chemistries including thyroid function.

A polysomnogram (PSG) is indicated in a

number of clinical situations. Polysomnography should be routine in the evaluation of unexplained daytime sleepiness and suspected sleep apnea. It should be considered for paroxysmal arousals. However, since most sleepwalking, sleep terror, and confusional arousal episodes in young children are benign and very characteristic, laboratory study usually adds little information. But a PSG may be helpful in children in whom the arousals are particularly frequent, violent, atypical, resistant to treatment, or continue or appear at older ages. Other diagnoses such as seizures and REM-behavior disorder must be considered. Even assuming only NREM arousal findings, the degree of sleep disruption may guide medication decisions. If the history does not provide complete information, a PSG may be helpful in determining whether rocking and headbanging are occurring in sleep, waking, or drowsiness. At times, a PSG is useful to discriminate between ictal and non-ictal events. It is occasionally helpful in enuresis, especially when seizures, snoring, sleep apnea, or other sleep disrupters are being considered. A PSG is not necessary in the evaluation of most sleepless children, but it may help when there are atypical features, a need for documentation, known neurologic impairment, or failure to respond to treatment.

Special channels added to a standard PSG, such as esophageal pH or end-tidal CO_2, may allow for additional diagnoses. For example, only by recording sleep and pH simultaneously can it be determined if gastroesophageal reflux precipitates arousal and perhaps apnea or whether the reverse occurs.

Continuous positive airway pressure (CPAP) calibration for the treatment of sleep apnea is also possible but is necessary less often in children than in adults since alternative treatment measures are usually available. Furthermore, the application of this equipment to young children may be difficult (although it is usually possible), but it is relatively easy to do by mid-childhood or adolescence.

Multiple sleep latency tests (MSLT) should be routine in the evaluation of every child with unexplained or persistent excessive sleepiness.[33] Even without a classic history for narcolepsy, an MSLT may prove diagnostic. Unfortunately, good norms do not exist and may make interpretation difficult. For example, when studying a 3-year-old child, do you measure sleep latency from the time lights are turned out or from the time the child stops bouncing around the bed? How do you interpret nap sleep latencies at an age when some daytime napping is considered appropriate? How much weight should be given to the natural wakefulness of mid-childhood that may overwhelm an underlying sleep tendency? Allowing for this wakefulness in the latency-age child, should nap attempts be allowed to go longer than 20 minutes?

Human leukocyte antigen (HLA) testing should also be considered in this group of children.[29] The full features of narcolepsy are usually not present in childhood, and a diagnosis made then will be carried throughout the child's life. A negative MSLT at such an inherently wakeful time of life may not rule out narcolepsy either. Positive HLA findings do not allow one to make a diagnosis but support it and give additional reason for follow-up sleep studies even if the initial studies were negative. Negative HLA findings suggest caution in interpretation of even suggestive MSLT results.

Toxic screens are an important consideration in the evaluation of an excessively sleepy child, especially an adolescent. Performing them at the time of the MSLT gives the desired information and helps assure the accuracy of the nap study.

Although a PSG may help distinguish ictal from non-ictal arousals, *long-term monitoring* with continuous EEG over many days may provide more information than the limited EEG montage at a relatively slow paper speed usually used in a PSG. This is particularly true when the events in question do not occur nightly. On the other hand, a PSG may be necessary to document that the apnea-related hypoxia was triggering the seizures (or even the cardiac arrhythmia). A PSG may also document recurrent discharge-related arousals (without full ictal events) causing severe sleep fragmentation, which may lead to daytime sleepiness and thus even to increased seizures.[34]

Cardiac studies may also be indicated. Electrocardiography (EKG) and echocardiography should be considered in patients with significant sleep apnea and, in addition, Holter monitoring may be required if worrisome arrhythmias have been detected or are suspected.

Laboratory PSG studies, occurring as they do in unusual settings, may not reflect what occurs nightly in the home. A number of devices are available to try to overcome this obstacle, but they are not yet part of routine pediatric sleep assessments in most settings. They include extended in-home video monitoring and actigraphy (perhaps including incident light measurement), which may help document a history that is questionable, telemetry, and other forms of unattended monitoring.[35-37]

Conclusion

Sleep problems in children occur frequently. To be of service to these children and their parents, a clinician must become sophisticated in the assessment of sleep-related complaints if intervention is to be made rationally, empathetically, and successfully.

References

1. Ablon SL, Mack JE: Sleep disorders. *In* Noshpitz JD (ed): Basic Handbook of Child Psychiatry, Vol 2. New York, Basic Books, 1979, pp 643–660.
2. Douglas J, Richman N: Sleep Management Manual. London, Department of Psychological Medicine, Hospital for Sick Children, 1982.
3. Ferber RA: Sleep disorders in infants and children. *In* Riley T (ed): Clinical Aspects of Sleep and Sleep Disturbance. London, Butterworths, 1985, pp 113–157.
4. Ferber RA: Solve Your Child's Sleep Problem. New York, Simon and Schuster, 1985.
5. Ferber R, Boyle MP, Belfer M: Initial experience of a pediatric sleep disorders clinic. Sleep Res 10:195, 1981.
6. Illingworth RS: Sleep problems in the first three years. Br Med J 1:722, 1951.
7. Jones DPH, Verduyn CM: Behavioral management of sleep problems. Arch Dis Child 58:442, 1983.
8. Richman N: Sleep problems in young children. Arch Dis Child 56:491, 1984.
9. Ferber RA: Assessment procedures for diagnosis of sleep disorders in children. *In* Noshpitz JD (ed): Basic Handbook of Child Psychiatry, Vol V. New York, Basic Books, 1987, pp 185–193.
10. Daws D: Through the Night. Helping Parents and Sleepless Infants. London, Free Association Books, 1989.
11. Ferber R: Childhood insomnia. *In* Thorpy MJ (ed): Handbook of Sleep Disorders. New York, Marcel Dekker, Inc, 1990, pp 435–455.
12. Cuthbertson J, Schevill S: Helping Your Child Sleep Through the Night. Garden City, NY, Doubleday & Co, 1985.
13. Ferber R, Boyle MP: Sleeplessness in infants and toddlers: sleep initiation difficulty masquerading as a sleep maintenance insomnia. Sleep Res 12:240, 1983.
14. Ferber R, Boyle MP: Sleeplessness in infants up to the age of 12 months: diagnosis and treatment. Sleep Res 13:79, 1984.
15. Ferber R, Boyle MP, Belfer M: "Insomnia" in toddlers seen in a pediatric sleep disorders clinic. Sleep Res 10:195, 1981.
16. Anders TF: Night-waking in infants during the first year of life. Pediatrics 63:860, 1979.
17. Ferber RA: Behavioral "insomnia" in the child. Psychiatr Clin North Am 10:641, 1987.
18. Ferber R: Boyle MP. Phase shift dyssomnia in early childhood. Sleep Res 12:242, 1983.
19. Ferber R: Sleep disorders. *In* Levine MD, Carey WB, Crocker AC (eds): Developmental-Behavioral Pediatrics, 2nd ed. Philadelphia, WB Saunders, 1992.
20. Ferber R: Sleep schedule-dependent causes of insomnia and sleepiness in middle childhood and adolescence. Pediatrician 17:13, 1990.
21. Ferber R, Boyle MP: Nocturnal fluid intake: a cause of, not treatment for, sleep disruption in infants and toddlers. Sleep Res 12:243, 1983.
22. Broughton R: Sleep disorders: disorders of arousal? Science 159:1070, 1968.
23. Thorpy MJ, Glovinsky PB: Headbanging (jactatio capitis nocturna). *In* Kryger MH, Roth T, Dement WC (eds): Principles and Practice of Sleep Medicine. Philadelphia, WB Saunders, 1989, pp 648–654.
24. Fraiberg S: On the sleep disturbances of early childhood. Psychoanal Study Child 5:285, 1950.
25. Anders TF, Carskadon MA, Dement WC, et al: Sleep habits of children and the identification of pathologically sleepy children. Child Psychiatry Hum Dev 9:56, 1978.
26. Carskadon MA, Harvey K, Duke P, et al: Pubertal changes in daytime sleepiness. Sleep 2:453, 1980.
27. Bakwin H: The genetics of enuresis. *In* Kolvin I, MacKeith RC, Meadow SR (eds): Bladder Control and Enuresis. Philadelphia, JB Lippincott, 1973, pp 73–77.
28. Kessler S: Genetic factors in narcolepsy. *In* Guilleminault C, Dement WC, Passouant P (eds): Narcolepsy. New York, Spectrum Publications, Inc, 1976, pp 285–302.
29. Billiard M, Seignalet J: Extraordinary association between HLA-DR2 and narcolepsy. Lancet 2:226, 1985.
30. Ferber R: Familial headbanging. Sleep Res 17:176, 1988.
31. Kelly DH, Shannon DC: Sudden infant death syndrome and near sudden infant death syndrome: a review of the literature, 1964 to 1982. Pediatr Clin North Am 29:1241, 1982.
32. Kales A, Soldatos CR, Bixler EO, et al: Hereditary factors in sleep walking and night terrors. Br J Psychiatry 137:111, 1980.
33. Carskadon MA, Dement WC, Mitler MM, et al: Guidelines for the multiple sleep latency test (MSLT): a standard measure of sleepiness. Sleep 9:519, 1986.
34. Erba G, Ferber R: Sleep disruption by subclinical seizure activity as a cause of increased waking seizures and decreased daytime function. Sleep Res 12:307, 1983.
35. Anders T, Sostek A: The use of time lapse video recording of sleep-wake behavior in human infants. Psychophysiology 13:155, 1976.
36. Sadeh A, Lavie P, Scher A, et al: Actigraphic home-monitoring sleep-disturbed and control infants and young children: a new method for pediatric assessment of sleep-wake patterns. Pediatrics 87:494, 1991.
37. Miles LE, Broughton RJ: Medical Monitoring in the Home and Work Environment. New York, Raven Press, 1990.

Monitoring of Sleep in Neonates and Young Children

EVELYN B. THOMAN and CHRISTINE ACEBO

Unlike adults, children do not and infants cannot complain about their sleep. An infant's sleep is a problem only if considered to be a problem by the parents (see Chapter 5). If a baby is "difficult" to get to sleep or awakens and cries frequently during the night, weary parents may seek help to improve the infant's sleep.

Consistent with this picture, the prevailing approach to assessing the sleep of the very young has been to rely on parents' perceptions of their baby's sleep patterns by using questionnaires, sleep logs, or diaries. If a parent's report becomes more positive during intervention, this can mean either that the baby's sleep has changed or that the parent's expectations or tolerance level has changed or some combination of these factors.

Limited success of efforts to improve the sleep of the very young may be, at least in part, a function of a lack of empirical information on their sleep. In a study combining sleep recordings with parental reports, we have found that mothers vary widely in the reliability with which they report their baby's sleep patterns.[1] Even when they report accurately for the daytime, they may be highly inaccurate for the nighttime because some infants awaken during the night and return to sleep without crying (see also Chapter 2). In such instances, parents may (happily) assume their baby is sleeping. Clearly, reliable description of a baby's sleep is needed to diagnose a possible problem and to follow changes in sleep patterns as a function of intervention (see Chapter 5).

A number of methods are available for objectively recording the sleep of infants and children. Those methods that have been reported in the literature most extensively and have been subjected to rigorous assessment for reliability and validity have been selected for description. They include direct behavioral observations, polysomnography, time-lapse video recording, actigraphic recording, and recording of motility patterns. Each of these has reasons for recommendation and each represents a degree of compromise. These procedures will be described, their advantages and limitations discussed, and suggestions as to purposes best suited for their use will be made.

Recording of Sleep in Infants from Behavioral Observation

Behavioral recording is described first because this is in a sense the "gold standard" for sleep monitoring in infants. This is in marked contrast to the acceptance of polysomnography as the most valid criterion for adult sleep. At the earliest ages, wakefulness and active sleep cannot be distinguished from EEG patterns alone, although these states are readily and reliably distinguished behaviorally. For this reason, behavioral observations are typically an adjunct to polysomnographic recordings of infants and young children.

A Behavioral Sleep Taxonomy

There are five states for behavioral sleep in infants,[2] which are described as they occur temporally after wakefulness.

Drowse or Daze. The infant's eyes are either

open but "heavy-lidded" or opening and closing slowly. The level of motor activity is typically low but may vary.

Active Sleep. The eyes are closed. Respiration is uneven and primarily costal in nature. REMs occur intermittently. Sporadic movements may occur, but muscle tone is low between these phasic movements. Active sleep corresponds to REM sleep in the adult.

Active-Quiet Transition Sleep. This state typically occurs between periods of active sleep and quiet sleep, and the baby shows mixed behavioral signs of the two states. The eyes are closed. There is little motor activity. Respiration is not as regular as in quiet sleep and more regular than in active sleep. Breathing may be abdominal or costal or mixed. Muscle tone may vary. Isolated REMs may occur.

Quiet Sleep. The eyes are closed. Respiration is relatively slow, regular, and abdominal in nature. A tonic level of motor tone is maintained, and motor activity is usually limited to occasional startles, sighs, or rhythmic mouthing. Brief periods of limb or body movements may occur, which are more frequent in premature infants. Quiet sleep corresponds to immature NREM sleep in the young infant.

Sleep-Wake Transition. The infant shows behaviors of both wakefulness and sleep. There is usually generalized motor activity. The eyes may be closed or they may open and close rapidly. Isolated fuss vocalizations may occur. This state generally occurs when the baby is awakening from sleep, following a bout of active sleep.

It should be noted that until about 6 months active sleep is the onset sleep state rather than quiet (NREM) sleep, as in the older child or adult. This sequencing of sleep states in infants can be disrupted by external, and possibly internal, stress.[3] That is, one can suspect that an infant is stressed if instead of progressing normally from wakefulness to active sleep, he or she enters quiet sleep directly from wakefulness.

A Behavioral Wakefulness Taxonomy

A major advantage of making behavioral observations is the possibility of recording the waking states as well as the sleep states. Waking and sleeping compose a system of state behaviors that are interrelated and serve common functions of regulating stimulus input, mediating social interactions, and modulating response output, as well as providing information on central nervous system (CNS) regulatory controls.[2]

The four waking states that are expressed from early infancy throughout early childhood may be defined as follows:

Alert. The infant's eyes are open, bright, and shining, and attentive or scanning. Motor activity is typically low during the first 2 weeks of life, but the infant may be active.

Non-Alert Waking. The infant's eyes are usually open but dull and unfocused. Motor activity may vary but is typically high. The eyes may be closed during periods of high-level activity. Isolated fuss vocalizations may occur.

Fuss. Fuss sounds are made continuously or intermittently at relatively low levels of intensity.

Cry. Intense vocalizations occur either singly or in succession.

A Summary State Set

For many research and clinical purposes, the states listed above are too numerous to differentiate and record. It is reasonable to combine the states into clusters to reduce the number of categories for observation.

The six sleep/wake categories in this state set are:

> Alert
> Non-alert waking
> Fuss or cry
> Drowse, daze or sleep-wake transition
> Active sleep
> Quiet sleep or active-quiet transition sleep

Note that this abbreviated classification scheme still includes all of the primary states.

Sleep-Specific Behaviors

Behaviorally, the sleep states during infancy are far more distinctive than they are at later ages. First, in infants, respiration is much more irregular in active sleep than in quiet sleep. REMs are primarily vertical rather than horizontal, as in adults. They may range from a brief, faint flicker of the eyelids to intense fluttering seen in REM storms, which may be accompanied by raising of the eyelids and occasional eye-opening.

Other phasic behaviors during active sleep include smiles, frowns, grimaces, mouthing; sighs and sigh-sobs; minor twitching of the extremities; gross motor movements, typically of a writhing or stretching nature; and even high-pitched cry vocalization. During quiet sleep occasional startles, brief limb or body movements, and rhythmic mouthing may occur. These sleep-associated behaviors diminish in frequency and intensity over the early months and then persist at a much lower level at later ages. Continuation at high levels beyond the early months is an indication of CNS immaturity. For example, we found that infants who show high frequencies of intense REMs (REM storms) at 6 months showed lower mental scores at 1 year of age.[4]

As with the waking states, phasic behaviors in sleep may provide important clues for the mother's care giving and social activities. There is also suggestive evidence that these behaviors provide indices of the infant's temperament.

Procedures for Observation

For making behavioral sleep/wake recordings, one needs an electronic timing device that will signal 10-second epochs through an ear microphone (preferably one that also signals the end of each minute), a pencil, and a form sheet marked off into 6-epoch minutes— and patience. Alternatively, states can be code recorded (paced by a time signal) into an electronic data-input device so the data can be entered directly into a computer. Minimal clothing and covering of the baby is preferred to provide a maximal view of the eyes, respiration, and limbs.

Simultaneous recording of respiration is a very useful adjunct to behavioral observations. This can be done by means of a small pressure-sensitive sensor pad placed under the infant and connected to a portable chart recorder. The analog signals from the infant's respiration provide ongoing information to the observer on the regularity of respiration, and they provide a permanent record of the occurrence of apneas. It is also possible to assess the regularity of quiet sleep respiration using a 4-point rating scale, as an index of maturation.[5, 6]

The 10-second epoch length for recording behavioral sleep states is appropriate even though sleep cannot be classified within such a short period. The 10-second epoch is used as a running probe for state change. Three epochs are required for a change from active sleep or quiet sleep; thus, the operational epoch for the sleep states is the traditional 30-second epoch. At the same time, by using a 10-second epoch, the occurrence of REMs and the other sleep-related behaviors can be recorded very precisely with respect to their temporal occurrence. In addition, 10-second epochs are requisite if also recording waking states, as wakefulness is much more volatile than sleep.

Any recording of sleep should also include the nature of wakefulness, at least insofar as whether the baby is quiescent or crying. Parents are not disturbed by a nonsleeping baby, only by a nonsleeping and *crying* baby.

Reliability

Each of the states defined above can be reliably judged after a period of training. In addition, reliability of measurement from the behavioral observations has been demonstrated.[5, 7–15] Reliability has been assessed in children[16] and babies,[14, 15, 17] including premature infants as early as 27-weeks conceptional age.[18]

Validity of Behavioral Observations

During the early postnatal weeks, infants spend 50% of the day (while in the crib) in active sleep, 28% in quiet sleep, 2% in active-quiet transitional sleep, 4% in drowse, and 1% in sleep-wake transition.[2] Over the first 6 months, active sleep diminishes, both in absolute amounts and as a percentage of sleep, and quiet sleep increases as a percent of sleep time only. In early infancy, active sleep–quiet sleep cycles are approximately 60 minutes rather than 90 minutes, as in adults.[19]

Predictive validity has been demonstrated in numerous studies of infants' behavioral sleep states. For example, inconsistency in the distribution of states over successive recordings has been repeatedly found to relate to developmental disabilities at later ages.[20–22] Infants who show stable sleep patterns when they are alone show stable waking state patterns when they are with their mothers.[7] Even in animals, active sleep from behavioral observations of infant rabbits is related to later social and exploratory behaviors.[23]

Critique of Behavioral Observations

Direct behavioral observations are obviously labor intensive, and the duration of an observation is constrained by the observer's attention span and endurance or the number of observers that can be used sequentially. Thoman and associates report up to 7-hour periods of observation in the home, with two observers recording for successive 3½-hour periods.[24] Why should such difficult procedures be used? The first reason is that sleep is a behavior, with manifestations in terms of sleep-state-specific behaviors that can only be recorded from direct observation. In addition, direct observations are minimally intrusive and can be made in the home, permitting assessment of the child's naturally occurring sleep.

An obvious drawback of direct observations is that it is not generally feasible to observe throughout the night, although it can be done using a dim light. In such instances, it is important to have a respiration recording to confirm the state judgments from respiration patterns.

Behavioral Observations Reveal Unique Characteristics of the Individual Baby

It is always a surprise to a new observer to learn how intimately one comes to know a baby just from watching him or her sleep. Although all babies show the commonality of behaviors prototypical for each sleep state, no two babies express their states identically. Each finds variations on the common themes. Some of these differences are quantifiable by data analyses (e.g., frequencies, recurrence times), but there are also qualitative differences that are unique to each baby—differences in their REMs; the way they move their limbs and body; whether their sighs are just sighs or deep, dramatic sigh-sobs; and the marked differences in their facial expressions. Some infants consistently frown more, while others smile more. One newborn was once seen to frown and smile at the same time! The clinical significance of these individual differences is not known, but one may speculate that these expressions reflect antecedents to temperamental differences that may be expressed in many ways at later ages.

Polygraphic Recording of Sleep

The states of very young infants cannot be recognized and reliably coded from EEG alone, in part because of a lack of concordance between individual physiologic parameters including patterns of EEG signals, respiration, eye movements, muscle tone, and cardiac rhythms.[25] These parameters can be recorded polygraphically, and they show unique developmental patterns and interrelationships,[26] with a gradual coalescence over the early months. Behavioral state classifications, as previously described, can be made from the earliest ages, and changing physiologic variables can be related to the developing behavioral characteristics.[27]

Procedures for Recording

In 1971, Anders, Emde and Parmelee, with a number of other infant sleep researchers, published *A Manual of Standardized Terminology, Techniques and Criteria for Scoring of States of Sleep and Wakefulness in Newborn Infants,* with the intent of providing some basis for standardization of recording procedures, coding of individual polygraphic parameters, and scoring states from such signals.[28] However, the emphasis for standardization was in terms of recording procedures and parameter coding, with specific flexibility given for state coding. Much of the description of recording procedures is based on recommendations from the Newborn Manual.

A number of environmental conditions and medical procedures have been shown to affect the expression of state and physiologic parameters including temperature and humidity, light and sound levels, handling and feeding schedules, and placement of electrodes.[29–33] Thus, the Newborn Manual recommends that nursery recording of infants should be done with infants loosely clothed and skin maintained at 32–34°C. They also recommend that the baby be recorded on a "typical day," that electrodes be applied before a feeding to minimize disturbances of sleep, that the feeding be observed and "judged normal," and then the subsequent sleep period recorded. Although recording of an entire interfeeding period was recommended, recording times have varied widely from 1 hour to 24-hour periods.[34–36]

For older infants brought into the sleep laboratory, arm restraints have been applied to prevent the infants from pulling the electrodes off.[37] Monitoring of older infants and children is typically carried out in a separate darkened room with a room temperature between 22 and 30°C. Behaviors and interventions are monitored by means of a low-illumination television camera and monitor and charted on the polygraph.

A variety of polygraph equipment and electrodes have been used in practice, as have a number of techniques of electrode application and placement. In general, however, the skin or scalp is cleansed thoroughly with acetone or alcohol, prior to electrode application, the superficial layer of the skin is abraded lightly, and electrode jelly is rubbed on to further abrade the skin. Electrodes are attached in a variety of ways, ranging from skin tape to collodion, which is removed with acetone. The number of scalp electrodes used has varied from study to study but can be as many as 11. The Newborn Manual recommends a minimum paper speed of 10 mm/second. In practice, paper speeds have varied from 3.0 to 30 mm/second.

Recording and Coding of Parameters

The parameters most often used in polygraphic studies of sleep in infants and children include behavior, respiration, eye movements (electro-oculogram [EOG]), brain electrical activity (EEG), muscle tone (EMG) or motor activity, and heart rate (electrocardiogram [ECG]).

Behavior. While the Newborn Manual states that "behavioral observations are crucial for the interpretation of polygraphic recordings in infancy" (p 2), some investigators observe and record behaviors as extensively as described previously for behavioral observations, while others utilize minimal behavioral observations (eyes open or closed and vocalizations).[37] Behaviors may be written directly on the polygraph record or recorded separately in a time-linked fashion elsewhere.

Respiration. Respiration has been monitored in a variety of ways: by strain gauges connected to a bellow's pneumograph around the infant's abdomen or thorax or both; mercury-filled tubing or graphite rubber around the thorax; inductance plethysmography; miniature cannulas taped under the nostrils to sample expired gas; thermistors and thermocouples taped in front of the nostrils; surface electrodes to record inspiratory diaphragmatic or intercostal muscle activity; or a combination of any of these. Artifacts and dislocation from movement are a problem with these methods.

Respiration may be coded into a regular or irregular pattern, either by gross visual categorization, hand measurement, or by computer analysis.[88] Dreyfus-Brisac[39] has coded respiration into three categories of regularity based on variability of rate, plus a fourth category for periodic respiration.

Eye Movements. These are typically recorded on two channels using at least one electrode placed lateral to the outer canthi of each eye, referenced to an ear or mastoid electrode, in order to obtain out-of-phase deflections on the two channels for conjugate horizontal eye movements. This array is a minimum for obtaining measures useful for scoring REMs in active sleep. If very precise measures of number and type of eye movements are needed, more electrodes may be used (above and below the eyes) and supplemented by direct observations.[40] Eye movements have also been monitored by mechanogram using a small piezoelectric crystal attached to one of the eyelids.[41]

The EOG may be coded in a variety of ways, including presence or absence of REMs during an epoch, or in terms of REM density per epoch. For scoring state, the epoch (usually 20 or 30 seconds) is coded as positive if REMs occur and negative if they don't.

Brain Electrical Activity. The Newborn Manual recommends a minimum of two channels for EEG recording: a scalp-to-scalp (C3-O1) and a scalp-to-ipsilateral mastoid or ear (C3-A1). In practice, a variety of derivations have been used.[42-44]

In premature infants less than 32 weeks of conceptional age, the EEG consists of a discontinuous pattern with bursts of mixed frequency waves alternating with long quiescent periods. The EEG pattern is similar during wakefulness and sleep (see Chapter 2).[43-45] After 32 weeks, the EEG consists of two main patterns—a discontinuous pattern (associated with wake and active sleep) and a continuous pattern (associated with quiet sleep). The continuous pattern consists of bursts of mixed sharp and slow waves alternating with a flattened background. With increasing age, the bursts lengthen and periods of quiescence shorten and increase in amplitude. The discontinuous pattern decreases with age, as do a number of other transient patterns.[43, 44]

Four patterns of activity have been identified during sleep in full-term infants: low voltage irregular (LVI); tracé alternant (TA); high voltage slow (HVS); and a mixed (M).[28] These patterns begin to be apparent by around 38 weeks of conceptional age in the premature infant.[46]

A number of changes in EEG patterning occur following the early post-term period.

The tracé alternant pattern begins to disappear after the first month post-term and is replaced by a continuous slow wave pattern that becomes the dominant pattern of quiet sleep.[44] Sleep spindles, which are characteristic of stage 2 NREM sleep in adults, develop from scattered, immature forms evident by around 4 weeks of age to a mature quality by about 8 weeks.[47] Other changes in NREM EEG patterns include the appearance of K-complexes, another landmark of stage 2 sleep, at around 6 months[46, 48] and high voltage, slow wave, delta activity characteristic of stage 3–4 NREM sleep, which begins to develop in the second half of the first year and then continues to change in form and amount through adolescence.

While the transition from waking to sleep through a drowsy state is not well differentiated by EEG changes in the newborn, a more distinctive pattern during drowse, termed hypnogogic hypersynchrony,[49] begins to be evident around 4 months of age. A similar pattern also begins to be seen during arousals.

Thus, there is a rapid maturation of EEG during the first year of life[46] and progressive changes and development of new rhythms throughout childhood and adolescence.[42, 50–52]

Muscle Tone. Muscle activity is recorded by electrodes placed over the mental or submental muscles on each side of the mandible, referred to each other, and recorded on one channel. Pressure on the electrodes may be increased by a strip of tape over them or by a rubber infant ECG strap around the head.

The EMG is coded as high if over half the epochs demonstrate tonic muscle activity and low with muscle suppression. This coding is most useful to help differentiate active sleep, the onset of active sleep from quiet sleep, and waking from active sleep.

In some studies, body movements have been registered by electrodes placed on the infant's limbs, by piezoelectric crystals on the limbs,[41] or by capacitor plates on the mattress surface under the crib sheet.[53] Measures of movement frequency or number of epochs with movements may be obtained.

Heart Rate. The ECG is generally recorded with two electrodes placed beneath the clavicles and the resulting signals may be classified as regular or irregular as in the case of respiration. Ground electrodes may be applied above the umbilicus, and a skin temperature probe may be applied to the abdomen.

State Classifications

A variety of ways of coding state in polygraphic studies of infants have been used, ranging from coding state from behavioral observations and then assessing relationships of physiologic measures within states, to coding state based on the concordance of specific measures obtained polygraphically, to a combination of both techniques. The variety of classification procedures is perhaps one reason for the variety of descriptions of state patterning, particularly in premature infants where the concordance of parameters is very low.

For full-term infants, the Newborn Manual categorizes three sleep states and describes them in terms of typical clusters of physiologic and behavioral parameters, while leaving decisions as to the actual parameter combinations and priorities to individual investigators.

Active-REM Sleep. The eyes are closed and there is considerable activity, consisting of facial movements, bursts of sucking, limb and body movements which are either slow and writhing or sudden and jerky, REMs and slow eye movements (SEMs), blinks, penile erections, and vocalizations. The EOG is positive for REMs, either singly or in bursts. The EEG is of the LVI, M, or (rarely) HVS pattern (only LVI is specific to active sleep). EMG is low when there are no movements and respiration is irregular.

Quiet Sleep. The eyes are closed and there is behavioral quiescence, with no body movements except for occasional startles and mouth movements. The EEG patterns are HVS, TA, or M (thus, only TA is specific to quiet sleep). Respiration is regular, the EOG is negative for REMs, and EMG is high.

Indeterminate Sleep. The eyes are closed and there are mixed criteria of active and quiet sleep. These epochs occur most often at sleep onset, during state transitions, and during sleep-wake transitions. Indeterminate sleep, defined for polysomnographic recordings, includes sleep-wake transition and active-quiet sleep transition when observed behaviorally.

The Newborn Manual also lists four waking states (crying, active awake, quiet awake, and drowse), judged by behavioral criteria. Sleep onset is also primarily dependent on behavioral observations.

Artifact time is scored when movements obscure the polygraphic record, and epochs so scored are sometimes deleted prior to analysis.

In infants older than 3 or 4 months, when EEG signals become more differentiated and contain landmarks similar to adult signals, sleep state criteria modified from adult standard criteria[54] have been used.[55] NREM sleep may be categorized into stages similar to adult sleep (infant stages 1, 2, and 3–4) based on the occurrence of spindles and delta waves.[55]

The Newborn Manual recommends epoch-by-epoch scoring with epoch lengths of 20 or 30 seconds, although epoch lengths have varied from 15 seconds to 1 minute. According to the Manual, "the investigator should code each physiological parameter independently for the entire recording" (p 4). Thus, the classification of physiologic activity should be made only on the basis of the isolated parameter. The authors agree, however, that in practice all parameters within an epoch are usually coded at once.

Methods for smoothing states have also varied. The Newborn Manual recommends smoothing states scored on an epoch-by-epoch basis by using the criterion of 1 minute of a new state to score a state change. In practice, states have been smoothed over a variable number of epochs. Prechtl and O'Brien[27] have recommended smoothing with a moving window of 3 minutes.

Measures

Variables measured have included quiet sleep, active sleep, and indeterminate sleep as a percent of sleep time and as a percent of observation time. Other measures include the longest sleep period, the number of sleep episodes, mean duration of episodes, mean interval between onset of quiet sleep or active sleep, number of state transitions, active sleep/quiet sleep ratio, frequencies of brief arousals in active sleep and quiet sleep. Measures of state-specific respiration and heart rate variability are also obtained.

Analyses have also included power-spectral analysis of EEG signals using the fast Fourier transform[56] to assess temporal sequencing of states and spectral densities of the EEG within states.[57, 57a]

Reliability

Stefanski and associates[40] have reported relatively high overall interscorer agreement (87.4%) in coding EEG patterns in premature and term infants, with the greatest disagreements occurring in records from infants less than 36 weeks of conceptional age. They also concluded that both behavioral observation and the EOG are necessary to detect REMs reliably.[40]

Hoppenbrouwers and associates[37] reported overall interscorer agreement for 12-hour overnight recordings made on normal infants from 1 week to 6 months of age. They found agreements in excess of 80% for active sleep, quiet sleep, and waking, while reliability of indeterminate sleep, which in this study occurred in 20% of the total recording session, was quite low. The unreliability in coding indeterminate sleep points to a limitation of their classification procedure, as indeterminate sleep occurs at all ages. In addition, they report significant reliability of measures (individual differences) for only active sleep and indeterminate sleep but not for quiet sleep or wake.

Validity

Measures of physiologic patterns show developmental trends.[6, 53, 58, 59] Maturational changes in states classified by polysomnographic methods very generally show the same trends described by behavioral observations, although important discrepancies exist.[18, 60] While results from EEG and polygraphic measures have been shown to differentiate grossly abnormal infants, predictive power for more subtle forms of poor developmental outcome has been low. Anders[61] has suggested that many of the conflicting results from polygraphic studies in infants may be attributed to the lack of standardized recording conditions and equipment, lengths of recording time, and choice of parameters used to define state.[62, 63]

Lombroso and Matsumiya,[21] using measures of state based on EEG, EMG, and EOG patterns along with observations of behavior, have replicated the finding of Thoman and associates,[20] using behavioral observations, that stability of state patterns over weeks in newborns may be related to later developmental dysfunction. These investigators, who categorized state in terms of three waking states and REM and NREM sleep, note that polygraphy is of doubtful value in terms of the waking states.

After 6 months of age there are relatively few research studies of children before adolescence, presumably because of the intrusiveness of the techniques, although some studies have been made at scattered ages.[64–71]

Critique of Polygraphic Recording

Effects of laboratory monitoring on sleep and waking in infants and children have been well documented.[32, 33, 37, 71] Laboratory procedures have generally been found to reduce active sleep and increase wakefulness. However, differences between normal sleep and sleep in the laboratory may vary depending on the status (e.g., premature, full-term) and ages of infants and children. For example, in a study of 2- to 6-year-old children recorded for 24-hour periods, Kahn and associates[69] noted that, "In the 2-year-olds, putting on EEG electrodes was so challenging that EMG recordings were not used."

All-night sleep recordings are expensive, time- and labor-intensive, and difficult to use. The quantity of data obtained may be more than is necessary for many questions. Thus, the collection of such enormous amounts of data, which must be somehow reduced, can be seen as both a strength and a limitation.

Sleep Monitoring Using Time-Lapse Video Recording

With the objective of providing an alternative to laboratory study of infants' sleep, Anders and collaborators[72, 73] developed another form of behavioral observation, time-lapse video recording.

General Procedures

In the afternoon or evening of the night of a recording, video equipment is brought to the home and set in place beside the crib. The camera is equipped with a wide-angle lens and an auto-iris, and it is sensitive to low levels of illumination. It is mounted on a tripod and placed as close to the infant's bed as possible. An infrared light source provides sufficient illumination for recording but does not interfere with the baby's sleep. A time-date generator superimposes continuous clock time and date on the video tape. Finally, a microphone, placed near the bed, records fussing and cry vocalization directly onto the tape.[73]

In the laboratory, the video tapes are played back at normal speed. In this mode, any movement occurs very rapidly, so that REMs, body movements, and facial grimaces are greatly exaggerated—the "Keystone Cops" effect. This speed-up of movements has the advantage of making quiet sleep, active sleep, and waking very distinctive.

The tapes are scored in 5-minute (real time) epochs for active sleep and quiet sleep. Waking and out-of-crib are scored on a minute-to-minute basis. The criteria for scoring the two sleep states are the same as those described in the earlier section on behavioral sleep. Periods of infant crying, the infant's mode of self-soothing, and parental interventions are also scored.

Anders has reported the use of 12:1[74] and 18:1[73] time-lapse ratios for 14- to 16-hour recordings. In video studies of premature infants by the authors' laboratory, a 60:1 ratio for 24-hour recordings were used (5 sec of replay is 5 min in real time).[75] The results of studies suggest that there is a wide latitude with respect to the time-lapse ratio that can be used for video recordings.

Developmental Indices

From multiple and prolonged recordings, it is possible to use a variety of descriptive statistics to characterize an infant's sleep. In addition to the usual measures, total amount of each state, percentages of time-in-bed for each state, and the active sleep/quiet sleep ratio, Anders and collaborators have suggested a number of indices, some of which have been shown to have predictive validity. The longest sleep period (LSP) during the night becomes a meaningful index of maturation.[73] The LSP increases from a little less than 4 hours at 2 weeks to about 7 hours at 5 months, then remains relatively constant throughout the remainder of the first year.

The portion of the LSP that occurs between midnight and 5:00 AM is an index of sleep consolidation and is considered to indicate the degree to which a baby has "settled." This percentage increases steadily from 46% at 2 weeks to 89% at 9 months, then decreases to 69% at 9 months when night waking emerges.[73]

Other measures on which Anders and collaborators have provided normative data include sleep onset latency and quiet sleep latency.[72–74, 76, 78] These measures are only relevant when the baby is put to bed before falling asleep. The predominance of quiet sleep throughout the night begins to emerge at 2 months and increases throughout the remainder of the first year. Anders also describes a holding time index and a transition probability index.[73, 76, 78] Tables of normative data for each of the measures are to be found in Anders' 1985 report.[73]

Reliability and Validity

Anders and Sostek established the validity of this procedure for infants at 2 and 8 weeks of age by comparing video recordings with polygraphic recordings.[78] Recordings by Thoman and associates of premature infants have been validated by comparing them with behavioral observations; significant observer reliability, as well as measurement reliability for each of the sleep states has been established.[75]

Critique of Video Recording

Video recording has a number of advantages. Because the procedure is relatively nonintrusive with respect to the parents as well as the baby, it is possible to record overnight in the home on repeated occasions. Unlike direct behavioral observations, constraints are not placed on the duration of an observation or the time of day during which observations can be made, but recordings are restricted to times when the infant is in the crib.

Video recordings are most appropriate if repeated nighttime monitoring is needed to evaluate the qualitative characteristics of sleep, the frequency and nature of wakeful periods (crying or noncrying) throughout the night, or the parents' frequency and timing of interventions.

There is some uncertainty with respect to the validity of video recordings after the early weeks. Anders and Sostek's validation study[78] was carried out with 2- and 8-week infants. During these early weeks, and even earlier in premature infants, active sleep is more distinctive from quiet sleep because of the level of activity, and active sleep is more distinctive from wakefulness because of the quality of the activity. However, from 3 to 6 months, the motor activity associated with active sleep diminishes markedly, and the distinctions are not as great. Thus, reliability and validity are somewhat uncertain after the early months.

In addition, there are times when an infant is covered up or curled up in a corner of the crib and the eyes and small movements are not visible. Such obstructions of visibility for state scoring are relatively rare. Another limitation is that the occurrence of specific phasic movements cannot be recorded from the fast-action replay.

Sleep/Wakefulness from Actigraphic Home Monitoring

Based on the notion that the level of body motility is the least common denominator for discriminating sleep and wakefulness, the wristogram was developed for adults. The actigraph has recently been miniaturized for infants and children, and Sadeh and collaborators[79, 79a] have carried out a number of studies using this device. The small solid-state computerized movement detector, weighing about 2 ounces, is worn on an arm or leg. The occurrence of limb movements was continuously registered, then summed over 1-minute periods. These values can be stored in memory over a period of at least a week. Thus, movements can be recorded for prolonged periods without interruption, except for bathing the baby and changing clothes.

Sadeh and collaborators[79] report that motility levels can be computer scored for sleep or wakefulness in 1-minute epochs by a specially developed algorithm. Thus, data on the total amount of sleep and distribution of sleep episodes can be obtained. Rates of agreement with conventional polysomnographic data range from 80 to 90% in babies 9 months and older.[79, 80] More recently, an algorithm has been developed to score active sleep and quiet sleep in infants.[79a] Agreement rates between observer-scored and algorithm-scored states are low during the newborn period (55–83%), good at 3 months (78–92%), and fair at 6 months of age (66–98%). Significant measurement reliability was reported for active sleep and quiet sleep only for 3-month-old infants. The sleep measures also differentiated sleep-disturbed and control children.

The actigraph is initiated by a software program and requires no further manipulation or installation, except for attaching it to the subject for the duration of the monitoring period. Clearly, this is an extremely simple, nonintrusive procedure for recording the naturally occurring sleep of infants and children in the home.

Critique of the Actigraph

When treating sleep problems of the very young, the primary information required is the frequency and duration of night wakenings. For this purpose, it is appropriate that the actigraph scores sleep as a single category. However, two categories of wakefulness are required: crying and noncrying wakeful periods during the night. Noncrying wakefulness provides information on the infant's ability to settle down by himself.[81]

Despite the high overall agreement between actigraph recordings and polysomnography, the actigraph is least reliable in distinguishing sleep from periods of quiet wakefulness.[79] In addition to signal similarity in these two states, signal artifacts can cause confusion between sleep and waking. For example, when the mother is rocking or carrying her baby during sleep, the recording of the baby would probably be coded as waking time. Documentation of sleep and waking by caregiver is requisite for elimination of artifacts due to monitor ''off'' times and periods of external motion.

For some older infants, the actigraph could not be attached by their parents until after they were asleep because of the child's reluctance or exaggerated interest in the monitor.[80] In such instances, it is not possible to record sleep-onset time. It is also not clear how long the monitor could be worn during the daytime.

For the most part, this procedure is very simple to use, relatively nonintrusive, and cost-effective. It can be used when no other recording procedure may be feasible or affordable and, especially, when global measures of sleep and waking are sufficient. Finally, this is the only procedure that permits continuous, prolonged recordings, and the only procedure, other than behavioral observations, that permits recordings when the baby is not in the crib.

Sleep Monitoring from Recordings of Motility Patterns

Another type of motility recording procedure is the Home Monitoring System (HMS), in which a thin, pliable, pressure-sensitive pad is placed under the baby's bedding.[2, 82, 83] The pad is 12″ × 24″ or 24″ × 24″, depending on the size of the crib. Motility signals are transmitted through a pre-amplifier to a small recorder; these components fit in a small briefcase that is placed on the floor under the crib. The recorder is slow-playing so that 24 hours of signals can be recorded on a 60-minute audio cassette tape. This system permits continuous recording in the home whenever the infant is in the crib.

Instead of recording the frequency and distribution of movements, as in the actigraph, analog signals from the baby's respiration and body movements are recorded. These motility signals vary in amplitude and rise-time as well as frequency and regularity of cycles (i.e., zero-crossings). The basic notion that guided the development of this procedure is that motility patterns are distinctive for each state. Figure 6–1 illustrates typical signals for four states. Whenever body movements occur, they predominate in the signal pattern; when there are no body movements, respiration patterns predominate; when respiration ceases (apneic events), the heart rate signal is apparent.

In the laboratory, the signals are demodulated, digitized (at 10 samples/sec), and entered into a computer. Using a pattern recognition algorithm developed for this purpose, the signals are computer coded, in 30-second epochs, for active sleep, quiet sleep, active-quiet transition sleep, sleep-wake transition, and wakefulness, as well as periods out of the crib. The full record is printed out and visually edited by a trained scorer. These are the sleep states that can be recorded from direct behavioral observations. Reliability (individual differences) has been demonstrated for measures of each of the sleep variables and wakefulness.[83]

Validity

The value of motility patterns for discriminating states has been documented in a series of studies. In a study of human infants,[84] state judgments from analog signals were compared and found to agree with the results from direct behavioral observations; then the same study design was carried out using infant rabbits with the same results.[85] Further, in a cross-species study,[86] observers trained only on behavioral states and their analog signals in animals were asked to judge analog signals in human infants. Their judgments showed high agreement with direct behavioral observations of the infants made by trained observers of humans. At the same time, an observer familiar only with human infant states was able to reliably score the analog signals from infant rats and rabbits. Thus, motility patterns expressed in the sleep states and wakefulness are distinctive, and these motor patterns show an invariance across species. Figure 6–1 shows the com-

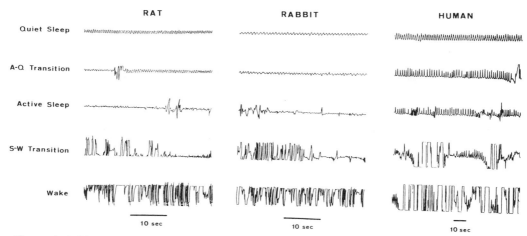

Figure 6–1. Motility patterns typical of quiet sleep, active-quiet (A-Q) transitional sleep, active sleep, sleep-wake (S-W) transition, and wakefulness in rat, rabbit, and human subjects. (From Thoman EB, Zeidner LP, Denenberg VH: Cross-species invariance in state-related motility patterns. Am J Physiol 10:R312, 1981.)

monality of motility patterns for young rats, rabbits, and humans. These findings indicate the fundamental nature of motility patterns and also address the issue of validity of the HMS procedure.

The sensitivity of measures from HMS recordings is indicated by findings of developmental changes in: active sleep, quiet sleep, wakefulness, sleep-wake transition, active sleep bout lengths, quiet sleep bout lengths, diurnal differences in wakefulness in the crib, and quiet sleep cyclicity within sleep episodes in premature and full-term infants.[1, 2, 19, 83] Predictive validity has also been demonstrated using this procedure. Sleep measures during the first postnatal day predict mental scores at 6 months.[87] Sleep patterns during the first 5 post-term weeks in premature infants predict specific forms of developmental disabilities that appear in the subsequent 3-year period.[1]

Critique of the Home Monitoring System

This procedure provides reliable and valid data on the sleep states of infants. Thus, it permits measurement of any of the sleep variables that can be obtained from behavioral observations. In addition, it is the least intrusive of recording systems. Unlike behavioral observations, it does not require the presence of an observer; unlike video recording, it does not require camera equipment and special lighting to be set up in the home; and unlike

the actigraph, nothing must be attached to the baby for the recordings.

However, in comparison with behavioral observations, phasic behaviors other than generalized movement cannot be recorded; in comparison with polysomnography, the stages 1–4 of NREM sleep cannot be differentiated when these appear in older babies and children; in comparison with time-lapse video recording, the nature of parental interventions is not apparent, nor are methods of self-soothing that the baby may use; and in comparison with the actigraph, it is possible to record all of the sleep states, but it is somewhat more expensive in terms of equipment required, personnel time, and complexity of signal processing. While the HMS is more reliable in determining all periods of wakefulness than the actigraph, like the actigraph, it does not permit a distinction between crying and noncrying wakefulness. Only behavioral observations, including video recording can make this important distinction. These comparisons highlight issues to consider in selecting a monitoring procedure. A final consideration for this procedure is that the system, including recording and computer processing, is not yet available as a commercial package.

Summary and Conclusions: Is There a Monitoring Procedure of Choice?

If the duration of monitoring is a critical parameter, consider the following: behavioral observations (made primarily in the daytime) have not been made for longer than 7 hours; polysomnography of infants is generally not used for longer than 12 hours; video recordings have not been made for more than 16 hours; motility recordings (using the HMS) cannot be made for longer than 24 hours (without a tape change); and the actigraph can record for as long as 8 days (with necessary interruptions only at bath and clothes-changing times).

If one is interested in cost-effectiveness, the actigraph is the procedure of choice. At the other extreme, laboratory recordings are clearly the most expensive in terms of equipment and personnel time. All of the procedures require training for behavioral and signal pattern recognition.

If one is interested primarily in noncrying wakefulness at sleep-onset and throughout the night, video recording is the procedure of choice. If nonintrusiveness is a major factor, motility (HMS) monitoring is the procedure of choice. If interested in the development of physiologic controls or neural correlates of sleep, or of sleep stages in the older infant or child, laboratory or home polysomnography is the only option. Finally, if interested in intensive study of sleep and state-related behaviors (as well as the waking states) or in validation of other procedures, behavioral observation is requisite.

Preparation of this chapter was supported by Grant 2RO1MH41244 from the National Institute of Mental Health, Center for Prevention Research, Division of Prevention and Special Mental Health Programs

References

1. Whitney MP, Thoman EB: Early sleep patterns of premature infants are differentially related to later developmental disabilities. Dev Behav Ped 14:71, 1993.
2. Thoman EB: Sleeping and waking states in infants: a functional perspective. Neurosci Biobehav Rev 14:93, 1990.
3. Papousek H, Bernstein P: The functions of conditioning stimulation in human neonates and infants. In Ambrose A: Stimulation in Early Infancy. New York, Academic Press, 1969, pp 229–247.
4. Becker PT, Thoman EB: Rapid eye movement storms in infants: rates of occurrence at 6 months predicts mental development at one year. Science 212:1415, 1981.
5. Thoman EB: Sleep and wake behaviors in the neonates: consistencies and consequences. Merrill-Palmer Quart 21:295, 1975.
6. Hoppenbrouwers T, Harper RM, Hodgman JE, et al: Polygraphic studies of normal infants during the first six months of life. II. Respiratory rate and variability as a function of state. Pediatr Res 12:120, 1978.
7. Becker PT, Thoman EB: Organization of sleeping and waking states in infants: consistency across contexts. Physiol Behav 31:405, 1983.
8. Thoman EB: Early development of sleeping behaviors in infants. In Ellis, NR: Aberrant Development in Infancy: Human and Animal Studies. New York, John Wiley & Sons, 1975, pp 122–138.
9. Thoman EB: A biological perspective and a behavioral model for assessment of premature infants. In Bond LA, Joffe JM (eds): Facilitating Infant and Early Childhood Development. (Primary Prevention of Psychopathology Series, Vol. 6). Hanover, NH, University Press of New England, 1982, pp 159–179.
10. Thoman EB: Affects of earliest infancy: the imperative for a biological model. In McDonald ET, Gallagher DL (eds): Facilitating Social-Emotional Development in Multiply Handicapped Children. Philadelphia, Home of the Merciful Saviour for Crippled Children, 1985, pp 9–27.
11. Thoman EB: The time domain in individual subject research. In Valsiner J: The Individual Subject and Scientific Psychology. Baltimore, Plenum Publishing Corp, 1986, pp 181–200.
12. Thoman EB, Korner AF, Kraemer HC: Individual consistency in behavioral states in neonates. Dev Psychobiol 9:271, 1976.
13. Thoman EB, Becker PT, Freese MP: Individual patterns of mother-infant interaction. In Sacket GP: Observing Behavior, Vol. I: Theory and Applications in Mental Retardation. Baltimore, University Park Press, 1978, pp 95–114.
14. Thoman EB, Acebo C, Dreyer CA, et al: Individuality in the interactive process. In Thoman EB (ed): Origins of the Infant's Social Responsiveness. Hillsdale, NJ, Lawrence Erlbaum Associates, 1979, pp 305–338.
15. Thoman EB, Becker PT: Issues in assessment and prediction for the infant born at risk. In Field T, Sostek A, Goldberg S, Shuman HH: Infants Born at Risk. New York, Spectrum, 1979, pp 461–483.
16. Guess D, Roberts S, Siegel-Causey E, et al: Investigations into the state behaviors of students with severe and profound handicapping conditions. Monograph funded under the Models Projects for the Most Severely Handicapped Children and Youth Program, University of Kansas, 1991.
17. Acebo C: Naturalistic observations of mothers and infants: description of mother and infant responsiveness and sleep-wake state development. (Dissertation) University of Connecticut, 1987.
18. Davis DH: The development of sleeping and waking states in high-risk preterm infants. Inf Behav Dev 13:513, 1990.
19. Thoman EB, McDowell K: Sleep cyclicity in infants during the earliest postnatal weeks. Physiol Behav 45:517, 1989.
20. Thoman EB, Denenberg VH, Sievel J, et al: State organization in neonates: developmental inconsistency indicates risk for developmental dysfunction. Neuropediatrics 12:45, 1981.
21. Lombroso CT, Matsumiya Y: Stability in waking-sleep states in neonates as a predictor of long-term neurologic outcome. Pediatrics 76:52, 1985.
22. Tynan WD: Behavioral stability predicts morbidity and mortality in infants from a neonatal intensive care unit. Inf Behav Dev 9:71, 1986.
23. Waite SP, DeSantis D, Thoman EB, et al: The predictive validity of neonatal state variables in the rabbit. Biol Behav 2:249, 1978.

24. Thoman EB, Davis DH, Denenberg VH: The sleeping and waking states of infants: correlations across time and person. Physiol Behav 41:531, 1987.

25. Prechtl HFR: Ultrasound studies of human fetal behavior. Early Hum Dev 12:91, 1985.

26. Parmelee A: Ontogeny of sleep patterns and assorted periodicities in infants. *In* Falkner F, Kretchmer N, Rossi E (eds): Modern Problems in Pediatrics. Basel, S Karger, 1974, pp 298–311.

27. Prechtl HFR, O'Brien MJ: Behavioral states of the full-term newborn. The emergence of a concept. *In* Stratton P (ed): Psychobiology of the Human Newborn. New York, John Wiley & Sons, 1982, pp 53–73.

28. Anders T, Emde R, Parmelee J: A Manual of Standardized Terminology, Techniques and Criteria for the Scoring of States of Sleep and Wakefulness in Newborn Infants. UCLA Brain Information Service, NINDS Neurological Information Network, 1971.

29. Parmelee A, Bruck K, Bruck M: Activity and inactivity cycles during the sleep of premature infants exposed to neutral temperatures. Biol Neonate 4:317, 1962.

30. Murray B, Campbell D: Sleep states in the newborn: influence of sound. Neuropediatrics 2:335, 1971.

31. Sander L: Regulation and organization in the early infant-caregiver system. *In* Robinson RJ (ed): Brain and Early Behavior. London, Academic Press, 1969, pp 311–322.

32. Bernstein P, Emde R, Campos J: REM sleep in four-month infants under home and laboratory conditions. Psychosom Med 35:322, 1973.

33. Sostek A, Anders T: Effects of varying laboratory conditions on behavioral state organization in two- and eight-week-old infants. Child Dev 46:871, 1976.

34. Ellingson RJ, Peters JF: Development of EEG and daytime sleep patterns in low risk premature infants during the first year of life: longitudinal observations. EEG Clin Neurol 50:165, 1980.

35. Coons S, Guilleminault C: Development of consolidated sleep and wakeful periods in relation to the day/night cycle in infancy. Dev Med Child Neurol 26:169, 1984.

36. Fagioli I, Salzarulo P: Sleep states development in the first year of life assessed through 24-hr recordings. Early Hum Dev 68:215, 1982.

37. Hoppenbrouwers T, Hadgman J, Arakawa K, et al: Sleep and waking states in infancy: Normative studies. Sleep 11:387, 1988.

38. Prechtl HFR: Polygraphic studies of the full-term newborn: II computer analysis of recorded data. *In* Bax M, MacKeith R (eds): Studies in Infancy. London, Heinemann, Clinics in Developmental Medicine, 1968, pp 22–40.

39. Dreyfus-Brisac C: Ontogenesis of sleep in human prematures after 32 weeks of conceptual age. Dev Psychobiol 3:91, 1970.

40. Stefanski M, Schulze K, Bateman D, et al: A scoring system for states of sleep and wakefulness in term and preterm infants. Pediatr Res 18:58, 1984.

41. Curzi-Dascalova L, Peirano P, Morel-Kahn F: Development of sleep states in normal premature and full-term newborns. Dev Psychobiol 21:431, 1988.

42. Westmoreland BF, Stockard JE: The EEG in infants and children: normal patterns. Am J EEG Technol 17:187, 1977.

43. Ellingson RJ: The EEG of premature and full-term newborns. *In* Klass DW, Daly DD (eds): Current Practice of Clinical Electroencephalography. New York, Raven Press, 1978, pp 149–177.

44. Werner SS, Stockard JE, Bickford RG: Atlas of Neonatal Electroencephalography. New York, Raven Press, 1977.

45. Dreyfus-Brisac C, Monod N: The electroencephalograph of full-term newborns and premature infants. *In* Remond A (ed): Handbook of Electroencephalography and Clinical Neurophysiology. Amsterdam, Elsevier, 1975, pp 6–23.

46. Dreyfus-Brisac C, Curzi-Dascalova L: The EEG during the first year of life. *In* Remond A (ed): Handbook of Electroencephalography and Clinical Neurophysiology. Vol 6: The Normal EEG Throughout Life. Part B: The Evolution of the EEG from Birth to Adulthood. Amsterdam, Elsevier, 1975, pp 24–30.

47. Metcalf D: EEG sleep spindle ontogenesis in normal children. *In* Smith JF (ed): Drugs, Development and Cerebral Function. Springfield, IL, Charles C Thomas, 1972, pp 125–144.

48. Metcalf D, Mondate J, Butler F: Ontogenesis of spontaneous K-complexes. Psychophysiology 8:340, 1971.

49. Kellaway P, Fox BJ: Electroencephalographic diagnosis of cerebral pathology in infants during sleep. I. Rationale, technique and the characteristics of normal sleep in infants. J Pediatr 41:262, 1952.

50. Karacan I, Anch M, Thornby JI, et al: Longitudinal sleep patterns during pubertal growth: four year follow-up. Pediatr Res 9:842, 1975.

51. Roffwarg HP, Muzio JN, Dement WC: Ontogenetic development of the human sleep-dream cycle. Science 152:604, 1966.

52. Smith JF, Karacan I, Yang M: Ontogeny of delta activity during human sleep. EEG Clin Neurophysiol 43:229, 1977.

53. Hoppenbrouwers T, Hodgman JE, Harper RM, et al: Temporal distribution of sleep states, somatic activity, and autonomic activity during the first half year of life. Sleep 5:131, 1982.

54. Rechtschaffen A, Kales A: A manual of standardized terminology, techniques and scoring systems for sleep stages of human subjects. Washington, DC, Public Health Service, Government Printing Office, 1968.

55. Guilleminault C, Souquet M: Sleep states and related pathology. *In* Korobkin R, Guilleminault C (eds): Advances in Perinatal Neurology. New York, Spectrum, 1979, pp 225–247.

56. Harper RM, Frostig Z, Taube D, et al: Development of sleep-waking temporal sequencing in infants at risk for the sudden infant death syndrome. Exp Neurol 79:821, 1983.

57. Prechtl HFR: Brain and behavioral mechanisms in the human newborn infant. *In* Robinson RJ (ed): Brain and Early Behavior: Development in the Fetus and Infant. New York, Academic Press, 1969, pp 115–131.

57a. Scher MS, Sun M, Steppe DA, et al: Comparison of EEG sleep state-specific spectral values between healthy full-term and pre-term infants at comparable postconcept ages. Sleep 17:47, 1994.

58. Harper RM, Hoppenbrouwers T, Sterman MB, et al: Polygraphic studies of normal infants during the first six months of life. I. Heart rate and variability as a function of state. Pediatr Res 10:945, 1976.

59. Sterman MB, Harper RM, Havens B, et al: Quantitative analysis of infant EEG development during quiet sleep. EEG Clin Neurophysiol 43:371, 1977.

60. Hoppenbrouwers T: Sleep in infants. *In* Guilleminault C (ed): Sleep and its Disorders in Children. New York, Raven Press, 1987, pp 1–15.

61. Anders TF: Annotation: Neurophysiological studies of sleep in infants and children. J Child Psychol Psychiatry 23:75, 1982.

62. Parmelee AH, Wenner W, Akiyama Y, et al: Sleep states in premature infants. Dev Med Child Neurol 9:70, 1967.

63. Monod N, Guidasci S: Sleep and brain malformation in the neonatal period. Neuropadiatrie 7:229, 1976.

64. Roffwarg HP, Dement WC, Fisher C: Preliminary observations of the sleep-dream pattern in neonates, infants, children and adults. *In* Harms E (ed): Problems of Sleep and Dreams in Children. International Monographs on Child Psychiatry. New York, Macmillan, 1964, pp 60–72.

65. Ross JJ, Agnew HW, Williams RL, et al: Sleep patterns in pre-adolescent children: an EEG-EOG study. Pediatrics 42:324, 1968.

66. Feinberg I, Koresko R, Heller N: EEG sleep patterns as a function of normal and pathological aging in man. J Psychiatr Res 5:107, 1967.

67. Carskadon MA: The second decade. *In* Guilleminault C (ed): Sleeping and Waking Disorders: Indications and Techniques. Redding, MA, Addison-Wesley, 1982, pp 99–125.

68. Carskadon MA, Orav EJ, Dement WC: Evolution of sleep and daytime sleepiness in adolescents. *In* Guilleminault C, Lugaresi E (eds): Sleep/Wake Disorders: Natural History, Epidemiology, and Long-Term Evolution. New York, Raven Press, 1983, pp 201–216.

69. Kahn E, Fisher C, Edwards A, et al: 24-hour sleep patterns: a comparison between 2 to 3 year old and 4 to 6 year old children. Arch Gen Psychiatry 29:380, 1973.

70. Coble PA, Kupfer DJ, Reynolds CF et al: EEG sleep of healthy children 6 to 12 years of age. *In* Guilleminault C (ed): Sleep and its Disorders in Children. New York, Raven Press, 1987, pp 17–27.

71. Kales JD, Kales A, Jacobson A, et al: Baseline sleep and recall studies in children. Psychophysiology 4:391, 1968.

72. Anders TF, Keener M, Bowe TR, et al: A longitudinal study of nighttime sleep-wake patterns in infants from birth to one year. *In* Galenson E, Call JD (eds): Frontiers of Infant Psychiatry. New York, Basic Books, 1983, pp 150–169.

73. Anders TF, Keener M: Developmental course of nighttime sleep-wake patterns in full-term and premature infants during the first year of life. Sleep 8:173, 1985.

74. Anders T: Home recorded sleep in two and nine month old infants. J Acad Child Psychiatry 17:421, 1978.

75. Thoman EB, Ingersoll EW, Acebo C: Premature infants seek rhythmic stimulation, and the experience facilitates neurobehavioral development. J Dev Behav Pediatr 12:11, 1991.

76. Bowe T, Anders T: The use of the semi-Markov model in the study of the development of sleep-wake states in infants. Psychophysiology 16:41, 1979.

77. Bowe T: A systems analysis of the maturation of sleep using a semi-Markov model. (Dissertation). Stanford University, Stanford, CA, 1981.

78. Anders TF, Sostek A: The use of time-lapse video recording of sleep-wake behaviors in human infants. Psychophysiology 13:155, 1976.

79. Sadeh A, Alster J, Urbach D, et al: Actigraphically based automatic bedtime sleep-wake scoring: validity and clinical applications. J Amb Monitor 2:209, 1989.

79a. Sadeh A, Acebo C, Scifer R, et al: Activity-based assessment of sleep-wake patterns during the first year of life. Inf Behav Dev, in press.

80. Sadeh A, Lavie P, Scher A, et al: Actigraphic home-monitoring sleep-disturbed and control infants and young children: a new method for pediatric assessment of sleep-wake patterns. Pediatrics 87:494, 1991.

81. Sadeh A, Lavie P: The capacity to sleep alone: actigraphic home-monitoring in children's sleep disorders. Israel Psychological Association Meeting, Jerusalem, Israel, 1988.

82. Thoman EB, Glazier RC: Computer scoring of motility patterns for states of sleep and wakefulness: Human infants. Sleep 10:122, 1987.

83. Thoman EB, Whitney MP: Sleep states of infants monitored in the home: individual differences, developmental trends, and origins of diurnal cyclicity. Inf Behav Dev 12:59, 1989.

84. Thoman EB, Tynan WD: Sleep states and wakefulness in human infants: profiles from motility monitoring. Physiol Behav 23:519, 1979.

85. Thoman EB, Zeidner LP: Sleep-wake states in infant rabbits: profiles from motility monitoring. Physiol Behav 22:1049, 1979.

86. Thoman EB, Zeidner LP, Denenberg VH: Cross-species invariance in state related motility patterns. Am J Physiol 241:R312, 1981.

87. Freudigman KA, Thoman EB: Infant sleep during the first postnatal day: an opportunity for assessment of vulnerability. Pediatrics 92:373, 1993.

CHAPTER

7

Culture and Family: Influences on Childhood Sleep Practices and Problems

BETSY LOZOFF

Cultural Influences on Children's Sleep Patterns

Cultural differences in childrearing strongly influence sleep patterns and practices and the definition of what constitutes a sleep problem. These points will be illustrated by three sleep-related issues: (1) thumbsucking and transitional object use, (2) breast-feeding, and (3) co-sleeping (the practice of children and parents sleeping in the same bed).

Transitional Object Use and Thumbsucking

Some child development authorities consider transitional object attachment to be an important part of normal, healthy emotional development.[1] However, cross-cultural studies document that there are major cultural differences in the prevalence of object attachment. For instance, fewer rural Italian children were attached to objects (4.9%) than were foreign children living in a large Italian city (61.5%).[2] Similarly, fewer Korean children compared with American children were object attached (18% vs 64%).[3] Differing rates of object attachment have also been documented in groups in the United States who differed in both ethnicity and socioeconomic status. The proportion of object attachment among black children seen at an outpatient pediatric clinic was lower than that among white children seen by private practitioners (44% vs 77%).[4]

Sleeping arrangements and breast-feeding are thought to be important in accounting for these differing rates of transitional object use. In the studies cited, Korean and Italian children were more likely than United States and other European children to sleep in the same bed or in the same room as their parents and to be breast-fed until an older age. Black children were also more likely than white children to sleep in the same room or bed as their parents.

How a child falls asleep may be even more important than *where* a child sleeps, and the pattern of parental interaction with the child at bedtime may be the critical factor. The relevance of adult company at bedtime is supported by a Turkish study of thumbsucking in which 96% of thumbsucking 1- to 7-year-old children had been left as infants to fall asleep alone, while all children in the nonthumbsucking comparison group had had adult company and body contact (rocking or nursing) as infants when falling asleep.[5] Even in the United States, children whose parents stayed with them at bedtime were less likely to use an attachment object or to suck their thumbs than were children who fell asleep alone (30% vs 57% for object attachment; 11% vs 32% for thumbsucking).[6]

These studies suggest that the use of attachment objects and thumbsucking are not universal components of healthy emotional or social development. Instead, they seem to be influenced by culturally determined parental behaviors, such as staying with children as they fall asleep versus leaving them to fall asleep alone.

Breast-feeding

The norms for infant sleep patterns were established in the United States and the United Kingdom when bottle feeding was widespread and breast-fed infants were generally weaned in the first few months of life. These feeding practices are so unusual from cross-cultural and historic perspectives that it is important to reflect on breast-feeding and its relationship to sleep patterns. The composition of human breast milk, with very low levels of protein and fat, is similar to that of mammalian species who feed their young continuously.[7, 8] In fact, nursing around the clock seems to have been the pattern during much of human evolution and is still the norm in many nonindustrialized societies.[9] For instance, the mean interval between nursing episodes among the !Kung of the Kalahari Desert was found to be 13 minutes,[10] and the number of nursings in rural Kenya averaged about 20 feedings per 24-hour period.[11] Nursing is prolonged in most of the world. In a representative sample of nonindustrial societies, 85% nursed their infants for 2 years or more.[12] Prolonged and frequent nursing clearly affect sleep. In the United States, a group of babies who were nursed on demand into the second year of life continued to wake and feed during the night.[13] Instead of having a long uninterrupted night sleep, they slept in short bouts with frequent wakings. This pattern was most pronounced in infants who nursed and shared a bed with their parents.

Because prolonged breast-feeding has been essential for infant survival for millennia, it could be argued that sleep/wake cycles among such nursing infants should be used to define "normal" sleep patterns. Although data from bottle-fed babies show that the human infant is *capable* of a long uninterrupted night sleep, defining normal or desirable behavior on the basis of such data seems questionable.

Co-sleeping

In the United States, pediatric professionals commonly recommend that children should sleep alone.[14, 15] It is interesting to note that this approach is relatively new in our culture, since until this century most families in the United States were co-sleeping.[16] Furthermore, with the exception of the industrialized West, few cultures expect young children to fall asleep by themselves and to stay asleep alone during the night. In one anthropologic sample of over 100 societies, the middle class in the United States was "unique in putting the baby to sleep in a room of his own."[17] McKenna and others have pointed out that when practices such as co-sleeping are longstanding and widespread, they may have been important for infant well-being during the course of human evolution.[18]

Despite pediatric advice, many parents in the United States currently do sleep with their children. Some degree of co-sleeping has been noted in approximately half of the families with young children. However, there are major ethnic differences in the prevalence and pattern of co-sleeping. In the United States, ethnic groups seem to differ most markedly in the proportion of regular all night co-sleeping (more than 2–3 times per week), with blacks highest (about 50%),[19, 20] then Hispanics (21%),[21] and whites the lowest (less than 10%).[19, 20] Social class has also been an important factor, with more co-sleeping among families of lower socioeconomic status, regardless of ethnicity.[19, 20] It should be emphasized that co-sleeping is not an isolated childrearing practice. Co-sleeping among both blacks and whites has been associated with an approach to sleep that includes parental involvement at bedtime as well as during the night.[19, 22]

In several recent studies in the United States, regular sleeping in the parental bed for all or part of the night was associated with children's sleep problems.[19, 22] In a study in Cleveland, 65% of co-sleeping white children 6- to 48-months-old had disrupted sleep, with protests at bedtime or night waking involving the parents three or more nights a week.[19] Only 28% of non-co-sleeping children showed such behaviors. Co-sleeping children were also more likely to be older and to have parents with lower levels of education and occupation, increased stress in the family, and mothers with more ambivalent attitudes toward them. Increased sleep problems have been reported among co-sleeping Hispanic-American children in New York,[21] and among both white and nonwhite (a mixture of black and Hispanic) children in Massachusetts.[20] In contrast, co-sleeping was not associated with sleep problems or such family factors among black children in the 1984 Cleveland study.[19] In a new, larger sample of black children in Cleveland, regular co-sleeping was associated with bedtime protests and frequent night waking.[22] However, the proportion of co-sleeping black families that considered these behaviors conflictual or frustrating was lower than that among whites (23% vs 55%). In summary, co-sleeping black families reported the same frequency of bedtime struggles and night waking as whites and Hispanics but not the same degree of distress and conflict. Similarly, breast-feeding La Leche League mothers did not report frequent night waking to be problematic.[13] Thus, pediatric professionals should not assume that an increase in bedtime protests or night waking associated with co-sleeping will be experienced as conflictual or stressful.

The issue of causality was not addressed by any of the studies to date. One cannot say whether co-sleeping *caused* the disrupted sleep or was a parental *response* to a child's sleeping difficulty. It is also conceivable that sleep problems might be worse without co-sleeping, but none of the studies could assess this possibility. However, it seems clear that bringing a child into the parental bed did not lead to *resolution* of sleep problems for most United States families, since in the cited studies sleep problems had lasted months to years despite co-sleeping.[19, 20]

Family Influences on Children's Sleep Problems

Background factors, such as socioeconomic status, ethnicity, and education, have generally been unrelated to children's sleep problems per se. Conflicting results regarding maternal employment have been obtained. An increase in sleep problems among young children whose mothers return to the workforce has been reported in some studies but not in others.[23, 24] If such an association exists, the interpretation is still not clear. It could be that the mother's work is stressful for the child and produces anxiety about separation, that the mother's fatigue makes her less tolerant of disruptions to her own sleep, or that the mother because of her own mixed feelings about leaving the child has trouble dealing firmly with the objections at bedtime and the night waking that can be expected in young children.

One of the more interesting directions in recent studies of sleep-disturbed children has been the inclusion of measures of family functioning and maternal mood. In every study in which family stress and maternal depression have been assessed, significant associations with early childhood sleep problems have been reported.[23–26] It seems that maternal depression may be part of an interrelated set of factors, such as the perception of the infant's temperament as difficult, parental sleep disturbances, or marital discord. These findings suggest at least two interpretations. Stressed families and/or depressed mothers may be more disturbed by and have difficulty handling what may be ordinary night waking or bedtime struggles in their child. Alternatively, the child may be aware at some level of the disturbance in the family and have trouble sleeping.

Applying Cultural and Family Perspectives to Pediatric Practice

Childrearing patterns, such as co-sleeping and prolonged breast-feeding, and child behaviors, such as night waking and night nursing, have been universal during human evolution. From this perspective it is hard to consider it "normal" for children to sleep alone and not to wake their parents during the night. Yet the distress many families in the United States experience when their child refuses to go to sleep alone or wakes during the night is very real. The following is a personal synthesis that applies cultural and family perspectives to pediatric practice.

With respect to breast-feeding, families may be provided with information about the expectable behavior of nursing babies and note that night waking will decrease with weaning. However, if parental fatigue and distress are interfering with the pleasure of the relationship with the baby and waiting for the weaning process does not seem comfortable, parents and pediatrician may consider a therapeutic approach that gradually increases the interval between nighttime feedings.[27] Putting babies to bed drowsy rather than allowing them to fall asleep at the breast may also be helpful.[28–30]

In response to questions about co-sleeping, share with families the fact that research on co-sleeping is limited and many issues remain unclear. Families may be told that co-sleeping children may wake more at night or have trouble falling asleep alone at bedtime. It is helpful to ask parents of young infants, regardless of cultural group, how they feel about co-sleeping with a toddler or preschooler or staying with their child at bedtime when he or she is older. If the parents do not like these ideas, it may be suggested that they avoid co-sleeping or plan to stop doing so well before the end of the child's first year, when attachment and separation issues become more intense. Thus, try to help parents match their sleep practices to their anticipated reactions to future sleep behaviors in their young child. In the case of a child who already has a sleep problem, it seems that regular co-sleeping is unlikely to solve the problem. Instead, be prepared to offer families a variety of other approaches that have been shown to be effective, again matching intervention to parental style and values.[27–37]

A developmental framework is also very useful in working with early childhood sleep problems. In addition to helping parents understand how their behavior may inadvertently reinforce certain undesired sleep patterns, the importance of separation and autonomy issues for both the child and parents may be discussed. After about 9 months of age, infants may cry for their parents at bedtime and on waking during the night as part of a normal separation response. After exploring their own discomfort with the child's separation distress, parents often can help their child master the normal age-related separation experiences. Fostering the use of a transitional object is one way in which parents may assist their child in mastering separation. However, in giving advice to encourage transitional object use, pediatric professionals should be aware of cultural differences and family values regarding childrearing. Although concerns with separation continue among older toddlers and preschool children, autonomy issues tend to become more prominent. Bedtime routines such as stories and saying good night to stuffed animals or pets may allow children in this age group to take charge of the process of going to sleep. Preschool- and school-aged children who are overly fearful at bedtime can also be helped with techniques of relaxation-imagery, self-hypnosis, and ''bravery'' training.[38, 39]

One should also routinely inquire about upsetting or stressful events in the family and try to assess the mother's mood and the degree of marital discord (see Chapter 5). Sometimes these concerns need to be addressed before parents can handle their child's sleep behavior effectively. Similarly, mothers who work outside the home often can handle bedtime protests and night waking once they voice their own concerns about the limited contact with their child and the multiple leave-takings that working entails.

Finally, it is important to keep in mind cultural influences on any advice given. Much of what comes to the pediatrician's attention as problematic sleep behavior—children who have difficulty falling asleep alone at bedtime, who wake at night and ask for parental attention, or who continue to nurse at night—is problematic only in relation to our society's expectations, rather than to some more general standard of what constitutes difficult behavior in the young child. Pediatric advice on transitional objects, breast-feeding, and co-sleeping may be unknowingly biased toward traditional Euro-American views of childrearing, especially those about bedtime and nighttime behavior. Thus, in giving advice about sleep, pediatric health professionals might do well to be aware of their own cultural values, to examine closely their patients' cultural and familial contexts, and to assess parental reactions to children's sleep behaviors.

References

1. Winnicott DW: Transitional objects and transitional phenomena. Int J Psychoanal 34:89, 1953.
2. Gaddini R: Transitional objects and the process of individuation: a study of three different social groups. J Am Acad Child Psychiatry 9:347, 1970.
3. Hong KM, Townes BD: Infants' attachment to inanimate objects. A cross-cultural study. J Am Acad Child Psychiatry 15:49, 1976.
4. Litt CJ: Children's attachment to transitional objects: a study of two pediatric populations. Am J Orthopsychiatry 15:344, 1981.
5. Ozturk M, Ozturk OM: Thumbsucking and falling asleep. Br J Med Psychol 50:95, 1977.
6. Wolf AW, Lozoff B: Object attachment, thumbsucking, and the passage to sleep. J Am Acad Child Adolesc Psychiatry 28:287, 1989.
7. Ben Shaul D: The composition of the milk of wild animals. Int Zoo Year Book 4:333, 1962.
8. Blurton Jones N: Comparative aspects of mother-child contact. In Blurton Jones N: Ethological Studies of Child Behaviour. London, Cambridge University Press, 1972, pp 305–328.
9. Lozoff B, Brittenham G: Infant care: cache or carry. J Pediatr 95:478, 1979.
10. Konner M, Worthman C: Nursing frequency, gonadal function, and birth spacing among !Kung hunter-gatherers. Science 207:788, 1980.
11. Super C, Harkness S: The infant's niche in rural Kenya and metropolitan America. In Adler LL (ed): Cross-cultural Research at Issue. New York, Academic Press, 1982, pp 47–55.
12. Lozoff B: Birth and bonding in non-industrial societies. Dev Med Child Neurol 25:595, 1983.
13. Elias MF, Nicolson NA, Bora C, et al: Sleep/wake patterns of breast-fed infants in the first 2 years of life. Pediatrics 77:322, 1986.
14. Spock B: Baby and Child Care. New York, Pocket Books, 1976.
15. Brazelton TB: Infants and Mothers: Individual Differences in Development. New York, Delacorte Press, 1969.
16. Thevenin T: The Family Bed: An Age Old Concept in Child Rearing. Minneapolis, Thevenin, 1976.

17. Burton RV, Whiting JWM: The absent father and cross-sex identity. Merrill-Palmer Q 7:85, 1961.
18. McKenna JJ, Mosko S, Dungy C, et al: Sleep and arousal patterns of co-sleeping human mother/infant pairs: a preliminary physiological study with implications for the study of sudden infant death syndrome (SIDS). Am J Phys Anthropol 83:331, 1990.
19. Lozoff B, Wolf AW, Davis NS: Cosleeping in urban families with young children in the United States. Pediatrics 74:171, 1984.
20. Madansky D, Edelbrock C: Cosleeping in a community sample of 2- and 3-year old children. Pediatrics 86:197, 1990.
21. Schachter FF, Fuchs ML, Bijur PE, et al: Cosleeping and sleep problems in Hispanic-American urban young children. Pediatrics 84:522, 1989.
22. Lozoff B, Askew G, Wolf AW: Cosleeping and early childhood sleep problems: effects of ethnicity and socioeconomic status. Submitted 1995.
23. Lozoff B, Wolf AW, Davis NS: Sleep problems seen in pediatric practice. Pediatrics 75:477, 1985.
24. Van Tassel EB: The relative influence of child and environmental characteristics on sleep disturbances in the first and second years of life. J Dev Behav Pediatr 6:81, 1985.
25. Richman N: A community survey of characteristics of one- to two-year-olds with sleep disruptions. J Am Acad Child Psychiatry 20:281, 1981.
26. Zuckerman BS, Stevenson J, Bailey V: Sleep problems in early childhood: continuities, predictive factors, and behavioral correlates. Pediatrics 80:664, 1987.
27. Pinilla T, Birch LL: Help me make it through the night: behavioral entrainment of breast-fed infants' sleep patterns. Pediatrics 91:436, 1993.
28. Ferber R: Solve Your Child's Sleep Problems. New York, Simon and Schuster, Inc, 1986.
29. Adair R, Zluckerman B, Bauchner H, et al: Reducing night waking in infancy: a primary care intervention. Pediatrics 89:585, 1992.
30. Anders TF, Halpern LF, Hua J: Sleeping through the night: a developmental perspective. Pediatrics 90:554, 1992.
31. Largo RH, Hunziker UA: A developmental approach to the management of children with sleep disturbances in the first three years of life. Eur J Pediatr 142:170, 1984.
32. Rickert VI, Johnson CM: Reducing nocturnal awakening and crying episodes in infants and young children: a comparison between scheduled awakening and systematic ignoring. Pediatrics 81:203, 1988.
33. Lozoff B, Zuckerman B: Sleep problems in children. Pediatr Rev 10:17, 1990.
34. Adams LA, Rickert VI: Reducing bedtime tantrums: comparison between positive routines and gradual extinction. Pediatrics 84:756, 1989.
35. Daws D: Through the Night: Helping Parents and Sleepless Infants. London, Free Association Books, 1989.
36. Douglas J, Richman N: Sleep Management Manual, Great Ormond Street Children's Hospital, London, 1982.
37. Weissbluth M: Healthy Sleep Habits, Happy Child. New York, Fawcett Columbine, 1987.
38. Tilton P: The hypnotic hero: a technique for hypnosis with children. Int J Clin Exp Hypn 32:366, 1984.
39. Graziano AM, Mooney KC: Family self-control instruction for children's nighttime fear reduction. J Consult Clin Psychol 48:206, 1980.

8

Colic

MARC WEISSBLUTH

The pattern of crying during the first year of life is independent of cultural differences in caretaking practices. Crying is always greater during the first three months of life. This pattern is present in industrialized societies and hunter-gatherer societies. Because the behavior is universal to infants, crying during the first 3 months may be viewed as a stage of development.[1-4]

Presentation

According to the criteria of Wessel,[1] babies may be divided into three groups, depending on the daily amount of crying and fussiness and its duration. About 51% of babies exhibit paroxysms of unexplained irritability, fussiness, or crying lasting less than 3 hours a day, occurring less than 3 days a week. Wessel labeled these infants as mildly fussy or contented. Often they are described by parents as unsettled, agitated, or unusually *wakeful*. The parents provide extra soothing caretaking during these paroxysms to prevent the crying, which would occur if not for the parent's extra effort. Sometimes these infants simply appear to be unusually "hungry" or "hard to feed" in the evening hours because the parent misinterpreted the soothing effects of non-nutritive sucking as meeting the infant's unmet hunger needs.

About 23% of healthy infants exhibit paroxysms of unexplained irritability, fussiness, or crying lasting more than 3 hours a day, occurring more than 3 days in any 1 week. Wessel called these babies "fussy."

A third group of about 26% of infants are differentiated because their spells of fussiness, or crying continue for more than 3 weeks. Wessel called these infants "seriously fussy" or

"colicky." British pediatricians labeled these infants as having "three months colic" or "evening colic."[5] Chinese parents may call this behavior "100 days of crying," the Vietnamese call it "3 months plus 10 days crying," and the Japanese call it "evening crying." The Asian view is similar to that of Shakespeare's description of infant crying as merely the first act in the play of life.

It appears that some degree of unexplained irritability, fussiness, or crying is universal. Even more important, perhaps, is the fact that there are no clear discontinuities in measurements of irritability, fussiness, or crying whether by direct observation in hospital nurseries,[6, 7] voice-activated tape recordings in homes,[3] or parent diaries.[1, 4] Thus, the grouping of infants or the attaching of labels based on these behaviors seems largely arbitrary.

The age of onset of these behaviors is characteristic. Crying spells begin a few days after delivery or a few days after the expected date of delivery regardless of the degree of prematurity.[1, 4, 5] Among the 26% of infants with the greatest amounts of crying, the crying begins by the second week in 80% and an additional 10% start by the third week. Only 2% of infants start their crying attacks during the first week.[8]

The age of termination of crying spells for infants with the most severe crying is also characteristic. By the third month, 60% have ceased their paroxysms, and, by the fourth month, the paroxysms have ended in all infants. Only 7% of infants stop crying in their second month. The time course of increasing then decreasing spontaneous crying during the first 3 months is paralleled by changes in reactivity to experimentally induced crying, e.g., snapping a rubber band against the infant's leg or foot.[9]

The time of day when these behaviors occur is also characteristic. Periods of crying appear to occur randomly during the first month, but later they occur predominantly in the evening hours.[1, 4, 5] Among those infants with the greatest amount of crying, spells start between 5:00 and 8:00 PM and end by midnight in 80% percent. An additional 12% have spells starting later (7:00 to 10:00 PM) and ending later (by 2:00 AM). Only 8% have their attacks randomly distributed throughout the day or night.[1, 5]

The state of the infant is also associated with these behaviors. Among those infants with the most crying, 84% begin their crying spell when they are *awake*, 8% have spells starting when asleep, and 8% have spells under variable conditions. When the crying spell ends, 83% of the infants fall *asleep*.[8]

Because the spells of unexplained irritability, fussiness, or crying are universal, differing only in degree among infants, because the occurrence of spells is related to post-conceptional age, and because the behaviors exhibit state specificity and a circadian rhythm, it is reasonable to think these behaviors reflect normally maturing physiologic processes—in particular those processes involving the development of arousal/inhibitory or wake/sleep control mechanisms. This impression is supported by the facts that consolidation of night sleep begins during the second month[10] and that stable periodic alternation of sleep and wake states is well-formed by 3 to 4 months of life.[11] From this perspective, it makes no more sense to say that an infant "has" colic than it does to say that a teenager "has" adolescence.

Differential Diagnosis and Evaluation

The diagnosis of "colic" is used when there are unexplained spells of crying in healthy infants. Infants who are not healthy and exhibit spells of crying receive the appropriate diagnosis describing their medical problem such as allergy to cow's milk protein or lactose intolerance. Any painful condition occurring in infants might produce crying, but these medical problems usually do not cause only evening crying. Furthermore, most medical problems are associated with other findings, such as poor weight gain or fever. A careful history and thorough physical examination is usually a sufficient evaluation for most colicky infants.

Management

Studies on colicky infants using reproducible subject selection criteria (such as occurring more than 3 hours per day, on more than 3 days per week, and for more than 3 weeks) have shown that only 3% *usually* respond to rhythmic rocking motions or similar soothing interventions, 18% *occasionally* respond, and 79% *rarely* or *never* respond.[8] "Supplemental" carrying or holding them more does not help these particular infants.[4, 5, 12] Therefore, there is an element of inconsolability in this group. There is no evidence that devices such as crib-vibrators, womb-sound recordings, heartbeat recordings, or antispasmodic medicines or drugs intended to decrease gastrointestinal gas reduce crying in this particular group. In general, drugs are not indicated in the treatment of colic because proof of effectiveness is lacking.

In other infants with lesser amounts of crying, management consists of rhythmic rocking motions, carrying more especially when awake, swaddling, and encouraging frequent sucking or feeding. The "effectiveness" of these strategies depends on the infant's age, the degree of consolability or "self-soothing" ability, and time of day or night.

Management strategies are aimed at helping parents cope with the stresses of caring for an infant who cries much of the time and effectively deal with the post-colic sleep disturbances.[8]

Parents and pediatricians can learn how to cope with infant crying by reading books and articles dedicated to crying and sleeping.[13–17] To care for the crying baby, soothing strategies include rhythmic rocking motions (cradles, swings, rocking chairs, buggy or car rides, or walking while carrying), swaddling or using a soft cloth carrier, and encouraging sucking. To care for the parents, educational strategies are aimed at helping them understand that crying is a normal developmental stage, that infant crying is not their fault, and that some babies will cry despite all their soothing efforts. Parents should be encouraged to take breaks from the baby to regain their strength and to not worry about spoiling the baby. The major pitfall to avoid is to dwell on medical or psychologic issues.

Post-colic sleep disturbances such as brief total sleep durations or fragmented night sleep respond to an age-appropriate sleep schedule.[16–20] Parents can be taught to use the child's naturally occurring daytime sleep rhythms as an aid to nap well. Most infants after 4 months of age will have two major nap periods, one occurring in the mid-morning and one in the early afternoon. Night waking may occur once or twice because the child is hungry. The first step is to teach parents a sense of timing: when wakeful be playful and pick him up; when sleepy, soothe him and put him down. The second step is to eliminate all the rhythmic rocking motions during sleep that may have helped during the first 3 or 4 months. It is important to teach parents that soothing efforts, such as rocking, lullabies, or massaging, are now more stimulating than soothing when continued too long at the time of biologic sleep onset. The third step is to teach parents the benefit of stimulus control. Terms such as healthy sleep habits, sleep learning, consistency, or "associations" help parents understand that the process of falling asleep is learned behavior. Parents need to be explicitly told that this learning process naturally occurs earlier in babies with lesser degrees of irritability, fussiness, or crying, but after 3 to 4 months of age, the learning process will also develop in their colicky babies. Unfortunately, parents of colicky babies have to put forth an extra effort in order to establish regular naps; for example, they may have to suffer the inconvenience of staying at home most of the day or returning quickly after brief outings, to create a quiet and dark sleep environment in anticipation of nap time. Also, if the child has learned to expect to be picked up with every cry, parents may have to ignore protest crying at sleep onset or during the night, except at one or two feedings.

Discussion

Even if their crying had been pharmacologically suppressed during the colicky period, post-colic infants tend to have brief sleep durations and fragmented sleep.[8, 13] This observation is compatible with the theory that infant crying represents the extreme end of high arousal states.[14] Inconsolability in the evening hours before 3 months of age might reflect circadian maturation of periods of high arousal similar to the circadian "forbidden zone" described in adults (a time period during which sleep onset and prolonged consolidated and restorative sleep states do not easily occur).[21] From this perspective, infant evening crying decreases after the second month be-

cause of the development of inhibitory sleep control mechanisms.

Recent research has shown that the incidence of colic increases as one moves farther away from the equator.[22] With increasing latitude, there is greater seasonal variation in the duration of day length. Melatonin is thought to code for the duration of the photoperiod. It has been hypothesized that the documented absence of a melatonin circadian rhythm during the first 3 months makes it difficult for infants to make the transition from wakefulness to sleep at the end of the day. At this transition from daylight to evening darkness neither wakefulness nor sleep is completely dominant. According to this hypothesis, the infant experiences a painful state, perhaps similar to sleep-inertia, and cries.

References

1. Wessel MA, Cobb JC, Jackson EB, et al: Paroxysmal fussing in infancy, sometimes called "colic." Pediatrics 14:421, 1954.
2. Emde RN, Gaensbauer TJ, Harman RJ: Emotional expression in infancy: a biobehavioral study. Psychol Issues 10:1, 1976.
3. Rebelsky F, Black R: Crying in infancy. J Genet Psychol 121:49, 1972.
4. Brazelton TB: Crying in infancy. Pediatrics 29:579, 1962.
5. Illingsworth RS: "Three months" colic. Arch Dis Child 29:167, 1954.
6. Aldrich CA, Sung C, Knop C: The crying of newly born babies. I. The community phase. J Pediatr 26:313, 1945.
7. Aldrich CA, Sung C, Knop C: The crying of newly born babies. II. The individual phase. J Pediatr 27:89, 1945.
8. Weissbluth M, Christoffel KK, Davis AT: Treatment of infantile colic with dicyclomine hydrochloride. J Pediatr 104:951, 1984.
9. Fisichelli VR, Karelitz S, Fisichelli BM, et al: The course of induced crying activity in the first year of life. Pediatr Res 8:921, 1974.
10. Coons S, Guilleminault C: Development of sleep-wake patterns and non-rapid eye movement sleep stages during the first six months of life in normal infants. Pediatrics 69:793, 1982.
11. Harper RM, Leake B, Miyahara L, et al: Temporal sequencing in sleep and waking states during the first six months of life. Exp Neurol 72:294, 1981.
12. Barr RB, McMullan SJ, Heinz S, et al: Carrying as colic "therapy": a randomized controlled trial. Pediatrics 87:623, 1991.
13. Weissbluth M, Davis AT, Poucher J: Night walking in 4 to 8-month-old infants. J Pediatr 104:477, 1984.
14. Lester BM: There's more to crying than meets the ear. *In* Lester BM, Boukydis CFZ (eds): Infant Crying. Theoretical and Research Perspectives. New York, Plenum Press, 1985, pp 1–27.
15. Weissbluth, M: Crybabies: What to Do When Baby Won't Stop Crying. New York, Berkley Press, 1983.

16. Weissbluth M: Healthy Sleep Habits, Happy Child. New York, Fawcett Columbine, 1987.

17. Weissbluth M: Sleep learning. The first four months. Pediatr Ann 20:228, 1991.

18. Weissbluth M: Sleep and the Colicky Infant. *In* Guilleminault C (ed): Sleep and Its Disorders in Children. New York, Raven Press, 1987, pp 129–140.

19. Weissbluth M: Colic. *In* Dershowitz RA (ed): Ambulatory Pediatric Care, 2nd ed. Philadelphia, JB Lippincott, 1993, pp 774–776.

20. Weissbluth M: Colic. *In* Burg FD, Ingelfinger JR, Wald EA (eds): Gellis & Kagan's Current Pediatric Therapy 14. Philadelphia, WB Saunders, 1993, pp 223–236.

21. Lavie P: Ultrashort sleep-waking schedule. III. "Gates" and "forbidden zones" for sleep. Electroencephalogr Clin Neurophysiol 63:414, 1986.

22. Weissbluth M, Weissbluth LT: Colic: sleep inertia, melatonin, and circannual rhythms. Med Hypotheses 28:224, 1992.

CHAPTER
9

Sleeplessness in Children

RICHARD FERBER

The causes and treatments of sleeplessness in children are often different from those in the adult. Differences even exist among infant, toddler, older child, and adolescent groups. The complaint of sleeplessness in the infant and young child usually comes from the parents, not the child; in fact, the child may be quite happy staying awake.[1, 2] On the other hand, the complaint of insomnia in an adolescent must come from the youngster; he or she must report an inability to sleep despite wanting and trying to do so. In general, the older and more self-sufficient the child is, the more an insomnia will resemble the adult disorder.

Although similar factors may be involved at different ages, their significance may be quite different. Stress, for example, must be considered a potential sleep disrupter at any age.[3] However, an inadequately nurtured, poorly sleeping infant is very different from a sleepless adolescent feeling school and peer pressures; and although the mechanisms of wakefulness triggered by pain are basically the same at all ages, the pre-verbal child is unable to describe what hurts.

The general differences between sleep difficulties in children (whether representing simple variations of normal or clearcut disorders of function) and those of adults are discussed in Chapters 1 and 5. In this chapter, and to some extent in Chapter 10, the causes and treatments of the major syndromes of childhood sleeplessness are outlined.

It will be useful to follow the broad terminology of the International Classification of Sleep Disorders.[4, 5] Most of the issues that need be considered in the context of sleeplessness in children may be classified as dyssomnias, in particular extrinsic sleep disorders and circadian rhythm disorders, and medical/psychiatric disorders. Extrinsic sleep disorders are those in which external factors are integral in producing the disorders, and removal of the external factors leads to resolution of the sleep disorder.[4] The one endogenous sleep disorder possibly relevant to pediatrics is psychophysiologic insomnia. However, this generally is not seen until adolescence, and its presentation and treatment are basically the same as in the adult.[6] The circadian disorders are discussed in Chapter 10. Most of the disorders reflecting psychiatric function are described in Chapter 16. Some complaints of nighttime wakings actually describe partial wakings or other paroxysmal events. The distinction between dyssomnia and parasomnia is critical because the latter reflect different etiology, imply different significance, and require different treatment. They are discussed in Chapters 11 and 13. Nighttime fears and nightmares, although technically classified as a psychiatric disorder or parasomnia, will be briefly discussed in this section because of the critical consideration of anxiety in the evaluation of the sleepless child and because the degree of anxiety causing such problems need not be pathologic.

The Infant and Toddler

Most infants "settle" or start sleeping through the night between 3 and 6 months of age.[7, 8, 9] Unfortunately, an increase in nighttime wakings is common in the second 6 months.[8–12] Such problems may still be present or not develop until after the first birthday. At least 23–33% of 1- and 2-year-olds are still waking at night to a degree that is worrisome to the parents.[9, 13-18] Nighttime wakings are still a problem in up to one-third of preschoolers.[19-21]

Although these numbers are large, the problem does not appear to be one of neurodevelopmental necessity,[10, 13, 22] nor does it usually suggest inherent central abnormalities of sleep initiation or maintenance (intrinsic sleep disorders). Studies trying to document increased sleep disturbances in male infants and toddlers have shown somewhat contradictory results.[8, 18, 19, 23-27] Similarly, a relationship between prematurity or perinatal distress and subsequent sleep difficulties is not clear.[8, 14, 15, 21, 22, 26, 28] Even attempts to associate co-sleeping (sharing the parents' bed) with good or bad sleep have had mixed results, possibly because of the importance of certain cultural variables (see Chapter 7).[9, 13, 26, 29] Most often these problems reflect certain established patterns of interaction between parent and child at times of sleep transition.[3, 13, 26, 30, 31]

The rapid development of these problems seems to be an expression of the extraordinary plasticity of the young organism. By 6 months of age a child generally has the potential (the "wiring") to be a sound and excellent sleeper. Although the neurologic connections required for such good sleep follow internal blueprints, other aspects of the development of sleep patterns suggest more of a *tabula rasa*. The child has the ability to learn new patterns, habits, and expectations of sleep very rapidly. For the parents, this is both bad news and good news. The bad news is that the child may learn a pattern of frequent nighttime wakings and parental interventions after only a few nights of disturbed sleep (caused by a transient sleep disrupter such as otitis or travel). Even worse, once this pattern of waking is established, it can continue for months or years. The good news is that this same child can learn a pattern of no apparent wakings and no needed interventions just as quickly.[30, 32-34] From the child's (or physiologic) point of view, these two patterns of sleep are variations of normal. From the parents' (or emotional) point of view, one pattern represents "good" sleep, the other "bad." Although it is not always appreciated as such, it is the child's superb adaptability that allows him to switch rapidly from being a "good sleeper" to being a "bad sleeper." However, it is this same ability that permits him, just as easily and just as rapidly, to switch back to "good."

Sleep-Onset Association Disorder

Although all infants, older children, and adults normally wake briefly a number of times across the night,[35, 36] particularly in association with REM sleep, generally they are unaware of most of these because a return to sleep is prompt. Perhaps for this reason adults do not expect such arousals to be a normal part of sleep patterns in the infant and toddler. When parents become aware of such wakings in their child, they may incorrectly conclude that the wakings are abnormal and help is required, and the parents may become intimately involved in the sleep transition process. Such "help," however, is more likely to become part of the cause of a chronic disturbance rather than a solution. The child learns this "help" pattern and becomes unable to make the transition back to sleep alone. From this point on a sleep problem may be said to exist.

Often exactly the same problem exists at bedtime as at times of waking during the night, although it is not always perceived as such. At both times the parents may be in contact with the child through the process of sleep transition, or they must supply something for it to occur, such as a bottle or pacifier. At bedtime, if sleep transition is accomplished easily without the child waking on transfer to the crib or when the parent leaves the room and requiring more intervention, this may not be considered a problem. But nighttime wakings may be viewed very differently even though the types of interventions required are exactly the same. The difference being at bedtime the parents are still awake; at nighttime wakings the parents are already asleep.

The child is now reliant on the parent to help complete the sleep transition.[13, 26, 30, 37, 38] Rather than simply associating things that are always there with the state of drowsiness and the act of falling asleep (such as the crib or bed, blanket, doll, or stuffed animal), the child learns to associate other environmental cues not always present. Therefore, the problem is that these patterns associated with falling asleep are broken once the child is asleep, and the parents must reestablish these patterns when the child wakes up. A child whose association with falling asleep is being held, rocked, or nursed, using a pacifier, having his back patted, or being driven around the block may be unable to fall asleep by himself at bedtime or when waking at night.

Even if the parents choose to have the

youngster sleep in their bed, the learned patterns may have to be repeated after nighttime wakings. This may seem easier, since parents usually do not have to get up to reinitiate the patterns. Still, the wakings continue and the parents are wakened. Only if the habit is simply one of parental contact or if the child has learned to go to sleep by himself even though in the parents' bed, will the child likely be able to return to sleep without much parental response.

Diagnosis is usually made by careful history (see Chapter 5). At bedtime if the usual associations are not established and on waking during the night if the conditions that were present at sleep onset have been changed, the child will call or cry. However, once a parent responds in the expected manner, the child calms quickly and returns to sleep (for example, when picked up and rocked, when given his pacifier, or when handed a bottle).[30, 37, 39–43] This rapid return to sleep when the habitual associations are reestablished helps to diagnose "associations" as the problem and to confirm the basic normality of the child and his or her sleep. Most other causes of sleep disruption will not respond as rapidly to such simple behavioral interventions.

Once the nature of the problem is clear, treatment is straightforward. The child must learn to make the transition from waking to sleep without the participation of a parent.[3, 16, 30–34, 37, 44–47] The patterns associated with sleep transitions must be ones that can be established and reestablished by the child. Gradual techniques are generally recommended, as they seem easier for both child and parents. Specific measures vary and usually treatment is not begun much before 6 months of age.[30, 32–34, 45, 48, 49] Generally, the child is put down while awake and allowed to be alone for progressively longer intervals between brief parental reassurances.[16, 30, 37, 41, 42, 45–47, 49–51] This procedure is repeated after nighttime wakings. The child gradually learns to fall asleep and not to expect or need the parents' help. Success rates are very high if the parents are given sufficient support, and the period of relearning is usually less than 1 week.[30, 45, 46]

The goal is to help the youngster learn a new set of sleep-associated habits. It is not to see how long he can cry, or how much he can tolerate or be frightened. For this reason, the parents' visits to the room are important. By starting with a few minutes, the child's expectations may change gradually without overwhelming confusion or sense of abandonment. The parents should be calm and reassuring, but they should not attempt to get the child back to sleep while in the room.

The milder the problem, often the harder it is to treat. A youngster who wakes twice a night needing only to be quickly covered to return to sleep (otherwise there is calling, crying, or getting out of bed) certainly has a minimal, if any, sleep disturbance. But if the parent is unable to return to sleep for a long time, the parent has a major sleep disturbance. Although the treatment is the same, since the problem was relatively small to begin with, the nighttime may become much worse before it gets better. It is hard enough listening to a child calling for an hour, but it is doubly hard when one knows that two seconds of intervention would get the child back to sleep. If the child is old enough and sufficiently verbal (age 3 yrs), a star chart may work in this setting (see Limit-Setting Sleep Disorder later in this chapter).

If parents have the child sleep in their bed or room by choice or necessity, association-related problems may still be solved but often with a bit more difficulty. The goals are the same. In this case the parents are present, but they must refuse the habitual demands. This may be harder to do because of the proximity. Enforcement may require having the parents leave the room for increasing amounts of time.

If separation issues are marked, a parent should consider sleeping in the same room with the child for several days, as new patterns are being learned. But if the problem is simply one of associations (and separation issues are minor), then instead of being reassured the child will be angry at the parent who is present for not doing what is "wanted." Consequently, being there "makes things worse." Enforcement of new patterns may be carried out as previously described.

The treatment presented is not a general treatment for infants and toddlers with nighttime wakings. It is a treatment for the specific problem of sleep-onset associations. Not only is it inappropriate therapy for the child who is awake because of fear or a schedule disorder, but in those settings it may also make matters worse. Similarly, associations involving parents need not be broken just because they exist. Some children may fall asleep rapidly in the parents' arms at bedtime, do not wake on transfer to the bed or crib, and "sleep through" the night (i.e., go back to sleep after nighttime wakings quickly, quietly, and by themselves). This ability to fall asleep quickly and easily under different conditions at different times is not shared by all children.

Nocturnal Eating (Drinking) Disorder

A number of studies,[8, 18, 26, 52–54] though not all,[14, 15, 25, 27, 55] have shown an increase in nighttime wakings among infants and toddlers fed during the night, either by bottle or at the breast. Similarly, some studies,[8, 54] though not all,[8] suggest that breast-fed babies settle (sleep through the night) at a later age than do bottle-fed infants. Infants brought to the breast throughout the day (for pacification, not nurturing) seem to settle later.[57, 58] Finally, infants fed large quantities at night (typically 8 to 32 oz) not only show continued wakings but frequent wakings, often three to eight per night.[8, 18, 26, 30, 52–54]

This last observation is perhaps the most important. The presence of only one or two wakings each night that require a brief period at the breast, with a bottle, or even a pacifier suggests that the association of the nipple with sleep onset is more important than the fluid consumed. However, when there are more frequent wakings with consumption of large volumes of fluid each time, the boundary is crossed from a normal sleep pattern to an abnormal one.

Extra fluid intake means wetter diapers, increased discomfort, and possible arousal. Hunger sensations become conditioned to occur during the night, and this may trigger a waking or interfere with return to sleep after a normal one waking. Certainly, by 6 months, all full-term, healthy, normally growing infants have the capacity to obtain satisfactory nutrition during the daytime only.[37, 38] The consolidation of sleep into a long period at night requires the expression of mature circadian physiology involving stable digestive, endocrine, temperature, and sleep-wake rhythms. Repeated wakings for ingestion of fluid, carbohydrates, fat, and protein directly disrupt the functioning of all circadian-modulated systems. These alterations of synchronous functions cannot help but cause further deleterious effects on sleep-wake stabilization.[9, 43, 58]

Diagnosis is made from a characteristic history: multiple nighttime wakings, return to sleep only with feeding, significant milk or juice intake during the night, and very wet diapers.

Treatment is straightforward and consists of decreasing the frequency of feedings at night in children who are being fed more than necessary for age or eliminating the feedings in children who are old enough to get all feedings during the day—certainly by 5 to 6 months. Conceptional age should be considered (i.e., expectations for a child born prematurely should not be based on chronologic age). However, just because there are feedings and wakings does not mean the feedings have to be stopped; this decision is based largely on the parents' preference and their desire for uninterrupted sleep (see Chapter 7). But when wakings are very frequent, perhaps three or more per night in a child over 6 months of age, it must be considered that this degree of sleep fragmentation may be deleterious to the child (although the effects of this remain somewhat speculative). When the night becomes too broken, to some extent the child remains on a neonatal pattern with sleep, wakefulness, and meals distributed around the clock. The child may sacrifice the chance for extended periods of wakefulness and learning during the day. At the same time, this child's parents may become sleep deprived and less able to relate consistently and positively to their child during the day.

Nighttime feedings may be substantially reduced or eliminated in various ways. Although these feedings could be eliminated very rapidly, at least when considering only the habitual component, for emotional reasons this approach makes little sense. Suddenly weaning a child from the breast or even from the bottle at night is not necessary and would be difficult for the parents as well as the child. In addition, conditioned hunger signals take some days to readjust. One does not want a child to be left hungry for hours.

Again, gradual programs work best. Most important is to increase the minimal time between nighttime feedings, perhaps by 30 minutes each night. This alone allows for elimination (or substantial reduction) of feedings within 1 week. Decreasing the amount of milk or juice per bottle by 1 ounce per night may be done simultaneously. Decreasing the amount of time at the breast as an estimation of volume may be done but is sometimes difficult. In any case, whether nursing or feeding by bottle, the child should be put down after the feeding is complete and not brought back to the breast or given another bottle if he cries on transfer to the crib. The hunger has been satisfied.

Some parents of bottle-fed children prefer to deal with the problems of hunger and associations separately. As a first step the feedings are progressively watered down (half-strength, quarter-strength) until only water is taken. What is left at this point is habit not hunger, and this can be dealt with as a sleep association problem.

Despite the fact that excessive feedings may cause some of the most severe problems of nighttime wakings, as feedings are decreased and associated habits eliminated over 1 to 2 weeks, sleep consolidation usually occurs promptly.[30, 52]

Colic

Colic, the most common medical condition affecting the sleep of very young infants, causes inconsolable fussiness and crying, especially in the late afternoon and evening (see Chapter 8). Although symptoms are generally gone by 3 to 4 months of age, continuing sleep disturbances are common. These disturbances are probably not biologically based but rather are secondary to altered sleep schedules and habitual patterns of parental responsiveness, which persist into the postcolicky period.[30, 59]

Food Allergy Insomnia

An allergy to cow's milk may also cause a very severe sleep disturbance in the early weeks and months of the infant, with markedly decreased total sleep.[60–63] Immunoglobulin E (IgE) levels are elevated, and radioallergosorbent testing (RAST) to cow's protein is positive. Sleep normalizes within 2 weeks of changing to a hydrolyzed milk-protein formula.

Associated with Medical Disorders

Certain medical problems affecting sleep in infants may not be obvious, particularly serous otitis media or gastroesophageal reflux. In both cases (as with colic or milk allergy insomnia), no intervention works quickly to reestablish sleep at times of nighttime wakings. If an upset child wakes (fully) frequently and if quick responses do little to assure rapid return to sleep, one must be concerned that the youngster is truly suffering discomfort. Careful history and examination may suggest a particular diagnosis. Tympanometry, esophageal pH probe, barium swallow, and endoscopy are some procedures that may be indicated. Treat-

ment would be for the underlying medical condition, not the sleep problem per se. If the medical problem resolves, a persisting sleep problem may reflect other diagnoses.

The Preschool and School-Aged Child

Nightly struggles in the preschool years remain common. However, the years between the start of elementary school and the start of high school are relatively calm in terms of sleep disturbances.[19] In these years, the child should have mastered the developmental hurdles of the early years and gained sufficient independence to handle sleep transitions. He or she has also not yet reached the stormy years of adolescence with its attendant anxieties, pressures, and independence.

Although problems of preschoolers may occur at bedtime or during the night, those of the school-aged child more often tend to be limited to bedtime. Important exceptions do exist.[19, 64, 65]

Limit-Setting Sleep Disorder

The move from crib to bed (or at least the ability to climb out of the crib) usually takes place at age 2 or 3. At this point, sleep problems may begin precipitously. Before then, the bars of the crib act as firm and consistent limit setters from bedtime until the morning. When no longer bound by these restraints, the youngster may test out his new-found "freedom." If parents are unable to find other ways to set limits at bedtime, sleep may deteriorate.

Typical bedtime struggles include various "curtain calls" with requests for water, more stories, use of the bathroom, adjustment of the lights, or more television.[30, 37, 43, 58] Frequently, the child will refuse to remain in bed and will simply follow the parents back to the living room or their bedroom.

A diagnosis of insufficient limit setting may be made from history when it is clear that parents are unable or unwilling to enforce nighttime rules with enough consistency to keep the child in bed and quiet so that sleep may come. It must be known, however, that the child is physiologically ready for sleep at the set bedtime; for example, if the child always falls asleep at the scheduled bedtime if allowed to remain in the living room, comes into the parents' bed, or is left with a sitter. If there are never struggles when bedtime is 2 hours later than usual, a schedule-related problem must be considered (see Chapter 10). Each time the child gets out of bed or calls, tension increases. Each time the parents give in, the child's behavior is reinforced. One parent (or even a sitter) may be much more successful getting the youngster to bed (and hence setting limits) than the other. Parents often use phrases such as "he insists" to describe their own reasons for giving in to their child's repeated and often irrational "demands." The inappropriate nature of their own responses is often completely unrecognized by the parents. The child may become progressively powerful as he directs his parents about the house, and the parents may become progressively impotent as they find themselves unable to keep the child in bed or even in the bedroom.

Parents may simply lack education in limit-setting techniques. They may be unaware of the importance of consistency and firmness in the care of their children and confuse "giving in" with being kind. Environmental settings may make limit setting difficult; for example, the sharing of a single room by parents and child in their own or another's home. Parents may also find it difficult to weigh the validity of certain of their child's nighttime complaints (thirst, fear).

Inability to set and enforce rules with supportive firmness may actually cause increased anxiety rather than provide reassurance, as a child, who is already having difficulty controlling his own impulses, sees his parents as too weak to take control over him. His self image is hurt since he knows his actions are displeasing to his parents. If his parents show an inability to maintain control themselves by losing their temper, screaming, threatening, and spanking, the child may become even more upset and be less able to control himself.[42, 66]

Psychosocial factors may interfere with limit setting. Thus, depression or alcoholism may preclude proper parenting. Not only does marital strife make limit setting difficult, but also the child's nighttime battles may provide an excuse for the parents to avoid facing their own issues. For this reason the child may get up and risk punishment just to keep his parents from fighting.

Treatment should be tailored to fit the cause. Education of the parents is most important. They must understand their child's need for consistency and firmness, and they must learn a limit-setting program they can carry out. Parents must enforce a regular bedtime ritual with a definite endpoint. Assuming the child is to sleep in his or her own room, then the youngster may be kept in that room with several techniques. The easiest way is to use a gate thus making a "crib" of the whole room. A gate with a fine nylon mesh or vertical bars is usually best, since these do not provide finger- or toeholds. If the child can climb this, a double gate may be necessary (at least initially). If this is not workable, then door closure may be necessary. The door is to be the passive limit setter that allows the parents to be supportive and controlled, not angry and punitive. Thus, parents should stay nearby when the door is closed (held closed if necessary), the door should be closed for only a short time at first and then increased gradually. When the door is open, a parent should remain on the same level of the house or apartment as the child, both for reassurance and to allow swift response. Once the child is convinced of the parents' ability to enforce these limits consistently, he usually relaxes and the nighttime disruption ceases rapidly. The tension that used to build nightly as bedtime approached disappears. The symbolic importance of the gate may be so important to the child in terms of control that he may remind his parents to close it each night.

If the child seems a bit fearful, then it may be necessary to sit in the child's room until sleep comes, enforcing the child's cooperation, if necessary, by temporarily leaving and shutting the door as described above. Once the situation has improved, parents may sit outside the door and later in their bedroom. If the child is more frightened, then it may be best to sleep in his room all night, temporarily leaving as described above if the child becomes too demanding.

If parent and child share a room or bed, it may be necessary for the parent to leave for periods of time, even to sleep on a sofa in the living room temporarily, until the child accepts the rules set forth about sleeping in the same room as the parent and the condition stabilizes. If the child shares a room with a sibling, that youngster may have to be moved to another room for several days.

A child over age 3, especially one with good verbal skills, may respond well to positive behavior modification using a star chart and prizes as rewards for staying in bed after the bedtime ritual is complete.[30, 37] This usually works best if the clinician negotiates the chart with the child and then has the child come back to see him or her to show the stickers and prizes.

Regardless of the specifics of the techniques chosen, it is often helpful to start with a bedtime that is somewhat later than usual for the first few nights. This helps assure the child's readiness for sleep, shortens the initial period of testing, and provides a sense of success to child and parent.

Psychosocial problems, if marked, may have to be dealt with first before trying to resolve the child's sleep difficulty. In fact, helping parents set firm limits at night if they are unable to provide satisfactory nurturing during the day may be contraindicated.[30, 51, 67] In such cases the nighttime struggles may be the only predictable (albeit negative) period of parent-child interaction during the entire 24-hours, and removal of this may leave the child with nothing. Therefore, in such situations, limit setting may actually have to be decreased initially and the child given more access to the parents at night instead of less.

Fears and Nightmares

"Fears," as a cause of insomnia, is technically a *medical/psychiatric sleep disorder associated with mental disorders (anxiety)*, and nightmares are technically *parasomnias*. They are discussed together because they are seen so frequently in early childhood, usually as part of intrinsically normal development.

Even the school-aged child may have significant worries and even fears. Concerns about masturbation or aggressive feelings toward parents or siblings may emerge when defenses are least able to cope, as in a dark room at night when parents are not nearby. This pattern is most likely to happen when parents have avoided facing these issues or have dealt with them poorly or inappropriately. Awareness of the significance of death, worries of dying in sleep, and confusion about death and ("eternal") sleep are also common.

Often these fears emerge indirectly, taking the form of monsters and robbers when the child is awake and of various villainous creatures when he or she is asleep. Thus, the psychologic causes of both nightmares[68, 69] and nighttime fears are the same. Therefore, a truly frightened or anxious child at night should be handled in the same manner whether these fears were initially expressed during waking or sleep.

If fears are marked, a strict limit-setting routine that requires the child to deal with the fears alone may not only be unsuccessful but harmful. The child needs full support and temporary compromises may be necessary, such as a parent sleeping in the child's room or the child sleeping in the parents' room on a cot or in a sleeping bag. Attempts to explore the underlying causes of these fears should be made in the daytime. If symptoms are chronic, then professional counseling should be considered.

Milder fears often respond to supportive firmness, at least in a stable social setting. With clearcut reassurance and consistent enforcement of the nighttime rules, a child may be able to deal satisfactorily with mild concerns that otherwise might become unmanageable. Positive reinforcements with rewards for staying in bed may provide enough motivation for a youngster to deal with low-level anxiety and achieve a sense of mastery.

Fears arising in the context of an unrealistically early bedtime may disappear immediately upon schedule correction (see Chapter 10). Progressive relaxation,[70] group instruction in self-control,[71] and progressive desensitization[10] have all been reported useful in certain situations.

Adolescence

Across the teenage years, the sleepless adolescent progressively resembles the sleepless young adult. As the youngster becomes more independent, his sleep schedule often becomes more inappropriate (see Chapter 10). Anxieties during these turbulent years are often plentiful, with emotional maturation usually lagging behind the level of function at which the individual tries to operate. Peer, sexual, school, and family pressures are often paramount and certainly may be associated with difficulty falling asleep. Sleep disturbances may also be an early sign of major emotional disorders that can emerge at this time, such as schizophrenia, anorexia, or mania (see Chapter 16).[72]

Treatment of the insomniac adolescent requires the same approaches that are useful in the adult, including improved sleep hygiene, normalization of sleep schedules, decreased use of alcohol and other drugs, sleep restriction therapy, relaxation training, biofeedback, chronotherapy, and psychotherapy.[6, 73–80] Successful intervention does require direct discussion with the adolescent. Parents are no longer able to take on full responsibility for the enforcement of new and strict routines.

Sleep Problems Affecting Children at All Ages

Environmental-Induced Sleep Disorder

Even though children can sleep well in more settings and under more circumstances than adults, their ability to ignore disrupting influences from the environment has a limit. This limit decreases with increasing age.

The biggest problems occur in cramped and chaotic settings. There may be noise from the outside (planes, cars, or people) or from the inside (parents laughing or fighting, people coming and going). There may be distractions in the child's room from his or her own personal television or telephone used without restrictions. A child can be inadvertently wakened by a parent who comes home from work late each night as the child is about to fall asleep or who gets up early each morning before the child would be waking naturally. Children, especially of similar age, sharing a room may play and talk instead of sleeping. One child is often the most guilty. When they share the same bed, the restless, and, possibly enuretic, patterns of one child may easily disturb the other. When they share the same room or bed with the parents, the television, parents' talking, and even sexual encounters may be disruptive.

Although these problems pose great challenges, they can be handled. Televisions and phones can be removed or restricted; bedrooms can be switched or re-arranged to move a child away from the noisy street or to give an enuretic child his own bed or mattress; room dividers can be added for privacy; room darkening shades and drapes can be used to decrease morning light and sounds; and constant sound producing devices, such as fans, humidifiers, radios, or white noise machines, may be left on to help block out uncontrollable intermittent noises. Schedules for bedtime can be changed to earlier or later to avoid evening or early morning disruption. Bedtimes may be staggered so one child is already asleep when the other goes to bed. Children may be put down in separate locations at bedtime and moved later when asleep, and separate mats on the floor may allow for better sleep than a single bed for several children.

Sometimes because of lack of cooperation from a family member or simply because of lack of control of the outside environment, treatment remains unsatisfactory.

Associated with Medical Disorders

Many medical conditions can influence sleep and most are easily recognized, particularly when pain, discomfort, or fever is present. In these cases, the treatment is of the medical disorder and not the secondary sleep problem. Even temporary use of hypnotics is rarely needed in the child, unlike in the adult.

Respiratory difficulties in sleep secondary to tonsilloadenoidal enlargement, maxillofacial abnormality, or obesity may disrupt sleep even if respiratory impairment is not so severe as to qualify for a diagnosis of obstructive sleep apnea (see also Chapters 17, 18, 19).

All medications must be considered possible causes of sleep disruption. Theophylline and other stimulants are known to have this effect. Phenobarbital and other drugs with sedative properties may show paradoxical effects. (Actually the sleep problems seen with such sedatives may not be so paradoxical since they resemble patterns seen in "overtired" children.) Even relatively benign medications, such as antibiotics, may be associated with daytime behavioral changes and nighttime sleep disturbances. This most often occurs with liquid preparations, suggesting that the antibiotic is not the cause.[81] In the teenage years, nonprescription and "street" drugs must also be considered, including alcohol.

At times, a medical condition, such as leukemia, diabetes, or cystic fibrosis, may present multiple factors that can potentially affect sleep. These may include the direct effects of the child's illness on central systems controlling sleep, the effects of multiple medications, the consequences of repeated hospitalizations and sleep schedule disruptions, the impact of the child's apprehension, the parents' anxiety, and altered patterns of interactions between parents and child. Assigning relative weights to these various factors may be difficult, and attempts to treat these specific causes in such a complicated context is quite a challenge.

Associated with Neurologic Disorders

Most children with sleep difficulties have completely normal brain function. However, some children with very poor sleep have suffered severe central insults, such as cerebral injury, malformation, or metabolic dysfunction (see Chapter 15). One may find marked developmental delays, spasticity, autistic behaviors, and sensory deficits. Total sleep time is often dramatically reduced (perhaps 7 hours total for a 3-year-old child) and circadian function may be abnormal.[42, 82] During the hours the child is awake he may be loud and disruptive, demonstrate self-injurious behaviors, and require constant parental supervision.

The assumption here is that the poor sleep reflects abnormalities in central sleep systems; it is not behavioral or related to other medical or neurologic factors. Hence, other disorders must be ruled out. This means that no behavioral intervention should improve sleep significantly. If the child sleeps fine when in the parents' bed, then central systems are fully functional. Decreased nocturnal sleep must not be secondary to multiple catnaps or even long sleep during the day. Electroencephalography and polysomnography may be necessary to rule out disorders such as sleep-associated seizures, apnea, or gastroesophageal reflux. It will also show if the youngster's sleep stage formation and pattern of cycling appear normal or if REM and NREM cannot even be identified or distinguished.

From the youngster's viewpoint, increased sleep may bring only minimal direct benefits. But it may make the difference between the parents being able to keep him at home or needing to place him in an institution.

When all is taken into account, pharmacologic trials are often warrented. Drugs useful in adults, such as the benzodiazepines, are of limited use in these children. However, chloral hydrate in large doses (500–3000 mg) may be very beneficial. The dose can be adjusted to allow for a satisfactory increase in sleep at night without residual effects during the day (in fact, daytime function may even improve). This usually can be given as a single dose at bedtime, but occasionally it must be split giving some at bedtime and some halfway through the night. Promethazine (25–100 mg) or clonidine (0.25–1.0 mg) is sometimes a useful alternative, and preliminary studies suggest possible therapeutic benefit of evening administration of melatonin.

If medication is necessary, then the lowest dose achieving satisfactory results should be chosen; it should be periodically tapered to check for its continued need; and liver functions and blood counts are followed. Increasing the dose over time is usually not necessary except as may be required for growth.

Associated with Mental Disorders (Social Stresses)

Social stresses may affect any child at any age, even when the attendant anxiety does not seem marked. When there is stress in the home, there may be little sleep at night. Marital discord, separation or divorce, financial or professional difficulties, parental affective illness, medical disorder or death, family move, start of school, toilet training, and birth of a sibling are all possible causes.[5, 31, 66] In these settings, the parents' ability to support, nurture, and interact with children may be altered, limits may not be set, consistent schedules may not be followed, and understandable fears and anxieties may not be dealt with appropriately.

Brief disturbances may be handled with support, but more chronic ones require psychosocial intervention, the specifics of which are dependent on the particulars of the family's difficulties. Direct help for the child's sleep problem is sometimes possible during this intervention, which may help reduce the overall tension and anger. At other times this help has to be delayed until the underlying stressful issues are in better control.

The major psychiatric disorders are discussed in Chapter 16.

Conclusions

Insomnia in the young child is phenomenologically different from insomnia in the adult. This is because it is the caretakers' complaint that usually must be addressed and the interaction between caretaker and child is critical. Although the specifics of the problem in later childhood and adolescence still reflect the child's age and neuropsychologic development, the characteristics progressively resemble those seen at older ages. Treatment must take all of these factors into account. In general, the younger the children, the more adaptable are their habits and routines, the more their environment is under the control of others, and the better their potential sleep ability. Because of this, most of the causes of sleeplessness in young children can respond to rapid intervention. As the children grow older, their habits become more fixed, they gain more independent control over their environment, and their sleep becomes less deep. As they cross adolescence, they make the final transition to adulthood and with this comes increased resistance to therapy.

Although this means that it is usually possible to resolve a problem of sleeplessness in a young child faster than a problem of insomnia in an adult, it does not mean that the task is an easy one. Proper diagnosis and carefully designed intervention are necessary and must take into account the specifics of the child and his or her problem in the context of the entire family and psychosocial setting.

References

1. Illingworth R: The child who won't sleep and whose parents won't let him. Mims Magazine, November 1976, pp 71–77.
2. Jackson H, Rawlins MD: The sleepless child. Br Med J 2:509, 1979.
3. Lozoff B, Zuckerman B: Sleep problems in children. Pediatr Rev 10:17, 1988.
4. Diagnostic Classification Steering Committee, Thorpy MJ, Chairman. International Classification of Sleep Disorders: Diagnostic and Coding Manual. Rochester, MN, American Sleep Disorders Association, 1990.
5. Thorpy MJ: Classification of sleep disorders. *In* Kryger MH, Roth T, Dement WC (eds): Principles and Practice of Sleep Medicine, 2nd ed. Philadelphia, WB Saunders, 1994, pp 426–436.
6. Hauri P: Primary insomnia. *In* Kryger MH, Roth T, Dement WC (eds): Principles and Practice of Sleep Medicine, 2nd ed. Philadelphia, WB Saunders, 1994, pp 494–499.
7. Jenkins S, Owen CM, Bax M, et al: Continuities of common behavior problems in pre-school children. J Child Psychol Psychiatry 25:75, 1984.
8. Moore T, Ucko LE: Nightwaking in early infancy. Part 1. Arch Dis Child 32:333, 1957.
9. Ragins N, Schachter S: A study of sleep behavior in two-year-old children. J Am Acad Child Psychiatry 10:464, 1971.
10. Anders TF, Keener M: Developmental course of nighttime sleep-wake patterns in full-term and premature infants during the first year of life. I. Sleep 8:173, 1985.
11. Beal VA: Termination of night feeding in infancy. J Pediatr 75:690, 1969.
12. Shepherd F: Disturbed Sleep in Infancy and Childhood. Hatfield, England, 1948.
13. Bax MCO: Sleep disturbance in the young child. Br Med J 280:1177, 1980.
14. Bernal J: Night waking in infancy during the first 14 months. Dev Med Child Neurol 15:760, 1973.
15. Blurton Jones N, Rosetti Ferreira MC, Farquar Brown M, et al: The association between perinatal factors and later night waking. Dev Med Child Neurol 20:427, 1978.
16. Richman N: Sleep problems in young children. Arch Dis Child 56:491, 1984.
17. Roberts KE, Schoellkopf JA: Eating, sleeping, and elimination practices of a group of two-and-one-half-year-old children. Am J Dis Child 82:121, 1951.
18. Van Tassel EB: The relative influence of child and environmental characteristics on sleep disturbances in the first and second years of life. J Dev Behav Pediatr 6:81, 1985.
19. Klackenberg G: Sleep behavior studied longitudinally. Data from 4–16 years on duration, night-awakening and bedsharing. Acta Paediatr Scand 71:501, 1982.
20. Thomas JA, Bidder RT, Hewitt K, et al: Health visiting and pre-school children with behavioral problems in the County of South Glamorgan: an exploratory study. Child Care Health Dev 8:93, 1982.
21. Ungerer JA: Sleep behavior of preterm children at three years of age. Dev Med Child Neurol 25:297, 1983.
22. Anders TF, Keener MA, Kraemer H: Sleep-wake organization, neonatal assessment and development in premature infants during the first year of life. II. Sleep 8:193, 1985.
23. Carey W: Night waking and temperament in infancy. J Pediatr 84:745, 1974.
24. Jacklin CN, Snow ME, Gahart M, et al: Sleep pattern development from 6 through 33 months. J Pediatr Psychol 5:295, 1980.
25. Lozoff B, Wolf AW, David NS: Sleep problems seen in pediatric practice. Pediatrics 75:477, 1985.
26. Richman N: A community survey of characteristics of one- to two-year-olds with sleep disruptions. J Am Acad Child Psychiatry 20:281, 1981.
27. Weissbluth M, Todd Davis A, Poncher J: Night waking in 4- to 8-month old infants. J Pediatr 104:477, 1985.
28. Weissbluth M: Sleep duration, temperament, and Conner's ratings of 3-year-old children. J Dev Behav Pediatr 5:120, 1984.
29. Lozoff B, Wolf AW, Davis NS: Cosleeping in urban families with young children in the United States. Pediatrics 74:171, 1984.
30. Ferber RA: Solve Your Child's Sleep Problems. New York, Simon and Schuster, 1985.
31. Schmitt, BD: When baby just won't sleep. Contemp Pediatr, May:38, 1985.
32. Adair R, Zuckerman B, Bauchner H, et al: Reducing night waking in infancy: a primary care intervention. Pediatrics 89:585, 1992.
33. Adams LA, Rickert VI: Reducing bedtime tantrums: comparison between positive routines and graduated extinction. Pediatrics 84:756, 1989.
34. Rickert VI, Johnston CM: Reducing nocturnal awakening and crying episodes in infants and young children: a comparison between scheduled awakenings and systematic ignoring. Pediatrics 81:203, 1988.
35. Anders TF: Night-waking in infants during the first year of life. Pediatric 63:860, 1979.
36. Williams RL, Karacan I, Hursch CJ: EEG of Human Sleep. New York, John Wiley and Sons, 1974.
37. Douglas J, Richman N: Sleep Management Manual. London, Great Ormond Street Children's Hospital In-House Publication, 1982.
38. Illingworth RS: Sleep problems in the first three years. Br Med J 1:722, 1951.
39. Ferber RA: Assessment procedures for diagnosis of sleep disorders in children. *In* Noshpitz JD (ed): Basic Handbook of Child Psychiatry, Vol V. New York, Basic Books, 1987, pp 185–193.
40. Adair R, Bauchner H, Philipp B, et al: Night waking during infancy: role of parental presence at bedtime. Pediatrics 87:500, 1991.
41. Douglas J, Richman N: My Child Won't Sleep: A Handbook of Management for Parents. London, Penguin, 1984.
42. Ferber R: Childhood insomnia. *In* Thorpy MJ (ed): Handbook of Sleep Disorders. New York, Marcel Dekker, Inc, 1990, pp 435–455.
43. Ferber R: Sleeplessness, night awakening, and night crying in the infant and toddler. Pediatr Rev 9:1, 1987.

44. Ferber R, Boyle MP: Sleeplessness in infants and toddlers: sleep initiation difficulty masquerading as a sleep maintenance insomnia. Sleep Res 12:240, 1983.

45. Jones DPH, Verduyn CM: Behavioral management of sleep problems. Arch Dis Child 58:442, 1983.

46. Largo RH, Hunziker UA: A developmental approach to the management of children with sleep disturbances in the first three years of life. Eur J Pediatr 142:170, 1984.

47. Valman HB: Sleep problems. Br Med J 283:422, 1981.

48. Ferber RA: Sleep disorders in infants and children. *In* Riley T (ed): Sleep Disorders for the Clinician. London, Butterworths, 1985, pp 113–157.

49. Younger JB: The management of night waking in older infants. Pediatr Nurs 8:155, 1982.

50. Cuthbertson J, Schevill S: Helping Your Child Sleep Through the Night. Garden City, N.Y., Doubleday & Co, 1985.

51. Leach P: Babyhood: New York, Alfred A. Knopf, 1976.

52. Ferber R, Boyle MP: Nocturnal fluid intake: a cause of, not treatment for, sleep disruption in infants and toddlers. Sleep Res 12:243, 1983.

53. Osterholm P, Lindeke LL, Amidon D: Sleep disturbance in infants aged 6 to 12 months. Pediatr Nurs 9:269, 1983.

54. Wright P, MacLeod HA, Cooper MJ: Waking at night: the effect of early feeding experience. Child Care Health Dev 9:309, 1983.

55. Edgil AE, Wood KR, Smith DP: Sleep problems of older infants and preschool children. Pediatr Nurs 11:87, 1985.

56. Elias MF, Nicholson N, Bora C, et al: Effect of maternal care on social and emotional behavior of infants during the first year. Research report prepared for the Society of Research in Child Development, Detroit, April 1983.

57. Elias MF, Nicholson NA, Bora C, et al: Sleep/wake patterns of breast-fed infants in the first 2 years of life. Pediatrics 77:322, 1986.

58. Ferber RA: The sleepless child. *In* Guilleminault C (ed): Sleep and Its Disorders in Children. New York, Raven Press, 1987, pp 141–163.

59. Weissbluth M: Sleep and the colicky infant. *In* Guilleminault C (ed): Sleep and Its Disorders in Children. New York, Raven Press, 1987, pp 129–140.

60. Kahn A, Mozin MJ, Casimir G, et al: Allergy to cow's milk: a possible cause for chronic insomnia in infants. Sleep Res 14:16, 1985.

61. Kahn A, Mozin MJ, Casimir G, et al: Insomnia and cow's milk allergy in infants. Pediatrics 76:880, 1985.

62. Kahn A, Rebuffat E, Blum D, et al: Difficulty in initiating and maintaining sleep associated with cow's milk allergy in infants. Sleep 10:116, 1987.

63. Kahn A, Francois G, Sottiaux M, et al: Sleep characteristics in milk-intolerant infants. Sleep 11:291, 1988.

64. Beltramini AU, Hertzig ME: Sleep and bedtime behavior in preschool-aged children. Pediatrics 71:153, 1983.

65. Ferber R, Boyle MP: Six year experience of a pediatric sleep disorders center. Sleep Res 15:120, 1986.

66. Daws D: Through the Night. Helping Parents and Sleepless Infants. London, Free Association Books, 1989.

67. Ferber RA: Behavioral "insomnia" in the child. Psychiatr Clin North Am 10:641, 1988.

68. Pivik RT: The psychophysiology of dreams. *In* Kryger MH, Roth T, Dement MD (eds): Principles and Practice of Sleep Medicine, 2nd ed. Philadelphia, WB Saunders, 1994, pp 384–393.

69. Hartmmann E: Nightmares and other dreams. *In* Kryger MH, Roth T, Dement MD (eds): Principles and Practice of Sleep Medicine, 2nd ed. Philadelphia, WB Saunders, 1994, pp 407–410.

70. Weil G, Goldried MR: Treatment of insomnia in an eleven-year-old child through self-relaxation. Behav Ther 4:282, 1973.

71. Hauri P, Olmstead E: Childhood-onset insomnia. Sleep 3:59, 1980.

72. Easson WM: The early manifestations of adolescent thought disorder. J Clin Psychiatry 2:469, 1979.

73. Anderson DR: Treatment of insomnia in a 13-year-old boy by relaxation training and reduction of parental attention. J Behav Ther Exp Psychiatry 10:263, 1979.

74. Hauri P: The Sleep Disorders. Kalamazoo, MI, Upjohn Scope Publications, 1977, pp 22–34.

75. Hauri P: Biofeedback techniques in the treatment of chronic insomnia. *In* Williams RL, Karacan I (eds): Sleep Disorders, Diagnosis and Treatment. New York, John Wiley and Sons, 1978, pp 145–149.

76. Hauri P: Behavioral treatment of insomnia. Med Times 107:36, 1979.

77. Saskin P, Spielman AJ, Jelin MA, et al: Sleep restriction therapy for insomnia: six month follow-up. Sleep Res 13:163, 1984.

78. Spielman AJ, Saskin P, Thorpy MJ: Sleep restriction and treatment of insomnia. Sleep Res 12:286, 1983.

79. Stepanski EJ: Behavioral therapy for insomnia. *In* Kryger MH, Roth T, Dement MD (eds): Principles and Practice of Sleep Medicine, 2nd ed. Philadelphia, WB Saunders, 1994, pp 535–541.

80. Zarcone VP, Jr: Sleep hygiene. *In* Kryger MH, Roth T, Dement MD (eds): Principles and Practice of Sleep Medicine, 2nd ed. Philadelphia, WB Saunders, 1994, pp 542–546.

81. Kumar A, Weatherly MR, Beaman DC: Sweeteners, flavorings, and dyes in antibiotic preparations. Pediatrics 87:352, 1991.

82. Okawa M, Sasaki H: Sleep disorders in mentally retarded and brain-impaired children. *In* Guilleminault C (ed): Sleep and Its Disorders in Children. New York, Raven Press, 1987, pp 269–290.

Circadian Rhythm Sleep Disorders in Childhood

RICHARD FERBER

Circadian physiology and schedule disorders in adults are discussed in detail in Kryger MH, et al: Principles and Practice of Sleep Medicine, 2nd ed, Chapters 21–25, 42–44, and 95. These chapters should be reviewed for explanations of basic concepts and definitions. General guidelines for evaluating a child in a circadian context are presented in Chapter 5 of this volume.

The circadian system is probably functional at birth, even though this is not initially apparent.[1] It may be that the circadian pacemakers in the neonate are slow to become entrained by external zeitgebers (partially because in the world of the very young infant, these zeitgebers are not very circadian). The pacemakers initially may not be fully coupled to the rhythms they ultimately will control or, perhaps, their effects are simply masked as the neonate responds to needs, stimuli, and feedings around-the-clock. Nevertheless, a (sometimes initially free-running) circadian pattern in sleep-wake alternation is usually apparent by 6 weeks of age and is quite stable by 3 months.[1-9] Although the ultradian REM/NREM cycle time is much shorter in young children than in adults,[10-12] the circadian clock seems to function near 25 hours from the start.[3, 4, 13]

These systems can be affected in various ways: there may be dysfunction of the clock at the hypothalamic level due to malformation or tumor; there may be lack of sufficient zeitgebers and subsequent inability to entrain because of blindness; or there may be inherently normal (potential) function but with problems occurring principally because a child's particular schedule comes into conflict with parental desires. The last is the most common. When this is the case in young children, the usual parental complaints are bedtime difficulties, naptime problems, nighttime wakings, or early morning wakings. Older children may complain of insomnia, and their parents may describe difficulty waking them for school. Sleepiness later in the day does not tend to be a common complaint until adolescence.[14-16]

Most diagnoses can be made from history alone, but the questioner needs to be astute (see Chapter 5).[17, 18] He or she must have a firm grasp of circadian physiology, understand the age-dependent variations in sleep patterns that may occur, be able to differentiate a child's biologic needs from the parents' desires, and know how to recognize and treat coexisting problems that may be affecting sleep.

General Considerations

Certain features of a child's sleep schedule must be considered during the initial evaluation, regardless of the complaint. The specifics may have important implications to the understanding and treatment of various disorders.

Naps

It is important to carefully determine the timing, consistency, length, physical locations, and circumstances of all naps, and the wakings from naps should be characterized as induced or spontaneous. *All* daytime sleep should be described, including brief periods in the car or stroller.

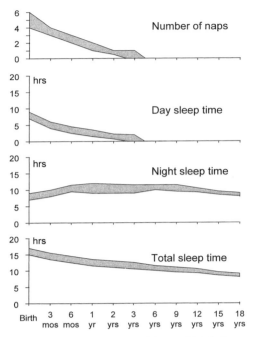

Figure 10–1. Amount of day, night, and total sleep and average number of daily naps across childhood. The number of naps decreases from 4 to 6 in the neonate to 0 by age 2 1/2 to 4 1/2. During the same time period daytime sleep decreases from about 8.5 hours to 0. Total sleep time decreases more slowly because part of the lost daytime sleep is initially replaced by an increase in nighttime sleep, which is maximal from late infancy into middle childhood. In the teenage years, actual sleep times are often less. (Data from Ferber R: Solve Your Child's Sleep Problems. New York, Simon & Schuster, 1985; Sheldon SH, Spire JP, Levy HB: Pediatric Sleep Medicine. Philadelphia, W.B. Saunders, 1992; Williams RL, Karacan I, Hursch CJ: Electroencephalography (EEG) of Human Sleep: Clinical Applications. New York, Wiley, 1975.)

Knowledge of normal or usual patterns helps the clinician interpret complaints and plan management. Children usually decrease from three to two naps a day by about 6 months of age and to one nap by about 1 year (see Chapter 2). They typically give up napping between their third and fourth birthdays (although this is quite variable). After the first 3 to 4 months, naps generally do not last over 2 to 2 1/2 hours (Fig. 10–1).

The total sleep time required per 24-hour day may be variably divided between night and day. One 18-month-old (with an 11-hour total sleep requirement) may still be taking two 1 1/2-hour naps each day and have only 8 hours of sleep left for the night. Another child with the same sleep requirement may take only a 30-minute nap each day but sleep 10 1/2 hours at night. One hour of daytime sleep is

worth roughly one hour of nighttime sleep and, to a degree, shifts between the two are possible. When a 1-year-old drops the second nap, the nighttime sleep and/or the remaining nap often increase by about the amount of time of the lost nap. However, the first minutes of a nap seem to be the most important for recuperation. A 10-minute nap may be worth more than 10 minutes of nighttime sleep. Thus, a child who falls asleep for 10–20 minutes two to three times a day may have his nighttime sleep reduced by more than this short actual nap time.

The youngster's age, current sleep patterns, concerns, and parental complaints, and desires must be taken into consideration when recommending changes in nap schedules (shortening, lengthening, addition/division, elimination/consolidation). Some situations are more clearcut than others. There may be little significant difference to a 1-year-old between taking two 1-hour naps and one 2-hour nap, but a 4-hour nap is sure to shorten the nighttime sleep, and six 15-minute catnaps are unquestionably inappropriate.

Naps must be taken into account when nighttime sleep is being adjusted. Appropriate napping for age may be permitted. However, if the child tries to nap excessively to make up for any sleep lost because of nighttime adjustment, efforts at correcting the sleep at night may be undermined.

Depending on their time of occurrence, certain early or late "naps" may not be viewed as naps by parents, and as a result they may not always be clearly distinguished from the nighttime sleep period. A child who retires at 7:00 PM, wakes at 2:00 AM, and goes back to sleep from 4:00 to 6:00 AM will usually be described as waking at night and then returning to sleep. The period of sleep from 4:00 to 6:00 AM is not considered a nap. But a child who retires at 10:00 PM, wakes at 5:00 AM, and goes back to sleep from 7:00 to 9:00 AM is generally said to have an early morning waking and an early morning nap. But these two schedules are exactly the same except for a 3 hour shift. Similarly, a period of sleep from 4:00 to 6:00 PM followed by 2 hours of waking before return to sleep is usually considered to be a late nap followed by the nighttime sleep, but a similar period of sleep from 7:00 to 9:00 PM followed by 2 hours of wakefulness is usually considered to be part of the nighttime sleep broken by a nighttime waking. Again, regardless of what they may be called, these two patterns are essentially the same.

It may also be that periods of sleep viewed

as early or late naps could be better viewed as part of the nighttime sleep. The last sleep cycle of the night may separate from the rest of the night by 1 or 2 hours and appear as an early morning nap while the nighttime sleep seems to be shortened and the child wakes early. Or the first sleep cycle of the night may appear broken off from the rest of the night as a late evening nap followed by 2 to 3 hours of wakefulness before the nighttime sleep continues and seems shortened with a late bedtime.

Schedule Options

Whether viewed as naps or nighttime sleep, the existence of the different patterns described above shows the ability of a child to divide his or her sleep into biphasic or multiphasic organization. This ability persists past the age such patterns are usually expected to occur (such patterns may be present in the older child but not recognized as such). Young children are particularly able to vary the timing of their sleep periods, dividing their sleep into epochs of various length occurring at various, though predictable, times of the day. Older children can do this to a lesser degree, but they certainly can change the time at which their nighttime sleep occurs. They are much less likely to pick options that divide their sleep into segments. The various schedules picked cannot necessarily be classified as normal or abnormal; most are probably normal variants. But certain schedules definitely are more problematic for the caretakers.

The clinician can help a youngster and the family switch from one option to another, but the choices must be within the range of physiologically normal function and necessity. Thus, nighttime sleep may be lengthened if long periods of daytime sleep are shortened, but naps cannot be eliminated in a child who still requires them. In fact, the elimination of a nap too early, before age 2 1/2 or 3 years, may leave the child overtired and physically stressed and may actually cause an increase in nighttime wakings. Similarly, rearrangements of sleep may allow for schedules that are more workable for the family, but do not expect a youngster to be able to adapt to any schedule the parents might want. A 9 + 2 schedule (9 hours at night, 2 in the day) is completely normal for a 15-month-old child. But the family may object to his staying up "late" until 9:00 PM or getting up "early" at 6:00 AM. An 8:00 PM to 5:00 AM or 10:00 PM to 7:00 AM schedule is a better option for some families and perhaps worse for others. A 7:00 PM to 4:00 AM schedule would be another option, one that is occasionally seen, but it is rarely an acceptable option for families. Instead of seeing this as normal but early sleep, parents view it as a normal bedtime and an abnormally early waking. The particular time at which this 9-hour period of sleep occurs can be moved somewhat, and perhaps it can be increased to 10 hours if the nap is shortened, but not much more is possible. But the parents may be requesting a 12 + 2 schedule, 7:00 PM to 7:00 AM at night plus a 2-hour nap. The child just cannot sleep that long.

All treatments involve making an estimation of the total sleep requirement, night plus day, and then negotiating with the parents the times that this sleep may be reasonably placed. The total sleep requirement is usually based on totalling actual sleep hours on days when all wakings are spontaneous.

It is usually fairly easy to find an acceptable option for a young child. But as the child gets older, sometimes no schedule is fully satisfactory: biologic and social needs cannot both be met.[14, 16] Generally the older the child, the earlier he or she must wake to get ready for school (school starts earlier, the bus comes earlier, the bus ride is longer). Some adolescents (boys more than girls) are willing to sleep until 5 minutes before the bus comes and then throw on clothes and run out of the house. Others (girls more than boys) insist on getting up at least 1 hour before leaving, no matter how little sleep they get, to allow enough time to take care of their personal appearance. Often this may mean getting up at 5:30 AM. If the child has a 9-hour sleep requirement, that would mean an 8:30 PM bedtime. This is unrealistic for even the most conscientious 16-year-old who only does homework in the evening and does not watch television or talk on the phone. After-school hours are usually busy and daily naps are not realistic options. This child will be sleep deprived during the week. On weekends makeup sleep will be needed, but on weekends social activities may also demand later bedtimes. So, later bedtimes and much later wake-up times on the weekends are the rule, resulting in considerable weekday/weekend schedule variability.[16, 19] The biologic needs for hours of sleep, the chronobiologic needs for sleep-schedule consistency, and the psychologic needs to interact in an educational/social world may make demands that appear to work at cross-purposes.

Early Feedings

The disrupting effect of multiple nighttime feedings is discussed in Chapters 7 and 9. However, there may only be a single feeding involved, coming in the early morning when the child wakes, perhaps at 5:00 AM. Although the child is usually fed because he is awake, regular feeding at this hour conditions hunger signals that may contribute to ongoing early wakings, whether or not the child has met his full sleep requirement for the night. To some degree the same can be said during the day. A child who takes his only nap in the late morning (before lunch) instead of the early afternoon (after lunch) may have his nap shortened as mid-day hunger stimulates waking.

Light Exposure

Since the timing of light exposure more than anything else determines the setting of the circadian clock, this must be taken into account. When aspects of children's schedules are changed (later bedtimes, earlier wakings), incident light exposure usually changes automatically in the process (when a child gets up earlier he is usually exposed to light earlier). Early wakings or later bedtimes may do little to reset the circadian clock if the child remains in a relatively dark room for several hours during those times (perhaps watching television). Opening shades, turning on all of the lights, and bringing in extra lights may be necessary. Similarly, if the child's bedroom is extremely well lit in the morning (lots of windows, no shades, sun exposure), then a later bedtime may not adjust the child's sleep to a later time in the morning.

Light boxes may be used to help shift sleep cycles, but it is difficult to get the cooperation needed from the child before age 6 or 7, and it usually is not even necessary before adolescence.

Sleep Charting

Sleep charting provides information crucial to the diagnosis of schedule-related problems. Parents often have difficulty accurately describing patterns that are not very stable. They may know the bedtime but are less sure of the time of sleep onset; they may know there are nighttime wakings but are unclear as to their number, timing, and length; they may know daytime sleep periods vary but are unsure as to how. Sometimes the patterns of fluctuation are only apparent on such charts. Estimations of the timing of sleep phases and total sleep requirements can often best be made with this information. Sleep charts may also show a tendency of naps to free-run to some extent during the day, merging into or emerging out of the morning or night, providing an explanation for apparently random variations in times of sleep onset and waking and in numbers of daytime naps.[13]

Sleep charting is a very important part of the treatment of schedule-related sleep disorders (in fact of most pediatric sleep disorders). Parents and older children are more likely to keep to a schedule if they plot it daily, and the day-to-day progress becomes more clearcut. People tend to exaggerate disturbances when they rely on memory because it may feel worse than it really is; the sleep charts are usually more accurate.

Second Wind (The Forbidden Zone)

The forbidden zone, described in adults as the period of least sleep tendency, occurring late in the day preceding the dip that leads to sleep-onset at bedtime, has an important counterpart in children.[20] Parents often describe with amazement that their child gets a "second wind" when the decided bedtime approaches. They find it strange that their child can seem and act so wide awake after almost falling asleep, or showing behavioral deterioration, in the late afternoon or at the dinner table. The reason: he is wide awake.

Parents, not understanding the physiology involved, often ignore the obvious and try to put the child to bed anyway. Such a youngster may stall or fight (behavior similar to a child with a limit-setting sleep disorder [see Chapter 9]) or he may go to bed cooperatively but be unable to fall asleep for some time. Even when struggles occur, the situation differs from a limit-setting problem, because on nights when bedtime is sufficiently late, struggles are completely absent. If there are no major bedtime struggles and the child remains in bed, wide awake for one to several hours until sleep readiness ("schlafbereitschaft") arrives, he may lie quietly, think, fantasize, and eventually end up scaring himself. Problems of schedule-related bedtime struggles, apparent insomnia, and bedtime fears generally resolve quickly and easily when bedtime is adjusted *later*. Moving the bedtime *earlier* would be totally incorrect and would only make matters worse. Yet this is exactly what happens when parents punish their wide-awake children for apparent bedtime problems one night by sending them to bed earlier the next.

Sleep Phase Shifts

Advanced Sleep Phase

As might be expected, an advanced sleep phase occurs mainly in infants and toddlers,[18, 21, 22] and even then it is relatively uncommon (see Kryger MH, et al: Principles and Practice of Sleep Medicine, 2nd ed, Chap 44). Although these children retire and wake early, the parents only complain about the early morning waking. These children may retire as early as 6:00 to 7:00 PM every night, and are likely to do so whether or not they are formally put to bed at that time. They simply get tired, recognize their sleepiness, and ask to go to bed. If they are not put to bed then, they likely will lie down somewhere and go to sleep anyway. It matters little what activity is going on about them. In fact, parents report difficulty keeping these children up late even when they try. These children are probably inherent "larks."[23, 24]

The timing of events across the whole day must be clarified. Typically, naps and mealtimes are shifted to an earlier time as well,[18, 22] and this, along with the early morning light exposure, only serves to reinforce an advanced sleep phase.

Once an acceptable schedule is decided upon, then it is achieved primarily through the gradual delay of bedtime. For some young children it is difficult to advance more than 15 minutes a day. Naps and mealtimes may have to be similarly delayed, especially early ones. Judicious light control may be helpful, for example, bright at night, dim in the morning.

Delayed Sleep Phase

A delayed sleep phase is a common cause of delayed sleep onset at all ages (see Kryger MH, et al: Principles and Practice of Sleep Medicine, 2nd ed, Chap 44).[25–28] The child is put down in the forbidden zone, wide awake, and the troubles previously described occur. Usually the child falls asleep about the same time each night regardless of bedtime. If the family is out very late, the child usually falls asleep in the car on the way home. There will also be late daily wakings for the child who is at home during the day, difficulty waking on weekdays for the child in daycare or school, and late weekend waking for all.[18, 22] (Some children actually get up early on the weekends spontaneously. In truth they have not really reached the end of their sleep phase and are only half-awake, and they sit dazed in front of the television for several hours watching cartoons in a dark room. The hour they get up, march into the kitchen, and announce that they are ready for breakfast is a better measure of the time of "spontaneous waking.") Naps are sometimes shifted to a late schedule as well.

Parents without morning obligations usually complain only about the bedtime struggles with a young child. They may appreciate the late morning sleep or simply allow it as catch-up; of course, this allows the sleep phase delay to persist or worsen. Morning wake-up battles and complaints of daytime sleepiness at school are described in older children and are particularly striking in adolescence.[15, 16, 18, 21, 22]

When the phase shift is large, perhaps 4 hours or more, and the youngster is older and independent, typically an adolescent, a progressive around-the-clock phase delay in which the youngster goes to bed 3 hours *later* each night until the desired schedule is reached works well (see Kryger MH, et al: Principles and Practice of Sleep Medicine, 2nd ed, Chap 44).[29] Occasionally, when the phase shift is quite marked, the same approach may be used in early or middle childhood, but a parent may have to stay up and "go around-the-clock" with the child. Increased light in the hours before sleep and decreased light in the first few hours after waking may help.[30–32]

In younger, less independent children who have smaller phase delays (usually 1 to 3 hours), a controlled phase advance is possible.[18, 22, 27] It is best to begin with a bedtime that is determined to be the start of the current sleep phase (i.e., the time he or she has actually been falling asleep). This way, bedtime struggles and tensions cease. For the child who has been sleeping late every morning, the time of waking must be gradually advanced, followed by a gradual advance of bedtime. If the youngster has been getting up (with difficulty) for school or daycare 5 days a week, the same early time of waking should be continued on the weekend, followed with gradual bedtime change. Bright morning light is important.

Since there may be decreased sleep during

the initial nights of phase advance, control of naps is particularly important. Children still at the age for napping should be allowed to continue doing so, but excessive daytime sleep should not be permitted. Older children must agree not to nap or should be kept from doing so; the increased pressure for sleep that follows shortening of the nocturnal sleep period should be allowed expression at bedtime.

The adolescent with a delayed sleep phase can be treated by phase delay or phase advance, as described above, but these techniques require motivation and cooperation. Where it is relatively easy to take control of a young child's schedule, it is very difficult to control an adolescent's schedule against his will. Furthermore, the delayed sleep phase is complicated by chronic sleep deprivation and schedule irregularities. During the correction phase, and even after correction, some degree of later "make-up" sleep on the weekends may have to be allowed, but, hopefully, without encouraging a greater (or recurrent) phase delay. If weekend schedules are too rigidly designed, the youngster may not cooperate. It is best to negotiate something acceptable, even if a gradually improved program emerges over a number of weeks. Use of a light box with 30 minutes early morning exposure (2500 to 10,000 lux) to correct significant phase delays rapidly and maintain stability after correction may be quite helpful (see Kryger MH, et al: Principles and Practice of Sleep Medicine, 2nd ed, Chap 95).[30, 32–34] This is assuming the youngster is cooperative and wants to correct his sleep problem. If there is no cooperation, there is little that can be done directly. Dragging the child out of bed is usually of limited benefit.

There are teenagers with apparent delayed sleep phase syndromes who use this as a means of avoiding school.[22, 28, 35] These youngsters are likely "owls" to begin with, predisposing them to this syndrome.[23, 24] A school refusal syndrome, often complicated by depression and significant family issues, is usually the true diagnosis (see Chapter 16). Certain aspects of these children's histories are characteristic. Unlike most adolescents with delayed sleep phases who get up for school even after only a few hours of sleep, these youngsters are often "unable to get up." They are frequently absent or tardy. Parents seem unable to wake them despite sometimes heroic efforts. Yet in the laboratory setting, their sleep seems normal and they have no difficulty waking at an early hour. If the school makes special arrangements to allow them to come in several hours late, their sleep phase shifts several hours later almost immediately. Furthermore, during the summer and winter holidays they show a "reversed vacation effect." Instead of a typical phase delay, which usually happens when morning wakings are not necessary, there is often a phase advance if the child has daytime activities that interest him. Treatment is often difficult. These children undermine measures aimed at directly correcting the timing of sleep, for example, by falling asleep too early when progressive phase delay is attempted, by taking long naps when they are supposed to stay awake and then staying up late, or by refusing to sit in front of a light box. Individual and family psychotherapy is important. For some, boarding or alternative schools is beneficial. Others seem to respond to antidepressants. When there is clear collusion from a needy parent who wants the child home during the day, treatment is even more difficult.

Regular But Inappropriate Schedules

Sleep disturbances can occur within the context of a regular sleep schedule even when phase shifts are not the problem.

Time in Bed Exceeds Total Sleep Requirement

This particular syndrome needs emphasis because it frequently occurs but often goes unrecognized, which leads to totally inappropriate management.[21, 22, 36] Some relevant concepts have been discussed in the section on Schedule Options.

The main problem is that the parents' estimation of sleep requirements and the child's actual sleep requirements differ. Usually this occurs because the estimation is based on convenience, not logic. It would be nice to have the children asleep early, wake late, and nap. The hours become unrealistic. Often there is a "children's bedtime" for all children regardless of their different ages, tendency to nap, and obvious individual and age-related differences.

Assume a child has a 10-hour nighttime sleep requirement (taking into account daytime sleep), but the family expects 12 hours (i.e., they want the child to sleep from 7:00 PM to 7:00 AM). There are three ways this can present.

1. Easy Bedtime, Early Waking

The child falls asleep at 7:00 PM but is wide awake at 5:00 AM, and the parents complain of an early waking. This is analogous to an advanced sleep phase and is corrected in the same manner but allowing for only 10 hours in bed.

2. Difficult Bedtime, But No Early Waking

There are bedtime struggles for 2 hours, sleep onset occurs at 9:00 PM, and the child wakes at 7:00 AM. This is analogous to a delayed sleep phase and is treated in the same manner but allowing for only 10 hours in bed.

3. Easy Bedtime, No Early Waking, But Extended Middle-of-the-Night Waking

This child goes to sleep at 7:00 PM, and he wakes in the morning 12 hours later. But he wakes at some point in the night, perhaps 2:00 AM, and he is wide awake. Nothing can get him back to sleep for 2 hours. Typically a parent gets up with him, lets him play, turns on the television or VCR, and dozes until the child falls back to sleep. Although playing with a child during the night may also reinforce extended nighttime wakings, the main problem is that the child is in bed longer than he or she can sleep. In this case, the nighttime sleep has become divided into a biphasic pattern.

Treatment consists of choosing a schedule in which bedtime and waking are 10 hours apart. It may require a later bedtime, earlier waking, or both. If this is enforced and nighttime play eliminated, resolution is usually rapid.

When a child is in bed too long, there is a set-up for trouble. He may find he cannot sleep and may begin to believe he is a poor sleeper. His parents may get angry at him for not sleeping, and his self-esteem may be hurt. He may use the time for fantasy and sexual activity, which may become scary. Some children occupy themselves by headbanging or bodyrocking (see Chapter 13). When time in bed is reduced appropriately, these behaviors decrease or disappear.

If parents feel that later bedtimes are not acceptable, then children at least of school age should be given options to read, listen to the radio, or play quietly until sleepy or on waking early in the morning. Discussion with parents as to possible changes in rigid expectations is a good idea.

Early Naps, Late Naps, Long Naps, Short Naps, or Early Feedings

The effects of excessive, inadequate, or inappropriate napping, poorly scheduled meals, and unrealistically early bedtimes can affect sleep. For example, early naps or feedings can cause early wakings, late naps can cause late times of falling asleep, and early bedtimes can cause bedtime struggles.

Irregular Sleep Schedules

Entrainment and stabilization of circadian rhythms can occur only if environmental cues and sleep schedules are kept consistent. As in the adult shift worker, frequently changing routines at any age means inconsistent sleep and less than optimal function during wakefulness (see Kryger MH, et al: Principles and Practice of Sleep Medicine, 2nd ed, Chap 43).[37, 38] In children, this is most commonly seen in the adolescent old enough to be setting (or not setting) his or her own schedule. Weekday/weekend variations and naps after school or in the evening may also occur. Besides a delayed sleep phase, there may be a more general breakdown of circadian synchronization so that even on weekends sleep timing is not normal, and there is tiredness or lack of energy during the day.

Younger children may show similar symptoms. For these children, the problem is the parents' failure to set and enforce consistent routines. Bedtime, naps, and mealtimes may vary. The home may be quite chaotic with little formal structure. Bedtime per se may not even exist; the child simply falls asleep whenever or wherever he or she chooses. In such an environment, the specifics of the sleep disturbance may also vary from child-to-child and day-to-day.

The absence of structure may reflect social instability, lack of parental education in child-rearing, or particular cultural patterns. Teaching parents the importance of consistent routines, helping to establish them, and working with the parents to assure successful follow-through is usually sufficient to resolve the sleep difficulties. Psychosocial issues may have to be addressed first or simultaneously.

Conclusions

Successful evaluation and treatment of many sleep problems in children require a sophisticated understanding of the rhythmic processes underlying good sleep and its potential disturbances. Schedule-related issues often partly or completely explain parents' and children's complaints, and if they are ignored, therapeutic efforts are likely to be ineffective.

References

1. Hellbrugge T: The development of circadian rhythms in infants. Cold Spring Harb Symp Quant Biol 25:311, 1960.
2. Ferber R, Boyle MP: Persistence of a free-running sleep-wake rhythm in a one-year-old girl. Sleep Res 12:364, 1983.
3. Kleitman N, Englemann TG: Sleep characteristics of infants. J Appl Physiol 6:269, 1953.
4. Kleitman N: Sleep and Wakefulness. Chicago, University of Chicago Press, 1939.
5. Davis RC: Ontogeny of circadian rhythms. In Aschoff J (ed): Handbook of Behavioral Neurobiology, Vol. 4, Biological Rhythms. New York, Plenum Press, 1981, pp 257–274.
6. Parmelee AH, Wenner WH, Schulz HR: Infant sleep patterns: from birth to 16 weeks of age. J Pediatr 65:576, 1964.
7. Parmelee AH: Ontogeny of sleep patterns and associated periodicities in infants. In Falkner F, Kretchmer N (eds): Pre- and Postnatal Development of the Human Brain. Modern Problems in Paediatrics, Vol. 13. Basel, Karger, 1974, pp 298–311.
8. Meier-Koll A, Hall U, Hellwig U, et al: A biological oscillator system and the development of sleep-waking behavior during early infancy. Chronobiologia 5:425, 1978.
9. Hellbrugge T: The development of circadian and ultradian rhythms of prematures and full-term infants. In Scheving LE, Halberg F, Pauly J (eds): Chronobiology. Tokyo, Igaku Shoin Ltd, 1974, p 339.
10. Anders TF: State and rhythmic processes. J Am Acad Child Psychiatry 17:401, 1978.
11. Stern E, Parmelee AH, Harris MA: Sleep state periodicity in prematures and young infants. Dev Psychobiol 6:357, 1973.
12. Stern E, Parmelee AH, Akiyama Y, et al: Sleep cycle characteristics in infants. Pediatrics 43:65, 1969.
13. Santacana P, Galofre I, Ferber R: Free-running nap rhythms in non-isolated infants. Sleep Res 21:386, 1992.
14. Carskadon MA: Patterns of sleep and sleepiness in adolescents. Pediatrician 17:5, 1990.
15. Carskadon MA, Keenan S, Dement WC. Nighttime sleep and daytime sleep tendency in preadolescents. In Guilleminault C (ed): Sleep and Its Disorders in Children. New York, Raven Press, 1987, pp 43–52.
16. Carskadon MA, Dement WC: Sleepiness in the normal adolescent. In Guilleminault C (ed): Sleep and Its Disorders in Children. New York, Raven Press, 1987, pp 53–66.
17. Ferber RA: Assessment Procedures for Diagnosis of Sleep Disorders in Children. In Noshpitz JD (ed): Basic Handbook of Child Psychiatry, Vol. V. New York, Basic Books, 1987, pp 185–193.
18. Ferber R: Circadian and schedule disturbances. In Guilleminault C (ed): Sleep and Its Disorders in Children. New York, Raven Press, 1987, pp 165–175.
19. Stone MD, Vieira CM, Carskadon MA: Circadian type in adolescents and their parents: impact on family functioning. Sleep Res 20:472, 1991.
20. Lavie P: Ultrashort sleep-waking schedule. III. 'Gates' and 'forbidden zones' for sleep. EEG Clin Neurophysiol 63:414, 1986.
21. Ferber R: Childhood insomnia. In Thorpy MJ (ed): Handbook of Sleep Disorders. New York, Marcel Dekker, 1990, pp 435–455.
22. Ferber RA: Solve Your Child's Sleep Problem. New York, Simon and Schuster, 1985.
23. Horne JA, Ostberg O: Individual differences in human circadian rhythms. Biol Psychol 5:179, 1977.
24. Horne JA, Ostberg O: A self-assessment questionnaire to determine morningness-eveningness in human circadian rhythms. Int J Chronobiol 4:97, 1976.
25. Moore-Ede MC, Sulzman FM, Fuller CA: The Clocks That Time Us. Cambridge, Harvard University Press, 1982.
26. Weitzman ED, Czeisler CA, Coleman RM: Delayed sleep phase syndrome: a chronobiologic disorder with sleep onset insomnia. Arch Gen Psychiatry 38:737, 1981.
27. Ferber R, Boyle MP: Phase shift dyssomnia in early childhood. Sleep Res 12:242, 1983.
28. Ferber R, Boyle MP: Delayed sleep phase syndrome versus motivated sleep phase delay in adolescents. Sleep Res 12:239, 1983.
29. Czeisler CA, Richardson GS, Coleman RM, et al: Chronotherapy: resetting the circadian clocks of patients with delayed sleep phase insomnia. Sleep 4:1, 1981.
30. Dijk DJ, Beersma DG, Daan S, et al: Bright morning light advances the human circadian system without affecting NREM sleep homeostasis. Am J Physiol 256(1 Pt 2):R106, 1989.
31. Lavie P, Tzischinsky O: The effects of two-hour bright light exposure on the 24-h sleep propensity function. Sleep Res 19:395, 1990.
32. Lewy A, Sack R, Frederickson R, et al: The use of bright light in the treatment of chronobiologic sleep and mood disorders: the phase-response curve. Psychopharmacol Bull 19:523, 1983.
33. Czeisler CA, Allan JS, Kronauer RE, et al: Strong circadian phase resetting in man is effected by bright light suppression of circadian amplitude. Sleep Res 17:367, 1988.
34. Czeisler CA, Allan JS, Strogatz SH, et al: Bright light resets the human circadian pacemaker independent of the timing of the sleep-wake cycle. Science 233:667, 1986.
35. Thorpy MJ, Korman E, Spielman AJ, et al: Delayed sleep phase syndrome in adolescents. J Adol Health Care 9:22, 1988.
36. Galofre I, Santacana P, Ferber R: The "tib>tst" syndrome. A cause of wakefulness in children. Sleep Res 21:199, 1992.
37. Monk TH, Folkard S: Individual differences in shift work adjustment. In Folkard S, Monk TH (eds): Hours of Work—Temporal Factors in Work Scheduling. New York, John Wiley and Sons, 1985, pp 227–237.
38. Rutenfranz J, Colquhoun WP, Knauth P, et al: Biomedical and psychosocial aspects of shift work. A review. Scand J Work Environ Health 3:165, 1977.

Sleepwalking, Confusional Arousals, and Sleep Terrors in the Child

GERALD ROSEN, MARK W. MAHOWALD, and
RICHARD FERBER

Sleepwalking, confusional arousals, and sleep terrors are seen much more commonly in children than adults. Together they constitute the prototypic NREM parasomnias. All are considered partial arousals from sleep because the underlying process appears to be one of incomplete arousal. Partial arousals from sleep result in nocturnal behaviors ranging from quietly sitting up in bed and engaging in some semi-purposeful activity to violent flight from bed associated with a blood curdling scream and heightened autonomic activity.

The symptoms of partial arousals occur along a spectrum, but for ease of description, they have been divided into three categories: (1) sleepwalking (calm or agitated), (2) confusional arousals, and (3) sleep terrors.

All the disorders of arousal share a number of important characteristics including timing in the nighttime sleep cycle, clinical features, genetics, and pathophysiology (Table 11–1).[1–4] Features common to all disorders of arousal include misperception of and unresponsiveness to the environment, automatic behavior, and variable retrograde amnesia. Family history of partial arousals in one or both parents is quite common, occurring in up to 60% in some studies.[5]

These disorders share a common pathophysiology. Figure 11–1 is an idealized sleep histogram describing the rhythmic cycling of wakefulness, NREM sleep, and REM sleep throughout the night. Slow wave sleep (SWS) occurs predominantly, but not exclusively, in the first one third of the night. The length of each cycle (REM–REM interval) is approximately 90 minutes with a range of 60 to 110 minutes. Within 15 minutes of sleep onset, most children will be in their deepest sleep of the night. This will last from 45 to 75 minutes, at the end of which there will be a transition to a brief period of wakefulness, a lighter stage of NREM sleep, or REM sleep before a return to deep NREM sleep (SWS) again. It is at this transition from SWS to the next sleep cycle that partial arousals most often occur. During this period children with partial arousals appear "caught" between deep NREM sleep and full arousal. Typically, the EEG during this dissociated state is characterized by a combination of alpha, theta, and delta frequencies without evidence of clear wakefulness.

Although only a single event usually occurs on a given night, some children may have two or three. When there are multiple events, some may occur in the second half of the night. Successive events on the same night tend to be progressively milder. Although return to SWS at the end of the night is common in young children, the occurrence of partial arousals near morning is rare. Some children may have partial arousals occasionally (or only) on waking from naps.

Children with disorders of arousal often have sudden arousals with complex motor activity and verbalizations that arise out of NREM 1 + 2 and REM sleep as well, though the number of arousals is most frequent out of slow wave sleep.[6]

Table 11–1. FEATURES IN PARTIAL AROUSALS

	Quiet Sleepwalking	Confusional Arousals	Sleep Terrors
Usual timing during night	First third	First third	First third
Duration	1–10 minutes	5–40 minutes	1–5 minutes
Agitation	None/mild	Moderate	Marked
Autonomic arousal	Mild	Moderate	Marked
Incidence	40%	5–15%	1%
Age of peak incidence	Middle childhood/pre-adolescence	Toddler/pre-school	Adolescence
Amnesia	Yes	Yes	Yes
Arousal threshold	High	High	High
Family history	Common	Common	Common

Sleepwalking

Calm

The stereotypical behavior of calm sleepwalking is fairly similar at all ages. The individual simply gets up and walks about calmly. The young child may walk or crawl about in the crib; but since he or she is quiet, these events often go unnoticed. An older child will usually get up and walk toward the light and/or parents. He or she often will be found simply standing in the living room or quietly next to the parents' bed. It is difficult to decide if the child is, in fact, asleep; that is, differentiation between drowsy wakefulness and walking about while not quite awake may be impossible and perhaps is only semantic. Some inappropriate behavior, such as urinating in the corner or next to the toilet, is common. Such a child may easily be led back to bed, perhaps with a stop at the bathroom, with little evidence of complete waking.

The older child may show similar behavior but may be more likely to walk about with his or her own agenda instead of following light, sound, and parents. Occasionally, the child may go to another room and return to sleep. Stairways are usually negotiated successfully, although perception is dulled, and slipping or tripping is quite possible. At times, the youngster will head toward the doorway and try to go outside. When successful, such children have been known to cross streets or walk barefoot

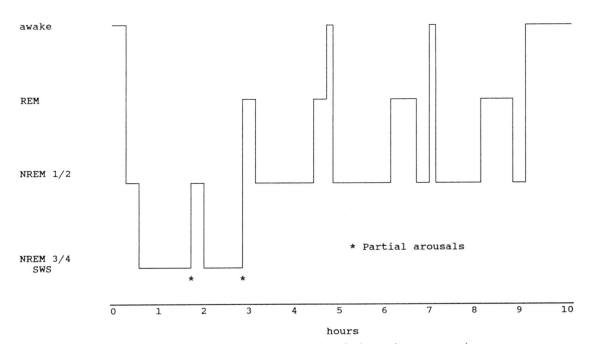

Figure 11–1. Sleep histogram showing timing of primary sleep parasomnias.

in the snow. Risks here are obvious. Older children usually do wake fully as the event terminates and often are embarrassed to find themselves out of their bedroom and possibly the center of attention or even of ridicule by other family members. Still, a return to bed and sleep at that point is usually rapid.

Sleepwalking is very common. In Klackenberg's longitudinal study of a group of 212 randomly selected children from Stockholm ages 6–16 years, the incidence of quiet sleepwalking was 40%.[5] The yearly prevalence varied from 6 to 17%, though only 2 to 3% had more than one episode per month. The sleepwalking persisted for 5 years in 33% of the children and for over 10 years in 12%.

Agitated

Agitated sleepwalking is seen more frequently in older children; the child gets up and walks about in an upset and agitated fashion. There may be more speech, but it is often garbled and unintelligible. The child recoils when touched or held, and the degree of agitation may increase. He or she is more likely to bump into a dresser or otherwise sustain a minor injury than the calm sleepwalker, but even this is not too likely. This type of sleepwalking also runs a course of a minute to a half-hour or so; the child then calms, wakes, and wants to return to bed.

Confusional Arousals

Although confusional arousals are often labeled "sleep terrors," they are actually a variation.[1, 7–9] Usually seen in infants and toddlers and, to a lesser degree, in school-age children, these arousals may seem quite bizarre and even frightening to observing parents. An arousal usually starts with some movement and moaning, progressing to crying and perhaps calling out, often associated with very intense thrashing about in the bed or crib. Wild thrashing is less often seen in the young infant, since physical movement is still limited; instead, such a child may simply be crying inconsolably. Eyes may be open or closed, and perspiration is usually marked. A look of "terror" is not described; rather the child is felt to look very confused, agitated, upset, or "possessed." Like sleepwalking episodes, these can last anywhere from 1 to 2 minutes up to 30 to 40 minutes, with 5 to 15 minutes being

typical. Even if the child calls for the parents, he or she does not recognize them and may appear to "look right through" them. Holding and cuddling do not provide reassurance; instead, the child often resists, arches the back, twists, pushes away, and becomes progressively more agitated. Even vigorous attempts to wake the child by shaking, taking him or her into the light, yelling, or using cold water may not be successful. Parents may report otherwise, but on closer questioning, it becomes clear that there is only the perception of success; that is, after 10 minutes of effort, "we finally succeeded in waking him." Actually, the event terminated spontaneously. In fact, the more the parents intercede, the longer the episode may run. Further, if they struggle sufficiently with their youngster, these efforts will succeed in fully waking and even scaring the child as the event terminates and may delay return to sleep.[6, 7]

Since these episodes vary so much in frequency, intensity, and duration, parental reports are often inaccurate; hence, despite various surveys, the true incidence is unknown.[10, 11] However, it seems fairly certain that almost all young children have at least a mild form of this from time to time, especially before age 5. Occasional events are often dismissed as "bad dreams," especially in the pre-verbal child, for whom dream reports are not yet possible.

Sleep Terrors

Sleep terrors, on the other hand, are uncommon in very young children; instead, they are seen more often in older children and young adults. Such events usually begin precipitously (not gradually as do confusional events), with the child bolting upright with a "blood-curdling" scream. He or she may continue to cry and scream. The eyes are usually wide open and bulging, the heart is racing, and there often is diaphoresis. The facial expression is now one of intense fear. In a full-blown episode, a youngster may jump out of bed and run blindly, as if away from some unseen threat. This may be very dangerous, and injury during this frenzied activity is quite possible. The youngster may knock over furniture or even break windows. Anyone attempting to intervene may also be injured.

These events are usually shorter than the confusional arousals, generally terminating within a few minutes. The child wakes before the autonomic storm has died down. Perhaps because this waking allows perception of the physical components of fear, the child may report some "memory." But it is most often brief and fragmented, not characteristic of imagery reported from typical dreams or nightmares, and it may well be that the "imagery" is constructed after the waking to fit or explain the residual feelings. Usually, descriptions are of "something" (or "it") that "is going to get me," "is after me," or "is closing in on me." The perception of attack may explain the resistance to attempts of restraint.

Etiology

Figure 11–2 is a schematic of the determinants and manifestations of partial arousals from sleep. At the end of a period of SWS there is a transition that leads to one of three possible state changes: (1) begin the next sleep cycle by switching to a different sleep stage, (2) continued arousal until full awakening, or (3) become "stuck"—unable to completely get out of deep sleep, unable to arouse fully, and unable to move onto the next sleep cycle. This is the state of partial arousal. Two major factors determine the occurrence of partial arousals: (1) constitutional or predisposing factors and (2) precipitating factors (Table 11–2).

Genetic and developmental factors are the most important constitutional determinants of partial arousals, but amount of sleep, schedule regularity, and psychologic factors must be considered. The nature of the genetic factors is not known. The important developmental factors appear to be depth and duration of

Table 11–2. CONSTITUTIONAL AND PRECIPITATING FACTORS FOR AROUSALS

I. Constitutional or predisposing factors
   1. Genetic
   2. Developmental
   3. Sleep deprivation
   4. Chaotic wake/sleep scheduling
   5. Psychologic
II. Precipitating factors
   1. Endogenous
      a. Obstructive sleep apnea
      b. Gastroesophageal reflux
      c. Seizures
      d. Fever
      e. Periodic movements of sleep
   2. Exogenous
      a. Stimulation-auditory, tactile, or visual
      b. Drugs

SWS. Partial arousals are most common in children who are young, when SWS tends to be very deep and long-lasting.

Sleep factors such as sleep deprivation and chaotic sleep scheduling that affect the depth, duration and consolidation of SWS are associated with partial arousals. Parents commonly report that events are most common on nights when their child is overtired (when arousal to full waking would understandably be difficult). Similarly, when schedules are irregular there may be poor synchronization between the circadian system's clock-based signal to switch out of SWS and the recuperative drive to maintain that state for a longer period.

Into the school years, and particularly as the child moves through adolescence, arousal from SWS becomes easier. In these years, continued arousal events may be associated with psychologic factors (although traumatic events

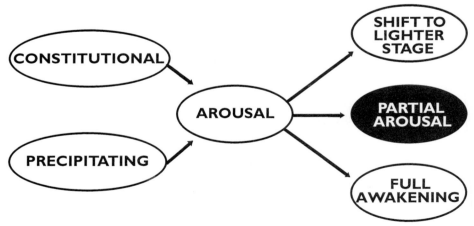

Figure 11–2. NREM sleep arousal determinants and manifestations.

at any age may be important) (see Chapter 16).[12, 13]

Some symptomatic older children are extremely well-behaved, at home and at school. In these children, emotions are over-controlled and withheld. There may be unexpressed feelings of anger, particularly regarding significant life events over which the youngster has little control (separation, divorce, parental discord, or family moves). These and other psychologic factors should be explored in the child with sleep terrors, and addressed by psychologic intervention where appropriate. Although such factors are less often relevant in young children, child abuse, surgery, and worries about a parent in a dangerous profession may all be important.

Precipitating sleep factors (occurring intermittently during sleep or otherwise directly affecting the sleep cycle) may disrupt sleep. In an individual predisposed to partial arousals due to one of the constitutional or predisposing factors, a partial arousal can be triggered by any strategically timed precipitating sleep factor (see Table 11–2). In the majority of children the arousals appear spontaneously. The fact that sleepwalking can be induced in normal children by standing them up during SWS[14] and that sleep terrors can be precipitously triggered in susceptible individuals by auditory stimulation (or even by just pulling up their blanket) in SWS, speaks against these

behaviors being the climax of complex, ongoing sleep mentation.[14–16]

In addition to the constitutional/predisposing and precipitating factors in some individuals, there appears to be a conditioned (perpetuating) component to their arousals. Some young children develop habits or become conditioned to call for or go to parents at each nighttime waking. This may become very automatic, with the child starting to call or to leave the bed before waking fully. When such a child only partly wakes from deep SWS early in the night, this automatic drive to complete a particular behavior pattern may push the child towards fuller and longer arousal, thereby triggering a full event.

Psychologic distress can function as a perpetuating factor in some older children and adolescents. In some cases, it is the fact that the child is having frequent arousals that is distressing. If the underlying stressor can be identified and eliminated and the child and family educated about partial arousals so the symptom is demystified, the perpetuating component can be eliminated. This often leads to a dramatic decrease in the number and severity of the arousals.[17]

Constitutional/predisposing, precipitating, and perpetuating factors all interact to determine the frequency, duration, and severity of the partial arousal disorder. This is illustrated in Figure 11–3, using a model developed by

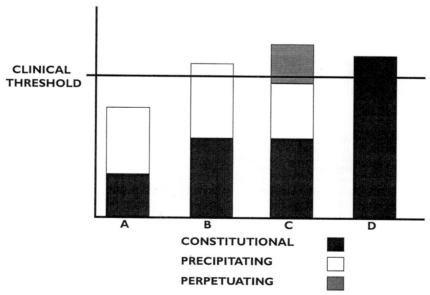

Figure 11–3. Factors in disorders of arousal. Group A: No partial arousals. Group B: Partial arousals only with precipitating factors. Group C: Partial arousals triggered by precipitating factors, perpetuated by conditioning factors. Group D: Partial arousals on a solely constitutional basis.

Spielman for insomnia.[18] In the majority of children, constitutional factors alone explain the occurrence of partial arousals (Group D). In a small number of children, the partial arousal disorder does not become manifest until the presence of a strategically timed precipitating factor (Group B). In some, the partial arousals appear to be maintained through some conditioning or perpetuating factors (Group C). Other children do not have any partial arousals (Group A). This model provides a framework for conceptualizing the factors contributing to partial arousals and may also suggest treatment modalities once the diagnosis has been established.

Differential Diagnosis of Nocturnal Arousals

The differential diagnosis of partial arousals includes nocturnal seizures, gastroesophageal reflux, obstructive sleep apnea, anxiety dreams, conditioned arousals, REM behavior disorders (RBD), post-traumatic stress disorder (PTSD), and dissociated states (see Chapter 13); each may present with unusual nocturnal behavior. The key to working through this differential diagnosis of unusual nocturnal behavior is obtaining a detailed history. In most cases this alone will establish the correct diagnosis. The key features of the history include timing during the sleep cycle; detailed description of the event; level of consciousness before, during, and after the arousal; daytime symptoms of sleepiness; injury associated with arousal; memory for the event; and personal and family history of partial arousal. The features distinguishing nocturnal seizures, anxiety dreams, and partial arousals are described in

Table 11–3. In most cases, formal PSG study is not necessary. The clinical indication for a PSG, possibly with an MSLT, would include: (1) rule out seizures—especially if the arousals are recurrent, stereotypical, or violent, (2) rule out apnea, (3) presence of daytime sleepiness, (4) violent arousals, and (5) rule out RBD.

Treatment

The most important aspect of the treatment of partial arousals is proper diagnosis, and then to offer reassurance. Both parent and child can be reassured of the benign, self-limited nature of the arousal in a majority of cases. The family should be instructed as to basic safety precautions. The bedroom should be cleared of obstructions, and the bedroom windows secured. In appropriate cases, additional locks or alarms need to be installed on outside doors. Sleep deprivation should be avoided, and the wake/sleep schedule made regular. A trial of sleep extension may be considered where appropriate. The parent should be instructed not to forcibly intervene during the arousal and not to wake the child, as this may serve only to prolong the event. Usually, the child responds best to being left alone, and the parents' job is simply to ensure that no injury occurs. In some cases, the child can be comforted and redirected by the parent. It is not uncommon for the frequency, severity, and duration of the arousals to diminish after employing these simple measures. When specific psychologic stressors are identified that appear to be related to the onset of the arousals, these should be addressed. Psychotherapy is indicated with children and in families where significant psychopathology is present.

Table 11–3. CHARACTERISTIC FEATURES OF NOCTURNAL SEIZURES, PARTIAL AROUSALS, AND ANXIETY DREAMS

	Nocturnal Seizures	Partial Arousals	Dream Anxiety Attacks
Time of the night	Anytime, often at sleep onset	First 1/3 of the night	Middle to last 1/3 of the night
Description of behavior	Repetitive, stereotypical, may be violent	Variable	Very little motor behavior
Level of consciousness	Unarousable during, confused but awake after	Unarousable or very confused if awakened	Asleep during attack, fully awake after
Memory of event	Amnesia	Amnesia	Vivid recall
Family history	Variable	Common	No
Potential for injury	Moderate	Usually low	Low
Prevalence	Rare	Common	Very common
Stage of sleep	NREM >> REM	Deep NREM > light NREM	REM
Daytime sleepiness	Often	Uncommon	Uncommon

In some cases, where the arousals are dangerous or disruptive to the child or the family and no obvious precipitant can be identified, symptomatic treatment is needed. Two successful interventions for partial arousals have been described: pharmacologic therapy (benzodiazepines and tricyclic antidepressants)[16, 19] and relaxation and mental imagery.[20–23] Use of medication in children is rarely necessary but may be considered when the arousals are felt to pose a significant risk to the child. Low-dose clonazepam, beginning at 0.25 mg 1 hour before bedtime, is often effective in controlling the partial arousals. The dose may need to be increased but should be done cautiously while monitoring for symptoms of daytime sedation.

Occasionally, 3 to 6 weeks of treatment may be "curative" with symptoms failing to return when the medication is discontinued (this is particularly likely in younger children in whom symptoms are not of long duration).

The major objection to drug therapy for partial arousals is the long-term nature of the disorder and the potentially adverse affects of chronic drug administration on behavior and learning.[24] Consequently, teaching children relaxation and mental imagery offers an attractive alternative. This form of treatment allows the child to utilize self-regulation techniques to control the previously uncontrolled nighttime behaviors. If the technique is to be effective, it must be performed by a competent, medically trained therapist, usually a behavioral psychologist or hypnotherapist. The mechanism of clinical improvement in partial arousals with pharmacologic therapy or with relaxation and mental imagery is poorly understood but currently under investigation. Possibilities include elimination of the precipitating or the perpetuating (conditioned) factors that supported the symptom or a change in underlying constitutional sleep factors resulting in a change in arousal frequency or characteristics. Scheduled awakenings 15 minutes prior to the onset of the partial arousal has been suggested as an intervention for night terrors and sleepwalking in several anecdotal reports.[25–27]

In summary, partial arousals from sleep represent a curious paradox, during which the individual may show an extraordinary level of endogenous arousal but is unarousable by exogenous stimuli. Clinically, there is a spectrum of behaviors that varies from quiet sleepwalking to sleep terrors, all arising from NREM sleep. In the milder forms, these disorders of arousal are quite common, especially in children, and require no intervention or only for safety. In difficult cases, formal, extensive PSG is mandatory. In some children, the arousals may be frequent, very disruptive, or dangerous, and pharmacologic treatment or relaxation and mental imagery training is often very effective.

References

1. Broughton RJ: Sleep disorders: disorders of arousal? Science 159:1070, 1968.
2. Guilleminault C: Disorders of arousal in children: somnambulism and night terrors. *In* Guilleminault C (ed): Sleep and Its Disorders in Children. New York, Raven Press 1982, pp 243–252.
3. The International Classification of Sleep Disorders. Diagnostic and Coding Manual. American Sleep Disorders Association 1990, pp 142–150.
4. Mahowald MW, Rosen GM: Parasomnias in children. Pediatrician 17:21, 1990.
5. Klackenberg G: Somnambulism in childhood—prevalence, course and behavioral correlations. Acta Paediatr Scand 71:495, 1982.
6. Naylor MW, Aldrich MS: The distribution of confusional arousals across sleep stages and time of night in children and adolescents with sleep terrors. Sleep Res 20:308, 1991.
7. Ferber R: Sleep, sleeplessness, and sleep disruptions in infants and young children. Ann Clin Res 17:227, 1985.
8. Ferber RA: Solve Your Child's Sleep Problem. New York, Simon & Schuster, 1985.
9. Ferber R, Boyle MP: Confusional arousals in infants and toddlers (not quite pavor nocturnus). Sleep Res 12:241, 1983.
10. Klackenberg G: Incidence of parasomnias in children in a general population. *In* Guilleminault C (ed): Sleep and Its Disorders in Children. New York, Raven Press, 1987. pp 99–113.
11. Richman N: Surveys of sleep disorders in children in a general population. *In* Guilleminault C (ed): Sleep and Its Disorders in Children. New York, Raven Press, 1987, pp 115–127.
12. Kales A, Soldatos CR, Caldwell AB, et al: Somnambulism: clinical characteristics and personality patterns. Arch Gen Psychiatry 37:1406, 1980.
13. Kales JD, Kales A, Soldatos CR, et al: Night terrors: clinical characteristics and personality patterns. Arch Gen Psychiatry 37:1413, 1980.
14. Fisher C, Kahn E, Edwards A, et al: A psychophysiological study of nightmares and night terrors. III. Mental content and recall of stage 4 night terrors. J Nerv Ment Dis 157:75, 1973.
15. Fisher C, Byrne J, Edwards A, et al: A psychophysiological study of nightmares. Monogr J Am Psychoanal Assoc 18:747, 1970.
16. Fisher C, Kahn E, Edwards A: The psychophysiological study of nightmares and night terrors. Arch Gen Psychiatry 28:252, 1973.
17. Dahl RE, Williamson DE: Aggressive partial arousals preceding competitive football games. Sleep Res 19:160, 1990.

18. Spielman AJ: Assessment of insomnia. Clin Psychol Rev 6:11, 1986.
19. Pesikoff RD, Davis PC: Treatment of pavor nocturnus and somnambulism in children. Am J Psychiatry 128:134, 1971.
20. Reid WH, Ahmed I, Levie CA: Treatment of sleep walking. A controlled study. Am J Psychother 35:27, 1981.
21. Gardner GG, Olness K: Hypnosis and Hypnotherapy in Children. Orlando, Grune & Stratton, 1981, pp 116–123.
22. Hurwitz TD, Mahowald MW, Schenck CH, et al: A retrospective outcome study and review of hypnosis as treatment of adults with sleepwalking and sleep terror. J Nerv Ment Dis 179:228, 1991.
23. Kohen D, Rosen GM, Mahowald MW: Sleep terror disorder in children: the role of self-hypnosis in management. Am J Clin Hypn 34:233, 1992.
24. Weissbluth M: Is drug treatment of night terrors warranted? Am J Dis Child 138:1086, 1984.
25. Lask B: Novel and non-toxic treatment for night terrors. Br Med J 297:592, 1988.
26. Lask B: "Waking treatment" best for night terrors. Br Med J 306:1477, 1993.
27. Tobin J: Treatment of somnambulism with anticipatory awakening. J Pediatr 122:426, 1993.

Nocturnal Enuresis in the Child

PATRICK C. FRIMAN

Nocturnal enuresis is one of the most prevalent and persistent sleep problems in children. Despite extensive clinical research many enuretic children in the United States remain untreated, mistreated, or treated ineffectively.[1, 2] For example, recent surveys suggest many parents use punishment and/or fluid restriction to treat their children's enuresis,[1] while many primary care physicians only recommend drug treatment or no treatment at all.[2] Effective skill-based alternatives are available, but they are described infrequently in medical journals and medical texts. This chapter will briefly discuss enuresis in terms of diagnosis, incidence, etiology, and bladder physiology and then more thoroughly discuss drug treatments, their limitations, and skill-based treatment alternatives.

Diagnosis

The most widely used criteria for enuresis specifies: (1) chronologic age of at least 5 years and mental age of 4; (2) two or more incontinent events in a month between 5 and 6 years of age and one or more events after 6 years; and (3) absence of a physical disorder associated with incontinence such as diabetes, urinary tract infection, or seizure disorder.[3] Enuresis is divided into primary, where the child has never had a long period of nocturnal continence, and secondary, where nighttime wetting recurs after one year of continence. This distinction is important because secondary cases are more likely to have a pathologic etiology.

Incidence

Research from several countries suggests enuresis is most prevalent in the United States.[4] Data from the United States National Health Examination Survey show that as many as 25% of boys and 15% of girls are enuretic at age 6 with as many as 8% of boys and 4% of girls still enuretic at age 12.[4] Primary enuresis accounts for up to 90% of these cases.[5]

Etiology

Family History. Family history is the most consistently supported etiologic variable. The probability of enuresis increases as a function of closeness and number of blood relations with a history positive for enuresis.[6–9] These findings suggest the importance of genetic factors, although some theorists argue that certain families convey tolerant attitudes toward bedwetting, not enuretic "genes."[10] But studies conducted in settings where family customs play a minimal role in determining a child's development (such as in Israeli kibbutzim) have also found a high correlation between a history of enuresis in the family and enuresis in the child.[9]

Maturation. Although family studies suggest the existence of a biologic factor, the identity of this factor, or factors, is uncertain. Certain evidence points to a maturational lag in enuretic youngsters.[5] For example, children with decreased developmental scores at 1 and 3 years of age are significantly more likely to develop enuresis than are children with higher scores.[11] There is also an inverse relationship between birth weight and enuresis at any age. Enuretic children tend to lag slightly behind their nonenuretic peers in Tanner sexual maturation scores, bone growth, and height.[4] Boys are not only more frequently enuretic than girls, but they generally have a slower rate of development throughout childhood and adolescence.[4, 11] Finally, enuretic children exhibit a 15% annual spontaneous remission rate, which is consistent with the notion that these youngsters are simply lagging behind in the acquisition of continence—a developmental milestone for all children.[12] Despite the apparent maturational lag in many (perhaps most) enuretic children, their scores on standardized intellectual tests are in the average range.[4] Thus, the maturational lag appears to be more anatomic and/or physiologic than intellectual, and one of its main features is reduced bladder control.[4, 13–15]

Functional Bladder Capacity (FBC). FBC refers to voiding capacity, that is, the volume of urine a bladder can hold before starting to contract and initiate emptying, as distinguished from true bladder capacity (TBC), which refers to actual bladder size.[16] FBC is established by the larger of the first two voidings after ingestion of a specified water load (e.g., 30 ml/kg body weight),[17, 18] the average of all voidings in 24 hours,[19] or the average of all voidings in 1 week.[18] Research suggests the FBC of enuretic children is generally lower than that of their nonenuretic siblings[17] and peers,[15–18] but their TBC is about the same.[16] Studies of FBC suggest many enuretic children urinate more frequently and in smaller volumes than do their nonenuretic peers and siblings. The urinary pattern of enuretic children is often similar to that of infants and toddlers.[14, 15]

Sleep Dynamics. Enuresis is regarded as a parasomnia by most sleep researchers,[19–21] as a manifestation of sleep disturbance by some sleep researchers,[22] and as an outcome of deep sleep by most parents.[1] Still, sleep dynamics have not been established as a cause of enuresis. Wetting episodes occur in all stages of NREM sleep and the probability that enuresis occurs in a given NREM stage appears to be a function of the amount of time spent in that stage.[21, 23] Enuretic episodes rarely occur during REM sleep; therefore, thematically related dreams (e.g., swimming) are more likely a result than a cause of wetting.[19, 24] Finally, despite parental reports, enuretic children are not more difficult to awaken than their nonenuretic peers.[25, 26]

Physical Pathology. There are numerous well-known potential physiopathologic causes of enuresis, which include urinary tract infection, urinary tract anomaly, bladder instability, occult spina bifida, epilepsy, diabetes mellitus, and sleep apnea. Most of these can be ruled out by the history, physical examination, and urinalysis. When unanswered questions remain, other, more elaborate laboratory examinations are available (e.g., voiding cystourethrogram, PSG).[4, 21, 24]

Psychopathology. The consensus of the current literature is that psychopathology is not a causal variable for primary enuresis.[5, 11, 20, 21, 27–35] Although some studies suggest enuretic children exhibit anxiety and/or problematic conduct,[29, 30] the research[27, 31] and prevailing position in the literature is that these symptoms are more likely a result of rather than a cause of enuresis.[5, 20, 21, 32–35] Recent longitudinal research showed that although maturational variables were predictive of enuresis, psychosocial variables, such as emotional disposition, were not.[11] If the underlying cause of enuresis were psychopathologic, then the elimination of the wetting presumably would give rise to other expressions of the pathology. Yet "symptom substitution" does not occur following successful nonpsychiatric treatment of enuresis.[27] Quite the contrary. In fact, enuretic children successfully treated with conditioning therapy actually exhibit improvement in psychologic status.[28]

Physiology of the Bladder and Continence Skills

The bladder is an elastic viscus with a complex arrangement of smooth muscle, blood vessels, and connective tissue. The body of the bladder is the detrusor muscle that joins the internal and external sphincters beginning at the bladder neck.[36] When empty the detrusor is relaxed and receptive and the sphincters are contracted and retentive. As the bladder fills, its stretch receptors are stimulated causing the bladder neck to descend. Descent of the bladder neck causes reflexive contraction of the detrusor, which opens the sphincters and urination occurs. Control of urination is established through the coordinated action of the thoracic diaphragm, abdominal wall, and levator ani. For urination to occur, these muscles lower the bladder neck and open the sphincters. To maintain continence, they keep the bladder neck elevated and the sphincters closed.[14, 15, 36]

Nocturnal continence involves several sequentially attained skills including awareness of urgency, initiation of urination, inhibition of urination while awake, and inhibition of urination while asleep. Establishing nocturnal continence requires repeated practice of these skills, day and night.

Pretreatment Assessment

The initial visit should include an interview with the child and parents. If the interview suggests emotional or psychologic abnormalities, consultation with a child psychologist or psychiatrist can be helpful. To rule out physical pathology, each enuretic child should receive a physical examination prior to treatment.[4, 32, 33, 35-37] The examination should include careful palpation of the abdomen for masses, motor and sensory testing of the lower extremities, assessment of anal sphincter function, and examination of the lower back and external genitalia for anomalies. The urine should be tested for specific gravity, glucose, protein, blood, and evidence of infection. In the absence of symptoms and findings other than simple sleep-associated incontinence (e.g., snoring, waking incontinence, infection), the more invasive diagnostic procedures are unnecessary (e.g., voiding cystourethrogram, PSG).

Drug Treatment

A recent survey[2] substantiates what much of the literature[11, 32-34, 37-39] on enuresis suggests: physicians prescribe drug therapy for enuresis more frequently than any other treatment. Historically, many types of drugs have been prescribed for enuresis, but two types comprise the majority of current prescriptions: antidepressants and antidiuretics.

Tricyclic Antidepressants

Until recently tricyclic antidepressants appeared to be the drugs of choice for treatment of enuresis with imipramine the most frequently prescribed.[2, 38-40] It is not known for certain how imipramine reduces bedwetting.[40] Most experts agree that its antidepressant and sleep effects, such as REM suppression, are not significant mechanisms responsible for the decrease in wetting, but the agreement ends there. Imipramine, perhaps by its anticholinergic effects, somehow reduces premature con-

tractions of the detrusor following partial filling of the bladder and thereby increases functional bladder capacity.[40]

Imipramine, in doses between 25 and 75 mg given at bedtime, produces initial reductions in wetting in the majority of children, often within the first week of treatment.[39] The primary therapeutic gain from imipramine, however, appears to be the respite from wetting obtained while the child is on the drug. Both short- and long-term studies show enuresis usually recurs when tricyclic therapeutic agents are withdrawn.[41] The permanent cure produced with imipramine is only about 25% (reports range from 5 to 40%).[39] Subtracting the annual spontaneous remission rate of 15%[12] leaves only about a 10% increment in cure rate using this medication. Thus imipramine is superior to no treatment or to placebo but not by much.

Use of imipramine does not teach continence skills. In fact, by diminishing detrusor contractions, it reduces the opportunity to learn sensory awareness of those contractions and to practice needed responses. This reduced opportunity to learn may account for the high relapse rate following termination of the medication and for reports showing that drug regimens may impair subsequent continence skill-training programs.[42] Imipramine can cause several untoward side effects ranging in severity from excessive sweating, irritability, nausea, and vomiting to convulsions, collapse, coma, and death.[32-34, 37, 43]

Given its low cure rate and high relapse rates, side effects, potential to diminish skill development, and potential toxicity, imipramine should not be used as a primary treatment for enuresis.[4, 5, 21, 32-34, 43] But, because its effects are seen so quickly, when they occur, it can be a valuable adjunct to treatment, especially when other methods are failing and a dry night is needed to heighten motivation or when a child plans to attend camp or a sleepover.[32-35, 43]

Antidiuretics

In 1985, Norgaard and colleagues reported on a small number of enuretic children who had abnormal circadian patterns of plasma vasopressin concentration, which should be highest at night.[44] Largely because of this report, desmopressin (DDAVP) became a popular treatment for enuresis. DDAVP concentrates urine, thereby decreasing urine volume and intravesical pressure, which makes bladder neck descent and detrusor contraction less probable. DDAVP also has far fewer side effects than imipramine.[44–49] Recommended dosages are 20 to 40 µg intranasally at bedtime (1–2 sprays in each nostril).

Research on DDAVP has yielded mixed results with success in some studies[45, 47, 48] and failure in others.[5, 49] Generally, its effects appear to last only as long as the drug is taken, i.e., when treatment stops, enuresis usually returns, and are less likely to occur in younger children or children who have frequent accidents.[47, 48] DDAVP is also very expensive. Finally, because DDAVP reduces urine output it also reduces opportunities to practice continence skills (similar to imipramine). Nevertheless, its effects, when they occur, are immediate and with fewer side effects than imipramine. Thus, DDAVP may be preferable to imipramine as a treatment adjunct.

Skill-Based Treatment

Skill-based treatment requires more effort than drug treatment, but it is safer and usually more effective. The superiority of skill-based treatment is probably due to its focus on two key components of toilet training: specific continence skills and the motivation to attain them.

Urine Alarm

The alarm works using a moisture sensitive switching system which, when closing allows the alarm to ring. Numerous safe, efficient, and effective alarms are available, many of which attach directly to the child's pajamas or underwear. Such proximity to the source of the urine permits alarm feedback to occur near the start of voiding.[35, 50]

The mechanism of action in alarm treatment was initially described as classic conditioning with the alarm as the unconditioned stimulus, bladder distention the conditioned stimulus, and waking as the conditioned response.[51] More recent literature emphasizes a negative reinforcement or avoidance paradigm in which the child awakens to the alarm, stops urinating, and either completes urination in the toilet or holds the urine until a more convenient time.[24, 52] Cures are obtained slowly, and during the first few weeks the child often awakens only after voiding completely.[35] However, the aversive quality of the alarm and subsequent arousal gradually strengthens

skills. These skills include becoming aware of the need to void, waking oneself in order to urinate, or contracting the external sphincter to postpone bladder emptying.

Reports of controlled comparative trials show the alarm is superior to imipramine,[53] DDAVP,[54] and other skill-based methods.[55] In fact, the literature has consistently described the urine alarm as the single most effective treatment for enuresis.[4, 20–24, 32–35, 37, 46, 52, 56] Reviews of the literature show its success rate is higher (approximately 75%), and its relapse rate lower (approximately 41%) than any other drug or skill-based treatment.[52, 56] Furthermore, by using an intermittent alarm schedule (e.g., alarm rings after every other accident), the relapse rate can be as low as 17%.[52]

Retention Control Training (RCT)

The emergence of RCT followed the observation that many enuretic children had reduced functional bladder capacities.[14, 15, 17] RCT expands functional bladder capacity by requiring children to drink extra fluids (e.g., 16 oz of water or juice) and delay urination as long as possible.[14, 15, 17, 57] In order to assess progress, at least once a week their parents should set up a game where the children urinate in an appropriate container and try to produce more urine than in previous weeks.

RCT is successful in as many as 50% of cases,[52, 57] but it is not as effective as the urine alarm. This lower effectiveness is not surprising, since RCT does not train nocturnal skills directly. It directly trains bladder control skills during the day, which indirectly affects such skills at night.

Stream Interruption

Stream interruption, a variation of a Kegel exercise, strengthens control of the external urethral sphincter and of the intra-abdominal muscles controlling bladder neck descent.[58] The exercise requires the children to start and stop their urine flow during at least one daytime urination. Stream interruption has not been evaluated as an intervention for enuresis, but the related Kegel exercises have been effective for stress incontinence in women.[58] Furthermore, stream interruption is frequently recommended for enuresis and is an integral component of some highly effective multicomponent treatments.[5, 35, 59]

Paired Association

Paired association involves pairing stream interruption with the alarm in a reinforcement paradigm. The parent stands outside the bathroom door with the alarm while the child urinates. The parent sounds the alarm and the child practices stream interruption. The parent praises and rewards accordingly. A more convenient version of this sequence involves making an audio tape of the alarm played intermittently. The child takes the tape and recorder into the bathroom and matches starts and stops of urine flow with the recorded alarm.

The paired association procedure has not yet been evaluated, but some basic literature supports its potential effectiveness. For example, sleeping persons can make discriminations between stimuli on the basis of meaningfulness and prior training[60] and the probability of a correct discrimination is significantly improved through contingent reinforcement.[61] Thus, reinforcing a relationship between stream interruption and the alarm while the child is awake may increase the probability that the child will interrupt urination in response to the alarm while asleep.

Waking Schedule

This component involves waking the child and guiding him or her to the bathroom for urination. Results obtained are attributed to a change in arousal, increased access to the reinforcing properties of dry nights,[62] and urinary urge in lighter stages of sleep.[5] In a representative study using a staggered waking schedule, four of nine children reduced their accidents to less than twice a week, suggesting a waking schedule may improve but is unlikely to cure enuresis.[63] A less effortful schedule involves waking the child just before the parents go to bed and systematically fading the schedule by waking him or her one-half hour earlier on nights following several successive dry nights (e.g., 1 week).[62]

Visual Sequencing

This procedure involves mentally rehearsing nighttime continence skills. Reports of its empirical evaluation have not yet been published, but it is included in several popular treatment programs.[59] The procedure involves visualization of either or both of the behavioral sequences leading to nocturnal continence. Both sequences include imagined detection of urgency and contraction of the external urethral sphincter followed by either holding urine throughout the night (in the first sequence) or rising and going to the bathroom (in the second). The procedure can be taught in the office. The provider should ask the child to sit in a comfortable chair, take three to four deep breaths, close their eyes, and relax fully. The provider should then discuss each detail of what will happen at night asking the child to focus on a mental picture of the details. The provider should demonstrate this procedure to the parents so they can assist the child with it at home.

Reinforcement Systems

Reinforcement systems may not cure enuresis, but they can sustain a child's motivation to participate in treatment, especially when the system reinforces success in small steps.[32–34] Various award systems, including the use of stickers or points and prizes may be used. One method uses a dot-to-dot drawing and a grab bag. The child identifies an affordable and desirable prize, and the parent draws or traces a picture of it using a dot-to-dot format with every third or fourth dot bigger than the rest. The child then connects two dots for each dry night. When the line reaches a larger dot, they earn access to a grab bag with small rewards (e.g., small toys, edibles, money, privileges, special time with parents). When all the dots are connected, the child is given the prize.[32, 33]

Responsibility Training

All the skill-based components mentioned above are designed to promote a mature voiding repertoire in the child. To be consistent with this design, the child should be treated in a way that promotes maturation.[20, 21] For example, they should not be left in diapers at night. They should be assigned household responsibilities associated with their accidents. In younger children this may merely mean bringing their sheets to the laundry basket. In older children, however, it may mean actually laundering the sheets. These responsibilities should not be presented as a punishment but as a correlate of increased responsibility and a demonstration of the parent's confidence and respect.

Optimal Treatment Plans

Historically, the choice of treatment for enuresis was governed more by the desire to establish continence than by concern for the child's health and well-being. Fortunately, medical care for enuretic children has evolved substantially. Nevertheless, the sustained reliance on drugs for primary treatment, the abiding parental use of punishment, and the often excessive restriction on fluid intake still places the health and well-being of many enuretic children at risk. The treatments most likely to cure enuresis with minimal risk to the child's health are those which specifically teach continence skills. Decades of behavioral research have generated several skill-based treatment components,[32–34] and the probability for cure increases with the number of components included in the treatment plan.[62]

Initially, the provider should inform the child and parents that numerous other children, many probably in the child's neighborhood and school, have the problem too. Then with the child in attendance, the provider should tell the parents to avoid blaming or shaming the child for wetting. The provider should then enthusiastically solicit the child's cooperation in treatment and work with the child and family on a plan.

The initial choice of components should be based on the provider's assessment of child readiness, child and parent willingness, and family resources. The components in the plan can be "titrated" over time in accordance with family resources and motivation until cure is obtained. For example, a two-parent, one-wage earner, middle-income family with a motivated 10-year-old bedwetting child and at least one motivated parent could be given a waking schedule, a motivational system, and the alarm on the initial visit. Over the course of one or two additional visits, other skill-based treatment components could be added as needed along with a small prescription of DDAVP or imipramine for sleepovers or campouts. Families with fewer resources and less motivation would be given fewer components. For example, a one-parent, low-income family with a motivated 10-year-old child and a nonmotivated parent could be given instructions on urine retention and stream interruption exercises. The chances for cure are lower in the second case than in the first, but they are still higher than if no treatment were used. Furthermore, the active involvement of the child may lead to increased involvement by the parent at which point the provider could add more components.

Developing an effective skill-based treatment plan for an individual enuretic child will require some extra time. But the investment of that time will more than offset the substantial decrease in potential harm to the enuretic child and the increase in potential for curing the enuresis.

References

1. Shelov SP, Gundy J, Weiss JC, et al: Enuresis: a contrast of attitudes of parents and physicians. Pediatrics 67:707, 1981.
2. Foxman B, Valdez RB, Brook RH: Childhood enuresis: prevalence, perceived impact, and prescribed treatments. Pediatrics 77:482, 1986.
3. American Psychiatric Association: Diagnostic and Statistical Manual of Mental Disorders (DSM-III-R), 3rd ed. Washington, D.C., American Psychiatric Association, 1987.
4. Gross RT, Dornbusch SM: Enuresis. In Levin MD, Carey WB, Crocker AC, Gross RT (eds): Developmental-Behavioral Pediatrics. Philadelphia, WB Saunders, 1983, pp 575–586.
5. Scharf MB, Jennings SW: Childhood enuresis: relationship to sleep, etiology, evaluation, and treatment. J Behav Med 10:113, 1988.
6. Bakwin H: The genetics of enuresis. In Kolvin I, MacKeith RC, Meadow SR (eds): Bladder Control and Enuresis. Philadelphia, JB Lippincott, 1973, pp 73–78.
7. Bakwin H: Enuresis in twins. Am J Dis Child 121:222, 1971.
8. Hallgren B: Enuresis: a clinical and genetic study. Acta Psychiatr Neuro Scand 32(suppl 114):73, 1957.
9. Kaffman M, Elizur E: Infants who become enuretics: a longitudinal study of 161 Kibbutz children. Monogr Soc Res Child Dev 42:2, 1977.
10. Kanner L: Child Psychiatry. Springfield, IL, Charles C Thomas, 1972.
11. Fergusson DM, Horwood LJ, Sannon FT: Factors related to the age of attainment of nocturnal bladder control: an 8-year longitudinal study. Pediatrics 78:884, 1986.
12. Forsythe W, Redmond A: Enuresis and spontaneous cure rate study of 1129 enuretics. Arch Dis Child 49:259, 1974.
13. Barbour RF, Borland EM, Boyd MM, et al: Enuresis as a disorder of development. Br Med J 5360:787, 1963.
14. Muellner RS: Development of urinary control in children. JAMA 172:1256, 1960.
15. Muellner RS: Obstacles to the successful treatment of primary enuresis. JAMA 178:147, 1961.
16. Troup CW, Hodgson NB: Nocturnal functional bladder capacity in enuretic children. J Urol 105:129, 1971.
17. Starfield B: Functional bladder capacity in enuretic and nonenuretic children. J Pediatr 70:777, 1967.
18. Zaleski A, Gerrard JW, Shokeir HK: Nocturnal enuresis: the importance of a small bladder capacity. In Kolvin I, MacKeith RC, Meadow SR (eds): Bladder Control and Enuresis. Philadelphia, JB Lippincott, 1973, pp 95–101.
19. Hauri P: The Sleep Disorders. Current Concepts. Kalamazoo, MI, Upjohn, 1982.

20. Ferber R: Solve Your Child's Sleep Problems. New York, Simon & Schuster, 1985.
21. Ferber R: Sleep-associated enuresis in the child. *In* Kryger MH, Roth T, Dement WC (eds): Principles and Practice of Sleep Medicine. Philadelphia, WB Saunders, 1989, pp 643–647.
22. Broughton RJ: Sleep disorders: Disorders of arousal. Science 159:1070, 1968.
23. Mikkelson EJ, Rapoport JL: Enuresis: psychopathology, sleep stage, and drug response. Urol Clin North Am 7:361, 1980.
24. Perlmutter AD: Enuresis. *In* Kelalis PP, King LR, Belman AB (eds): Clinical Pediatric Urology. Philadelphia, WB Saunders, 1985, Vol 1, pp 311–325.
25. Bostock J: Exterior gestation, primitive sleep, enuresis, and asthma: a study in aetiology. Med J Aust 2:185, 1958.
26. Boyd MM: The depth of sleep in enuretic school children and in non-enuretic controls. J Psychol Res 4:274, 1960.
27. Werry JS, Cohrssen J: Enuresis—an etiologic and therapeutic study. J Pediatr 67:423, 1965.
28. Moffatt MEK, Kato C, Pless IB: Improvements in self-concept after treatment of nocturnal enuresis: randomized controlled trial. J Pediatr 110:647, 1987.
29. Couchells SM, Bennet-Johnson S, Carter R, et al: Behavioral and environmental characteristics of treated and untreated enuretic children and match nonenuretic controls. J Pediatr 99:812, 1981.
30. Shaffer D: The association between enuresis and emotional disorder: a review of the literature. *In* Kolvin I, MacKeith RC, Meadow SR (eds): Bladder Control and Enuresis. Philadelphia, JB Lippincott, 1973, pp 118–136.
31. Morgan RT, Young GC: Parental attitudes and the conditioning of childhood enuresis. Behav Res Ther 13:197, 1975.
32. Friman PC, Warzak WJ: Nocturnal enuresis: a prevalent, persistent, yet curable parasomnia. Pediatrician 17:38, 1990.
33. Friman PC: A preventive context for enuresis. Pediatr Clin North Am 33:871, 1986.
34. Friman PC, Christophersen ER: Biobehavioral prevention in primary care. *In* Krasnegor N, Arasteh JD, Cataldo MF (eds): Child Health Behavior: A Behavioral Pediatrics Perspective. New York, John Wiley & Sons, 1986, pp 254–280.
35. Schmitt BD: Nocturnal enuresis. Prim Care 11:485, 1984.
36. Vincent SA: Mechanical, electrical and other aspects of enuresis. *In* Johnston JH, Goodwin W (eds): Reviews in Paediatric Urology. New York, Elsevier, 1974, pp 280–313.
37. Cohen MW: Enuresis. Pediatr Clin North Am 22:545, 1975.
38. Rauber A, Maroncelli R: Prescribing practices and knowledge of tricyclic antidepressants among physicians caring for children. Pediatrics 73:107, 1984.
39. Blackwell B, Currah J: The psychopharmacology of nocturnal enuresis. *In* Kolvin I, MacKeith RC, Meadow SR (eds): Bladder Control and Enuresis. Philadelphia, JB Lippincott, 1973, pp 231–257.
40. Stephenson JD: Physiological and pharmacological basis for the chemotherapy of enuresis. Psychol Med 9:249, 1979.
41. Ambrosini PJ: A pharmacological paradigm for urinary continence and enuresis. J Clin Psychopharmacol 4:247, 1984.
42. Houts AC, Peterson JK, Liebert RM: The effects of prior imipramine treatment on the results of conditioning therapy with enuresis. J Pediatr Psychol 9:505, 1984.
43. Herson VC, Schmitt BD, Rumack BH: Magical thinking and imipramine poisoning in two school-aged children. JAMA 241:1926, 1979.
44. Norgaard JP, Pedersen EB, Djurhuus JC: Diurnal antidiuretic hormone levels in enuretics. J Urol 134:1029, 1985.
45. Dimson SB: DDAVP and urine osmolality in refractory enuresis. Arch Dis Child 61:1104, 1986.
46. Novello AC, Novello R: Enuresis. Pediatr Clin North Am 34:719, 1987.
47. Post EM, Richman RA, Blackett PR, et al: Desmopressin response of enuretic children. Am J Dis Child 137:962, 1983.
48. Pedersen PS, Hejl M, Kjoller SS: Desamino-D-arginine vasopressin in childhood nocturnal enuresis. J Urol 133:65, 1985.
49. Ferrie BG, MacFarlane J, Glen ES: DDAVP in young enuretic patients: a double-blind trial. Br J Urol 56:376, 1984.
50. Mountjoy PT, Ruben DH, Bradford TS: Recent technological advancements in the treatment of enuresis. Behav Modif 8:291, 1984.
51. Mowrer OH, Mowrer WM: Enuresis—a method for its study and treatment. Am J Orthopsychiatry 8:436, 1938.
52. Doleys DM: Behavioral treatments for nocturnal enuresis in children: a review of the recent literature. Psychol Bul 84:30, 1977.
53. Wagner W, Johnson SB, Walker D, et al: A controlled comparison of two treatments for nocturnal enuresis. J Pediatr 101:302, 1982.
54. Wille S: Comparison of desmopressin and enuresis alarm for nocturnal enuresis. Arch Dis Child 61:30, 1986.
55. Fournier JP, Garfinkel BD, Bond A, et al: Pharmacological and behavioral management of enuresis. J Am Acad Child Adolesc Psychiatry 26:849, 1987.
56. Werry J: The conditioning treatment of enuresis. Am J Psychiatry 123:226, 1966.
57. Starfield B, Mellits ED: Increases in functional bladder capacity and improvements in enuresis. J Pediatr 72:483, 1968.
58. Kegel AH: Physiologic therapy for urinary stress incontinence. JAMA 146:915, 1951.
59. Scharf M: Waking Up Dry. Cincinnati, Writer's Digest Books, 1986.
60. Oswald K, Taylor AM, Treisman M: Discriminative responses to stimulation during human sleep. Brain 83:440, 1960.
61. Zung WW, Wilson WP: Responses to auditory stimulation during sleep. Arch Gen Psychiatry 4:548, 1961.
62. Bollard J, Nettlebeck T: A component analysis of dry-bed training for treatment of bedwetting. Behav Res Ther 20:383, 1982.
63. Creer TL, Davis MH: Using a staggered waking procedure with enuretic children in an institutional setting. J Behav Ther Exp Psychiatry 6:23, 1975.

Nonarousal Parasomnias in the Child

MARK W. MAHOWALD and MICHAEL J. THORPY

Parasomnias are undesirable motor, autonomic, or experiential phenomena that occur exclusively or predominately during the sleeping state.[1] Although the most common parasomnias in children are the disorders of arousal (confusional arousals, sleepwalking, and sleep terrors [see Chapter 11]), many other parasomnias exist, which may closely or exactly mimic them. Most of these other parasomnias can be readily diagnosed and treated. The purpose of this chapter is to briefly review these parasomnias which may occur in children and be confused with the disorders of arousal, with emphasis on clinical manifestation, diagnosis, and treatment. The overlapping nature of these parasomnias is illustrated in Figure 13–1. The parasomnias are divided into two major categories: primary—those disorders that are the manifestation of the sleep state per se and secondary—disorders that are symptoms originating in other organ systems and occur in or are precipitated by the sleeping state (Table 13–1).[2, 3]

Primary

Disorders of Arousal

These are the most common childhood parasomnias and are thoroughly discussed in Chapter 11.

REM Sleep Behavior Disorder

The REM sleep behavior disorder (RBD) is a recently described syndrome; the existence of which was predicted from animal experiments over 25 years ago (see also Kryger MH, et al: Principles and Practice of Sleep Medicine, 2nd ed, Chap 57.)[4] Normally, REM sleep is associated with somatic motor paralysis (sparing the diaphragm and extraocular muscles). This atonia may act as a protective measure by preventing the acting-out of dreams. In RBD, the expected REM-related atonia is absent, resulting in dramatic and occasionally injurious behavior during dreams.[5, 6] Although usually idiopathic and tending to affect older males, it has been reported in children[7, 8] and may be associated with a variety of primary neurologic diseases. RBD may be another manifestation of motor dyscontrol that occurs in children and adolescents with narcolepsy.[9] Treatment with low-dose bedtime clonazepam is very effective.[5]

Recurrent Hypnagogic Hallucinations/ Sleep Paralysis

Hypnagogic (occurring at sleep onset) and hypnopompic (occurring at end of sleep) hallucinations (HH) and sleep paralysis (SP) may occur spontaneously in otherwise healthy individuals. These experiences may be very frightening to the child, as there is the combination of dream mentation occurring during awareness of the true environment, thereby making differentiation between reality and dreaming impossible. For instance, a child may see dream people or animals in the bedroom, may be spoken to by dream images, think the phone is ringing, or hear imaginary conversations. All sensory modalities (visual, auditory, tactile, olfactory, and gustatory) may be in-

OVERLAPPING PARASOMNIAS

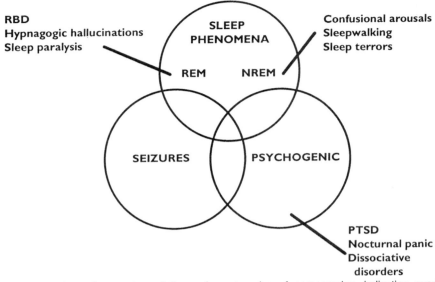

Figure 13–1. A schematic overview of the major categories of parasomnias, indicating overlapping boundaries.

volved. SP occurs when there is a persistence of REM sleep atonia into wakefulness, resulting in wakeful mentation associated with somatic paralysis, which spares eye movements and usually respiration. SP may be frightening, as it typically follows a conventional REM sleep period, accentuating and prolonging the fear that may have accompanied the preceding dream. It usually ends spontaneously but may be terminated by touching the child.[10] HH and SP frequently occur in combination. They are excellent examples of dissociated states, representing the admixture of wakefulness and isolated REM sleep phenomena (dreaming and paralysis).[11]

Although seen frequently in narcolepsy (see Chapter 14),[12, 13] HH and SP as isolated symptoms may be experienced by non-narcoleptic patients[14–16] (particularly following sleep deprivation) and are occasionally familial in nature.[17, 18] In the absence of other symptoms of narcolepsy, further evaluation is usually unnecessary and reassurance is sufficient.

Table 13–1. DIFFERENTIAL DIAGNOSIS OF CHILDHOOD PARASOMNIAS

Primary
Disorders of arousal
REM sleep behavior disorder
Recurrent hypnagogic hallucinations/sleep paralysis
Bruxism
Rhythmic movement disorder
Periodic limb movement disorder
Sleep starts
Sleeptalking
Secondary
Neurologic
  Seizures
  Headaches
  Muscle cramps
Arousals triggering parasomnias
  Apnea
  Gastroesophageal reflux
  Seizures
Sleep-related expiratory groaning
Psychiatric
  Post-traumatic stress disorder
  Nocturnal panic
  Psychogenic dissociative states/malingering

Bruxism

Bruxism is a parafunctional grinding or clenching of the teeth which may occur during sleep. Differing definitions and population samples result in the reported prevalence of bruxism in children ranging from 7 to 88%.[19] It may occur during any stage of sleep, both REM and NREM, and is not associated with any specific mentation.[20, 21] The force of nocturnal bruxing may actually exceed that obtainable with conscious clenching[22] and, in severe cases, may result in damage to the teeth and surounding structures.[23]

Many etiologic factors have been proposed, including: local (malocclusion), systemic, psychologic, occupational, and developmental, but none has been established as prominent. A genetic component is present.[24] A popular concept of bruxism is that it is a primary disorder of sleep, and therefore centrally mediated—but, as with other centrally mediated conditions, it may be precipitated or exacerbated by stress.[25] Recent studies indicate that bruxism may actually represent the symptom of a number of different disorders, including simple bruxism, orofacial dyskinesia, mandibular dystonia, and tremor.[26] Sleep bruxism may be the manifestation of mild RBD[27] or part of a more generalized sleep movement disorder.[28] In many cases, the etiology may be multifactorial.

As would be expected in a condition of diverse etiologies, the proposed treatments are legion, and usually lack scientifically validated objective results. Therapy has included occlusal adjustment and splints, psychotherapy, and medications—without predictable or significant improvement.[29, 30] The response to interocclusal appliances is variable, and there appears to be a greater subjective than objective response. Other treatment options include nonsteroidal anti-inflammatory agents, stress management (such as diurnal and nocturnal biofeedback, counseling, avoidance conditioning, hypnosis and progressive relaxation, and occupational and life-style changes), physical therapy, or muscle relaxants such as diazepam.[31] Suggestive hypnotherapy has been found to be subjectively effective.[32]

The recent trend to subclassify bruxism according to documented etiology is to be encouraged. Now that more is known about bruxism, more treatments are available and will depend upon the identified cause. For instance, promising results have been obtained with contingent afferent electrical stimulation of the lip for common bruxism and with botulinum toxin for bruxism associated with orofacial dystonia and dyskinesia.[33] Formal sleep studies to rule out nocturnal seizures are indicated in individuals who experience significant oral damage.

Rhythmic Movement Disorder

Rhythmic movement disorder (RMD) applies to a group of stereotyped movements occurring at sleep onset or at the end of sleep. These movements occur on a broad spectrum, including headbanging, headrolling, and bodyrocking. Headbanging is the most prominent form, characterized by occasionally violent anteroposterior head movements. These movements are usually into a pillow but may be into the side of the crib or wall. Headrolling is associated with side-to-side movements of the head, with the subject usually in the supine position. Bodyrocking is often performed while on the hands and knees, with anteroposterior thrusting of the entire body into a pillow or other object.[34] These repetitive movements may be associated with rhythmic "humming" sounds, which may be quite bothersome to other household members.

RMD usually begins during the first 9 months of life, and rarely after the age of 2 years. RMD tends to decrease with increasing age; rarely, it persists into adolescence or adulthood. Klackenberg's[35] study indicates a combined incidence of all rhythmic movements of 60% at 9 months, 22% at 2 years, and 5% at 5 years of age. Although the majority of children experiencing RMD have episodes just prior to sleep onset, up to one-third have movements that continue into lighter stages of NREM sleep, and rarely during slow wave (Fig. 13–2) or REM sleep. The duration of a given episode is typically less than 15 minutes but may last up to several hours. Injuries are infrequent, although soft-tissue injury to the forehead and eyes (in the form of corneal abrasions and cataracts) have resulted from headbanging in mentally retarded children.[36]

There is no apparent association between RMD and neuropsychiatric conditions except in individuals with severe neurologic dysfunction. Rarely, headbanging may the sole manifestation of a seizure disorder.[37] In most cases, no specific treatment is needed, and the parent and child can be reassured as to the benign and usually self-limited nature of the events.[34] In children whose rocking behaviors appear to be attention-getting, behavioral contracts may be effective. Sometimes, RMD occurs during wakefulness in bed and can be reduced by restricting the time in bed. In difficult cases, behavioral techniques such as overpracticing of rhythmic behavior[38] or the judicious use of benzodiazepines may be effective.[36]

Periodic Limb Movement Disorder

The periodic limb movement disorder (PLMD) occasionally occurs in childhood, but its prevalence and significance are unknown

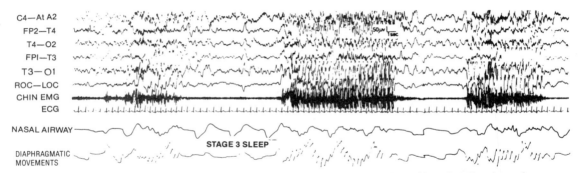

Figure 13–2. Three headbanging episodes occurring during stage 3 sleep. Note that the deep sleep continues without interruption. CHIN EMG, Chin electromyogram; ECG, electrocardiogram.

(see also Kryger MH, et al: Principles and Practice of Sleep Medicine, 2nd ed, Chap 58). PLMD is characterized by the *periodic* (every 20–40 sec) and *sustained* (0.5–4.0 sec in duration) contractions of one or both anterior tibialis muscles often associated with unperceived arousals.[39] Although PLMD is typically benign, it can be associated with metabolic disorders and has been reported in association with childhood leukemia.[40] PLMD should not be confused with the motor sleep start, which occurs infrequently during sleep (discussed below). Some cases of PLMD are very dramatic, involving the four extremities and the trunk. Rarely, similarly prominent limb jerks represent repetitive myoclonic seizures.

Sleep Starts

Sleep starts, or hypnic jerks, are common experiences, usually occurring during the transition between wakefulness and sleep. The most common is the motor sleep start—a sudden body jerk that may awaken or startle the subject or bedpartner.[41] Other less common but occasionally frightening types include: (1) visual—a sudden, blinding flash of light, (2) auditory—a loud cracking or snapping noise in the head, and (3) somesthetic—pain or flowing sensations. The mechanism of sleep starts is uncertain. One suggestion is that they represent a sudden intrusion of an isolated REM sleep event into light NREM sleep.[42] Although they rarely cause sleep-onset insomnia, sleep starts generally are of no clinical significance. They should not be confused with PLMD, myoclonic seizures, or other neurologic phenomena. Reassurance of their usually benign and ubiquitous nature is usually sufficient treatment. Neurologic or psychiatric evaluation is unwarranted.

Sleeptalking

Sleeptalking (somniloquy) is a common disorder which may arise from either REM or NREM sleep. Sleeptalking occurring in REM sleep more often is associated with recall of sleep mentation.[43, 44] There may be a genetic component.[45] Sleeptalking is rarely of clinical significance unless unusually frequent or loud but may be problematic in situations where two or more children share a bedroom. No treatment studies are available.

Secondary

Neurologic

Seizures

Nocturnal seizures represent the most common masquerader of disorders of arousal and are commonly misdiagnosed. Although infrequent, they must be considered in any case of recurrent, unusual nocturnal behaviors. They may take many forms.

Recurrent Dreams, Nightmares, or Sleepwalking (Episodic Nocturnal Wanderings).[46–55] Although in the laboratory, these episodes may be diagnosed as seizures, they may be indistinguishable clinically from disorders of arousal. They do respond to anticonvulsants.

Recurrent Isolated Arousals.[56–60] Such symptoms may be the sole manifestation of seizures. Affected children often do not experience diurnal seizures and present with complaints of sleep-maintenance insomnia or excessive daytime sleepiness resulting from the seizure-induced sleep fragmentation. These arousals may be the manifestation of seizures arising from deep foci.[61]

Unusual Autonomic Symptoms.[62–64] Virtually

any isolated autonomic symptom may be the manifestation of a seizure (i.e., pain,[65] apnea,[66–68] stridor,[69] coughing,[70] choking,[71] emesis,[72–74] laryngospasm,[75, 76] chest pain and arrhythmias,[77–80] piloerection,[81] paroxysmal flushing, and localized hyperhidrosis[82, 83]). Such spells are routinely misdiagnosed as being symptoms of non-neurologic organ-system dysfunction.

Nocturnal Paroxysmal Dystonia (NPD). This condition is characterized by predominantly or exclusively nocturnal episodes of coarse, occasionally violent, movements of the limbs associated with tonic spasms and often occurring multiple times nightly. There are often no scalp EEG abnormalities seen during the clinical spell, and the diagnosis may be suspected by the fact that the arousals, when captured on videotape, are extremely stereotypic in nature. NPD most likely represents an epileptic phenomenon, probably emanating from the frontal lobe.[84, 85]

Seizures must be considered in *any* sleep-related behavior that is recurrent, stereotyped, or inappropriate regardless of the specific nature of that behavior. These unusual seizure syndromes have been recently reviewed.[86] Prevalence data are not available. Nocturnal seizures with unusual presentations are undoubtedly more common than generally realized; however, they are often underdiagnosed and may be misdiagnosed because of certain features occasionally found: (1) absence of scalp EEG abnormalities, (2) bizarre nature of the clinical manifestations, leading to the suspicion of psychiatric disorders or isolated autonomic phenomena that are misattributed to disorders of other organ systems, and (3) preservation of consciousness during the seizure.[86] The treatment of all nocturnal seizures is similar to that of diurnal seizures.

Other apparently primary parasomnias such as RMD[87] and PLMD may actually be the manifestation of a seizure disorder. The converse is also true that nocturnal seizures may be epiphenomena of secondary parasomnias. Obstructive sleep apnea may be present and be misdiagnosed as a nocturnal seizure disorder.[88, 89] Diffuse esophageal spasm in infants may result in clinical behaviors that can be confused with seizures.[90]

Headaches

Although rare in children, cluster headaches, chronic paroxysmal hemicrania, and migraine have been shown, in some cases, to be REM sleep related, explaining the common report of sleep-related headaches in these conditions (see also Kryger MH, et al: Principles and Practice of Sleep Medicine, 2nd ed, Chap 49).[91–93] The obstructive sleep apnea syndrome[94] and carbon monoxide intoxication may also present with sleep-related headaches.[95]

Muscle Cramps

The complaint of muscle cramping, frequently nocturnal, is common in children. The true incidence and etiology are unknown, as there has been no systematic study of this phenomenon. There may be a familial component.[96]

Arousals Triggering Parasomnias

A wide variety of stimuli may trigger a clinical disorder of arousal in susceptible individuals. In this context, arousals induced by other sleep disorders such as apnea,[3] gastroesophageal reflux,[90] or seizures may present as typical confusional arousals, sleepwalking, or sleep terrors.

Sleep-Related Expiratory Groaning

Anecdotal cases of sleep-related dyspnea, choking, and expiratory groaning have been reported. The etiology and treatment are unclear.[97] It must be remembered that paroxysmal nocturnal choking may be the sole manifestation of a nocturnal seizure, masquerading as primary gastrointestinal or pulmonary disease.[98]

Psychiatric

Post-Traumatic Stress Disorder

Post-traumatic stress disorder (PTSD) is often associated with prominent sleep complaints and nightmares.[99–101] PTSD may be seen following any "psychologically distressing event that is beyond the range of usual human experience."[102] PTSD occurs in children who have experienced catastrophic trauma such as physical or sexual abuse.[103–105] No formal sleep studies in children with PTSD have been reported, but studies in adult PTSD patients indicate that nocturnal PTSD episodes represent neither conventional REM anxiety attacks nor simple sleep terrors.[106] Prevalence data are not available. Because some children presenting with apparent sleep terrors or sleepwalking may be experiencing PTSD, a history of severe physical or psychic trauma should be sought in all cases. Treatment may be difficult and protracted. Counseling or pharmacologic treatment with imipramine or alprazolam has been reported to be effective in adults.[107–109] Propranolol has also been reported effective in acute PTSD in children.[110]

Nocturnal Panic

It is clear that symptoms of panic disorder may occur during sleep. In some individuals, panic attacks occur exclusively during the sleeping state; in others, the diurnal symptoms may "spill over" into the sleeping state.[111, 112] Prevalence data are not available, but panic disorder does occur in children and adolescents.[113] Adults with panic disorder often report onset in childhood.[114, 115] Little data are available regarding treatment of childhood panic, but tricyclic antidepressants or benzodiazepines may be effective.[116, 117] The simultaneous onset of panic and SW/ST has been reported.[118] The overlap of symptoms of nocturnal panic and other parasomnias (sleep terrors, gastroesophageal reflux, obstructive sleep apnea, nocturnal asthma, and seizures with fear/autonomic symptoms) dictates caution in diagnosis and case reporting.[86]

Psychogenic Dissociative States/ Malingering

Bizarre, violent, or injurious behaviors due to psychogenic dissociative states occurring during the sleep period have been described both in adults and adolescents.[119–121] Childhood physical or sexual abuse is a common historic feature.[122] Psychogenic dissociative disorders are rare and should be diagnosed only after exclusion of all other parasomnias. PSG evaluation reveals complex motor behavior arising from a period of clear EEG wakefulness during the sleep period. Treatment requires specialized psychiatric intervention.[122]

Evaluation

The clinical presentation of these unusual parasomnias may be distressingly similar, and it is often impossible to differentiate among them by history alone. Disorders of arousal will account for the vast majority of childhood parasomnias and usually do not require formal evaluation or treatment when the diagnosis appears to be clear. Indications for evaluation and/or treatment are: (1) potentially violent or injurious behaviors, (2) disruption of other household members, (3) resultant excessive daytime sleepiness, (4) atypical features (nature of the behaviors, time of night, age of onset, frequency), or (5) history of known seizures. In these situations, a detailed history and physical examination (with particular emphasis on the neurologic and psychiatric components) followed by exacting PSG evaluation is indicated. Such evaluation must include extensive PSG monitoring with a full scalp EEG montage, a paper speed of at least 15 mm/second, and continuous audiovisual monitoring with detailed technician observation performed in a center experienced in evaluating these disorders. Prolonged video-EEG (long-term monitoring [LTM]) with a full headset may be helpful. Ambulatory studies are not adequate.

Treatment

Treatment of parasomnias depends on the identified etiology. Once the proper diagnosis is established, the vast majority are treatable by either behavioral or pharmacologic means.[3, 123] There may be daytime behavioral consequences of parasomnias in the form of hypersomnia, irritability, or embarrassment. Environmental safety measures may be needed (securing doors, sleeping on the first floor, the use of door/window alarms, removal of furniture with sharp corners from the bedroom). The potentially adverse psychologic or pharmacologic consequences of erroneous diagnosis and treatment may be significant (i.e., psychotherapy for enuresis due to nocturnal seizures or obstructive sleep apnea, or chronic administration of anticonvulsant medication for "spells" representing disorders of arousal).

Summary

Although disorders of arousal constitute the majority of unusual behavioral and experiential phenomena occurring during sleep, it must be remembered that there are many other conditions that mimic them. In enigmatic cases, appropriate clinical and sleep laboratory evaluation will usually result in a correct diagnosis, with effective therapeutic implications. Erroneous diagnosis may lead to ineffective and potentially detrimental behavioral or pharmacologic treatment. Continued evaluation of unusual or difficult cases will undoubtedly lead to greater understanding of these disorders. The overlap of symptoms dictates the use of exacting diagnostic criteria in case reporting.

References

1. Diagnostic Classification Steering Committee, Thorpy MJ, Chairman. International Classification of Sleep Disorders: Diagnostic and Coding Manual. Rochester, MN, American Sleep Disorders Association, 1990, p 141.
2. Mahowald MW, Ettinger MG: Things that go bump in the night: the parasomnias revisited. J Clin Neurophysiol 7:119, 1990.
3. Mahowald MW, Rosen GM: Parasomnias in children. Pediatrician 17:21, 1990.
4. Jouvet M, Delorme F: Locus coeruleus et sommeil paradoxal. C R Soc Biol 159:895, 1965.
5. Schenck CH, Bundlie SR, Ettinger MG, et al: Chronic behavioral disorders of human REM sleep: a new category of parasomnia. Sleep 9:293, 1986.
6. Schenck CH, Bundlie SR, Patterson AL, et al: Rapid eye movement sleep behavior disorder. A treatable parasomnia affecting older adults. JAMA 257:1786, 1987.
7. Schenck CH, Bundlie SR, Smith SA, et al: REM behavior disorder in a 10-year-old girl and aperiodic REM and NREM sleep movements in an 8-year-old brother. Sleep Res 15:162, 1986.
8. Herman JH, Blaw ME, Steinberg JB: REM behavior disorder in a two-year-old male with evidence of brainstem pathology. Sleep Res 18:242, 1989.
9. Schenck CH, Mahowald MW: Motor dyscontrol in narcolepsy: REM sleep without atonia and REM sleep behavior disorder. Ann Neurol 32:3, 1992.
10. Schneck JM: Sleep Paralysis. Am J Psychiatry 108:921, 1952.
11. Mahowald MW, Schenck CH: Status dissociatus—a perspective on states of being. Sleep 14:69, 1991.
12. Bowling G, Richards NG: Diagnosis and treatment of the narcoleptic syndrome. Cleve Clin Quart 28:38, 1961.
13. Parkes JD, Baraitser M, Marsden CD, et al: Natural history, symptoms, and treatment of the narcoleptic syndrome. Acta Neurol Scand 52:337, 1975.
14. Snyder S, Hams G: Serotonergic agents in the treatment of isolated sleep paralysis. Am J Psychiatry 139:1202, 1982.
15. Snyder S: Isolated sleep paralysis after rapid time zone change ("jet lag") syndrome. Chronobiologia 10:377, 1983.
16. Penn NE, Kripke DF, Scharff J: Sleep paralysis among medical students. J Psychol 107:247, 1981.
17. Roth B, Bruhova S, Berkova L: Familial sleep paralysis. Arch Suisses Neurol Neurochir Psychiatrie 102:1321, 1968.
18. McDonald C: A clinical study of hypnagogic hallucinations. Br J Psychiatry 118:543, 1971.
19. Attanasio R: Nocturnal bruxism and its clinical management. Dent Clin North Am 35:245, 1991.
20. Glaros AG: Incidence of diurnal and nocturnal bruxism. J Prosthet Dent 45:545, 1981.
21. Rugh JD, Harlan J: Nocturnal bruxism and temporomandibular disorders. Adv Neurol 49:329, 1988.
22. Clarke NG, Townsend GC, Carey SE: Bruxing patterns in man during sleep. J Oral Rehabil 11:123, 1984.
23. Ware JC, Rugh JD: Destructive bruxism: sleep stage relationship. Sleep 11:172, 1988.
24. Abe K, Shimakawa M: Genetic and developmental aspects of sleeptalking and teeth-grinding. Acta Paedopsychiatr 33:339, 1966.
25. Satoh T, Harada Y: Tooth-grinding during sleep as an arousal reaction. Experientia 15:785, 1971.
26. Clark GT, Koyano K, Browne PA: Oral motor disorders in humans. Calif Dent Assn J 21:19, 1993.
27. Tachibana N, Yamanaka K, Kaji R, et al: Sleep bruxism as a manifestation of subclinical rapid eye movement sleep behavior disorder. Sleep 17:555, 1994.
28. Sjoholm T, Polo O, Ikkala C, Alihanka J: Body movements during sleep in teethgrinders. In Horne J (ed): Sleep '90. Pontenagel Press, Bochum, 1990, pp 226–228.
29. Nadler SC: Bruxism, a classification: critical review. J Am Dent Assoc 54:615, 1957.
30. Gallagher SJ: Diagnosis and treatment of bruxism: a review of the literature. Gen Dent 28:62, 1980.
31. Attanasio R: Nocturnal bruxism and its clinical management. Dent Clin North Am 35:245, 1991.
32. Clarke JH, Reynolds PJ: Suggestive hypnotherapy for nocturnal bruxism: a pilot study. Am J Clin Hypn 33:248, 1991.
33. Clark GT, Koyano K, Browne PA: Oral motor disorders in humans. Calif Dent Assn J 21:19, 1993.
34. Thorpy MJ, Glovinsky PB: Parasomnias. Psychiatr Clin North Am 10:623, 1987.
35. Klackenberg G: Rhythmic movements in infancy and early childhood. Acta Pediatr Scand 224:(Suppl)74, 1971.
36. Thorpy MJ: Rhythmic movement disorder. In Thorpy MJ (ed): Handbook of Sleep Disorders. New York, Marcel Dekker, 1990, pp 609–629.
37. Guilleminault C, Sylvestri R: Disorders of arousal and epilepsy during sleep. In Sterman MB, Shouse MN, Passouant P (eds): Sleep and Epilepsy. New York, Academic Press, 1982, pp 513–531.
38. Decatanzaro DA, Baldwin G: Effective treatment of self-injurious behavior through a force arm exercise. Am J Ment Defic 82:433, 1978.
39. Montplaisir J, Godbout R, Pelletier G, Warnes H: Restless legs syndrome and periodic movements during sleep. In Kryger MH, Roth T, Dement WC (eds): Principles and Practice of Sleep Medicine, 2nd ed. Philadelphia, WB Saunders, 1994, pp 589–597.
40. Kotogal S, Chu J-Y, O'Connor DM: Nocturnal myoclonus—a sleep disturbance in children with leukemia. Ann Neurol 16:392, 1984.
41. Parkes JD: The parasomnias. Lancet 8514:1021, 1986.
42. Carskadon MA, Dement WC: Normal human sleep: an overview. In Kryger MH, Roth T, Dement WC, (eds): Principles and Practice of Sleep Medicine, 2nd ed. Philadelphia, WB Saunders, 1994, pp 16–25.
43. Arkin AM, Toth MF, Baker J, et al: The frequency of sleep talking in the laboratory among chronic sleep talkers and good dream recallers. J Nerv Ment Dis 151:369, 1970.
44. Arkin AM, Toth MF, Baker J, et al: The degree of

concordance between the content of sleep talking and mentation recalled in wakefulness. J Nerv Ment Dis 151:375, 1970.

45. Abe K, Shimakawa M: Genetic and developmental aspects of sleepwalking and teeth grinding. Acta Paedopsychiatr 33:339, 1966.

46. Epstein AW, Hill W: Ictal phenomena during REM sleep of a temporal lobe epileptic. Arch Neurology 15:367, 1966.

47. Boller F, Wright DG, Cavalieri R, et al: Paroxysmal "nightmares." Neurology 25:1026, 1975.

48. Snyder CH: Epileptic equivalents in children. Pediatrics 21:308, 1958.

49. Epstein AW: Recurrent dreams. Their relationship to temporal lobe seizures. Arch Gen Psychiatry 10:49, 1964.

50. Fuster B, Castells C, Etcheverry M: Epileptic sleep terrors. Neurology 4:53, 1954.

51. Montplaisir J, Laveriere M, Saint-Hilaire JM: Sleep and temporal lobe epilepsy: a case study with depth electrodes. Neurology 31:1352, 1981.

52. Drake ME, Jr: Cursive and cursing epilepsy. Neurology 34:267, 1984.

53. Halbreich U, Assael M: Electroencephalogram with sphenoidal needles in sleepwalkers. Psychiatr Clin (Basel) 11:213, 1978.

54. Spire J-P, Maselli R: Episodic nocturnal wandering: further evidence of an epileptic disorder. Neurology 33(Suppl 2):215, 1983.

55. Popoviciu L: Frontier states between sleep incidents and nocturnal epileptic attacks. In Koella WP, Levin P (eds): Sleep 1976. Third European Congress of Sleep Research. Montpellier. Basel, S. Karger, 1977, pp 65–74.

56. Niedermeyer E, Walker AE: Mesio-frontal epilepsy. Electroencephalogr Clin Neurophysiol 31:104, 1971.

57. Erba G, Cavazzuti V: Pure tonic seizures with arousal. Sleep Res 10:164, 1981.

58. Benner RP, Atkinson R. Generalized paroxysmal fast activity: electroencephalographic and clinical features. Ann Neurol 11:386, 1982.

59. Peled R, Lavie P: Paroxysmal awakenings from sleep associated with excessive daytime somnolence: a form of nocturnal epilepsy. Neurology 36:95, 1986.

60. Erba G, Ferber R: Sleep disruption by subclinical seizure activity as a cause of increased waking seizures and decreased daytime function. Sleep Res 12:307, 1983.

61. Montagna P, Sforza E, Tinuper P, et al: Paroxysmal arousals during sleep. Neurology 40:1063, 1990.

62. Mulder DW, Daly D, Bailey AA: Visceral epilepsy. Arch Intern Med 93:481, 1954.

63. Brown RW, McLeod WR: Sympathetic stimulation with temporal lobe epilepsy. Med J Aust 2:274, 1973.

64. Van Buren JM: Some autonomic concomitants of ictal automatism. A study of temporal lobe attacks. Brain 81:505, 1958.

65. Trevathan E, Cascino GD: Partial epilepsy presenting as focal paroxysmal pain. Neurology 38:329, 1988.

66. Sanmarti FX, Estivill E, Campistol J, et al: Apneic episodes in an infant: exceptional epileptic seizures. Electroencephalogr Clin Neurophysiol 60:16, 1985.

67. Walls TJ, Newman PK, Cumming WJK: Recurrent apnoeic attacks as a manifestation of epilepsy. Postgrad Med J 57:575, 1981.

68. Monod N, Peirano P, Plouin P, et al: Seizure-induced apnea. Ann N Y Acad Sci 533:411, 1988.

69. Maytal J, Resnick TH: Stridor presenting as the sole manifestation of seizures. Ann Neurol 18:414, 1985.

70. Winans HM: Epileptic equivalents, a cause for somatic symptoms. Am J Med 7:150, 1949.

71. Brown LW, Fry JM: Paroxysmal nocturnal choking: a newly described manifestation of sleep-related epilepsy. Sleep Res 17:153, 1988.

72. Kramer RE, Luders H, Goldstick LP, et al: Ictus emeticus: an electroclinical analysis. Neurology 38:1048, 1988.

73. Panayiotopoulos CP: Benign nocturnal childhood occipital epilepsy: a new syndrome with nocturnal seizures, tonic deviation of the eyes, and vomiting. J Child Neurol 4:43, 1989.

74. Panayiotopoulos CP: Benign childhood epilepsy with occipital paroxysms: a 15-year prospective study. Ann Neurol 26:51, 1989.

75. Ravindran M: Temporal lobe seizure presenting as "laryngospasm." Clin Electroencephalogr 12:139, 1981.

76. Amir J, Ashkenazi S, Schonfeld T, et al: Laryngospasm as a single manifestation of epilepsy. Arch Dis Child 58:151, 1983.

77. Devinsky O, Price BH, Cohen SI: Cardiac manifestations of complex partial seizures. Am J Med 80:195, 1986.

78. Kiok MC, Terrence CF, Fromm GH, et al: Sinus arrest in epilepsy. Neurology 36:115, 1986.

79. Gilchrist JM: Arrhythmogenic seizures; diagnosis by simultaneous EEG/ECG recording. Neurology 35:1503, 1985.

80. Hockman CH, Mauck HP, Hoff EC: ECG changes resulting from cerebral stimulation. II. A spectrum of ventricular arrhythmias of sympathetic origin. Am Heart J 71:695, 1966.

81. Brogna CG, Lee SI, Dreifuss FE: Pilomotor seizures. Magnetic resonance imaging and electroencephalographic localization of originating focus. Arch Neurol 43:1085, 1986.

82. Metz SA, Halter JB, Porte D Jr, et al: Autonomic epilepsy: clonidine blockade of paroxysmal catecholamine release and flushing. Ann Intern Med 88:189, 1978.

83. Kuritzky A, Hering R, Goldhammer G, et al: Clonidine treatment in paroxysmal localized hyperhidrosis. Arch Neurol 41:1210, 1984.

84. Tinuper P, Cerullo A, Cirignotta F, et al: Nocturnal paroxysmal dystonia with short lasting attacks: three cases with evidence for an epileptic frontal lobe origin of seizures. Epilepsia 31:549, 1990.

85. Kotagal P, Luders H, Morris HH, et al: Dystonic posturing in complex partial seizures of temporal lobe onset: a new lateralizing sign. Neurology 39:196, 1989.

86. Mahowald MW, Schenck CH: Parasomnia purgatory—the epileptic/non-epileptic parasomnia interface. In Rowan AJ, Gates J (eds): Non-epileptic Seizures. Boston, Butterworth–Heinemann, 1993, pp 123–139.

87. Guilleminault C, Silvestri R: Disorders of arousal and epilepsy during sleep. In Sterman MB, Shouse MN, Passouant P (eds): Sleep and Epilepsy. New York, Academic Press, 1982, pp 513–531.

88. Cirignotta F, Zucconi M, Mondini S, et al: Cerebral anoxic attacks in sleep apnea syndrome. Sleep 12:400, 1989.

89. Wyler AR, Weymuller EA, Jr: Epilepsy complicated by sleep apnea. Ann Neurol 9:403, 1981.

90. Wyllie E, Wyllie R, Rothner AD, et al: Another paroxysmal disorder of the differential diagnosis of seizures in infants: diffuse esophageal spasms. Ann Neurol 24:328, 1988.

91. Dexter JD, Weitzman ED: The relationship of nocturnal headaches to sleep stage patterns. Neurology 20:513, 1970.
92. Dexter JD, Riley TL: Studies in nocturnal migraine. Headache 15:51, 1975.
93. Kayed K, Godtlibsen OB, Sjaastad O: Chronic paroxysmal hemicrania. IV: "REM sleep locked" nocturnal headache attacks. Sleep 1:91, 1978.
94. Guilleminault C: Obstructive sleep apnea in children. *In* Guilleminault C (ed): Sleep and its disorders in children. New York, Raven Press, 1987, pp 213–224.
95. Thompson AE: Environmental emergencies. *In* Fleisher G, Ludwig S (eds): Textbook of Pediatric Emergency Medicine. Baltimore, Williams and Wilkins, 1983, pp 582–603.
96. Jacobsen JH, Rosenberg AS, Huttenlocher PR, et al: Familial nocturnal cramping. Sleep 9:54, 1986.
97. DeRoeck J, Van Hoof E, Cluydts R: Sleep-related expiratory groaning: a case report. Sleep Res 12:237, 1983.
98. Brown LW, Fry JM: Paroxysmal nocturnal choking: a newly described manifestation of sleep-related epilepsy. Sleep Res 17:153, 1988.
99. Van Der Kolk B, Blitz R, Burr W, et al: Nightmares and trauma: a comparison of nightmares after combat with lifelong nightmares in veterans. Am J Psychiatry 141:187, 1984.
100. Lavie P, Hefez A, Halperin G, et al: Long-term effects of traumatic war-related events on sleep. Am J Psychiatry 136:175, 1979.
101. Ross RJ, Ball WA, Sullivan KA, et al: Sleep disturbance as the hallmark of posttraumatic stress disorder. Am J Psychiatry 146:697, 1989.
102. American Psychiatric Association: Diagnostic and Statistical Manual of Mental Disorders, 3rd ed, revised. Washington, DC, American Psychiatric Association 1987, p 247.
103. Terr L: Children of Chowchilla: study of psychic trauma. Psychoanal Study Child 34:547, 1979.
104. Pynoos RS, Frederick C, Nader K, et al: Life threat and posttraumatic stress in school-age children. Arch Gen Psychiatry 44:1057, 1987.
105. Kiser LJ, Ackerman BJ, Brown E, et al: Post-traumatic stress disorder in young children: a reaction to purported sexual abuse. J Am Acad Child Adolesc Psychiatry 27:645, 1988.
106. Kramer M, Schoen LS, Kinney L: The dream experiences in dreaming-disturbed Vietnam veterans. *In* Van Der Kolk BA (ed): Post-traumatic Stress Disorder: Psychological and Biological Sequelae. Washington, DC, American Psychiatric Press, 1984, pp 82–95.
107. Modlin H: Posttraumatic stress disorder—no longer just for war veterans. Postgrad Med 79:26, 1986.
108. Brett EA, Ostroff R: Imagery and posttraumatic stress disorder: an overview. Am J Psychiatry 142:417, 1985.
109. Marshall JR: The treatment of night terrors associated with the posttraumatic stress syndrome. Am J Psychiatry 132:293, 1975.
110. Famularo R, Kinscherff R, Fenton T: Propranolol treatment for childhood posttraumatic stress disorder, acute type. A pilot study. Am J Dis Child 142:1244, 1988.
111. Mellman TA, Uhde TW: Sleep panic attacks: new clinical findings and theoretical implications. Am J Psychiatry 146:1204, 1989.
112. Craske MG, Barlow DH: Nocturnal panic. J Nerv Ment Dis 177:160, 1989.
113. Bradley SJ: Panic disorder in children and adolescents: a review with examples. Adolesc Psychiatry 17:422, 1990.
114. Vitiello B, Behar D, Wolfson S, et al: Diagnosis of panic disorder in prepuberal children. J Am Acad Child Adolesc Psychiatry 29:782, 1990.
115. Black B, Robbins DR: Panic disorder in children and adolescents. J Am Acad Child Adolesc Psychiatry 29:36, 1990.
116. Ballenger JC, Carek DJ, Steele JJ, et al: Three cases of panic disorder with agoraphobia in children. Am J Psychiatry 146:922, 1989.
117. Biederman J: Clonazepam in the treatment of prepuberal children with panic-like symptoms. J Clin Psychiatry 48(Suppl):38, 1987.
118. Garland EJ, Smith DH: Simultaneous prepuberal onset of panic disorder, night terrors, and somnambulism. J Am Acad Child Adolesc Psychiatry 30:553, 1991.
119. Fleming J: Dissociative episodes presenting as somnambulism: a case report. Sleep Res 16:263, 1987.
120. Braun BG (ed): Multiple personality. Psychiatr Clin North Am 7:1–198, 1984.
121. Schenck CH, Milner D, Hurwitz TD, et al: Dissociative disorders presenting as sleepwalking: polysomnographic, video, and clinical documentation (8 cases). Dissociation 2:194, 1989.
122. Putnam FW: Diagnosis and treatment of multiple personality disorder. New York, Guilford Press, 1989.
123. Kohen DP, Mahowald MW, Rosen GM: Sleep-terror disorder in children: the role of self-hypnosis in management. Am J Clin Hypn 34:233, 1992.

Narcolepsy, Kleine-Levin Syndrome, and Other Causes of Sleepiness in Children

LAWRENCE W. BROWN and MICHEL BILLIARD

If one of the main criteria for "good" sleep is the maintenance of daytime alertness, then children are generally extremely successful. Prepubertal children as a group are very resistant to sleepiness during the waking state; this has been confirmed by means of the Multiple Sleep Latency Test (MSLT) in support of conventional wisdom.[1] Children beyond the toddler age are typically fully alert throughout the day, fall asleep readily when tired, sleep soundly through the night with few brief arousals, and awaken refreshed in the morning. They do not usually require constant prodding from their parents or from alarm clocks to get out of bed. For these prepubertal children, total sleep time on school nights is actually longer than on weekend nights.[2] However, there has been too little attention to the potential problems when excessive sleepiness in children does occur.

Normal sleep requirements in young children are not completely understood and adequate objective measures of daytime alertness are problematic. Sleep in normal children has been adequately described only recently.[1–3] How does one interpret a 12-hour nightly sleep period in a 4-year-old, a 6-year-old who consistently falls asleep on brief car trips, an 8-year-old who naps regularly, or the high school freshman who nods off in English class? Objective measures such as the MSLT can be difficult to interpret in young children since it is hard to be certain that he or she understands and is compliant with instructions. A more difficult problem in clinical practice is the recognition of sleepiness in the overtired

child who demonstrates increased motor activity and irritability rather than the adult-like somnolence. Even less is known about sleep in children when handicaps, chronic illness, or medications must be taken into account.

The most common cause of sleepiness at all ages is insufficient sleep. Working parents may find it difficult to provide adequate "quality time" in the evening and still get their infant or toddler to day care in the early morning without compromising the sleep time their child needs. Homework, television, telephone, video games, and after-school employment compete with the need to sleep. According to a survey by Carskadon, parental influence on bedtime hour diminishes dramatically in early adolescence from more than 50% at 10 years to less than 20% at 13 years.[4] She reported that the battle over sleep timing between parents and teenagers shifts from bedtime to arousal in the morning. Despite later bedtime hours and earlier school openings in many high schools, teenagers often report that they need at least an hour to shower and dress, sometimes rising by 5:30 AM in order to satisfy their hygiene and fashion demands. Compensatory sleep on weekends only aggravates the natural tendency toward delayed sleep phase in many youngsters. Carskadon also emphasized the discontinuity between the pattern of decreasing total sleep time of teenagers with the laboratory finding that they often demonstrate a physiologic need for more sleep than prepubertal children as measured by MSLT.

While there are many causes for daytime sleepiness in children, this discussion will not focus on some of the most common ones, including inadequate sleep or schedule disorders (Chapter 10), obstructive sleep apnea syndrome (Chapters 18 and 19), or consequences of epilepsy (Chapter 13).

Narcolepsy

Narcolepsy is a clinical syndrome, first described more than 100 years ago, involving abnormalities of normal regulation of wakefulness and sleep (see also Kryger MH, et al: Principles and Practice of Sleep Medicine, 2nd ed, Chap 54).[5, 6] In addition to excessive daytime sleepiness, there are pathologic intrusions of REM sleep into wakefulness including episodic motor weakness (cataplexy, sleep paralysis) and perceptual distortions (hypnagogic hallucinations). Narcolepsy is currently diagnosed by a combination of these clinical findings and characteristic features on an overnight PSG with subsequent MSLT. It is a biologically based hereditary disorder with close genetic linkage to the HLA DR2 class II antigen on chromosome 6.[7] Onset of overt symptoms, although most often occurring between midadolescence and young adulthood, can vary from early childhood to full maturity.[8] Many investigators believe that the physiologic changes of puberty, altered sleep schedules often associated with adolescence, or other psychologic stressors may allow the expression of an underlying tendency to excessive sleepiness and narcolepsy in the susceptible individual.

Genetics

Despite the common perception that narcolepsy is a rare disorder, current estimates suggest a prevalence of about 1 in 2000.[9, 10] There is a strong genetic component, still not completely understood, that may be necessary but insufficient to cause the clinical syndrome.[11] Even if most individuals with narcolepsy have one particular HLA haplotype (i.e., DR2), the prevalence of narcolepsy is far less than the prevalence of the HLA marker in the general population (0.05% compared to 35%). Furthermore, clinically indistinguishable cases without DR2 positivity have been described.[12, 13]

The concept of a genetic basis for narcolepsy has been firmly established, but the search for the specific gene locus has proved elusive. Numerous independent reports over the past decade have confirmed Honda's finding of a narcolepsy susceptibility gene on chromosome 6 in the region of the major histocompatibility complex: the worldwide incidence of HLA DR2 and DQw1 or both exceeds 90% in narcolepsy compared to the 35% frequency in the general population. Since there are well-documented cases of narcolepsy with cataplexy negative for these particular alleles, it is likely that this region may not be the exact locus for a single gene controlling the disease.

The literature on HLA nomenclature is confusing and has been undergoing continual revision. New techniques have improved the discriminate powers of HLA typing but increased its complexity. The HLA DR and DQ molecules are heterodimers formed by the association of an alpha and beta chain and are encoded by specific and largely polymorphic genes. In the most recent nosology,[13a] what used to be known as DR2 is now identified as DR15 and DR16 and is represented by 11 different alleles at the DRB1 locus (such as DRB1-1501, -1502, and -1503). Similarly, DQw1 is now identified as DQ5 and DQ6 and is represented by 16 different alleles at the DQB1 locus (such as DQB1-0601, -0602, and -0603). Under the old nosology, almost all white and Japanese, but only about 70% of black, narcoleptics were positive for DR2 although most were positive for DQw1.[13b–e] To date, the best single association has been with the DRB1-0602 allele which is present in almost all white, black, and Japanese narcoleptic patients.[13a, b]

Pathophysiology

The precise pathophysiology of narcolepsy has not been completely determined. Considerable advances have been made since the first descriptions of sleep-onset REM periods in narcoleptics in 1963.[14] Subsequently, the development of the MSLT allowed a quantitative index of the narcoleptic patient's pathologic sleepiness and abnormal tendency to achieve REM sleep during planned daytime naps.

A profound alteration of motor and proprioceptive systems occurs during normal REM sleep. This is the basis for cataplexy and the other associated phenomena of narcolepsy. Nearly total atonia of the skeletal musculature during REM is produced by hyperpolarization of alpha motor neurons of the spinal cord and lower brainstem through inhibition of reticulospinal and reticulobulbar pathways. Gamma motor neurons are also inhibited. In association with REMs during this phase of sleep, there is presynaptic inhibition and reflex suppression. The pathophysiologic changes during cataplexy in both human and canine narcolepsy are identical to features of normal REM sleep. The paralysis induced by the inhibition of both alpha and gamma motor neurons can lead to the terror reported by narcoleptic patients with sleep paralysis. These wakeful episodes can be accompanied by overt hallucinatory experiences (hypnagogic hallucinations).

In addition to intrusions of REM phenomena into the waking state, prolonged PSG over several days have demonstrated disruption of normal sleep-wake rhythms with intrusions of wakefulness into sleep and vice versa. Although narcoleptic patients are pathologically sleepy, chronobiologic studies under free-running and entrained conditions have not shown that they sleep excessively compared with normal individuals.[15] Rather, there are far more transitions between sleep and wakefulness leading to fragmentation of the normal circadian cycle.

Neuroanatomic studies of brainstem transections have shown that the pons is the most critical area for the generation of REM sleep, especially the tegmentum pontis rostral to the locus coeruleus and nucleus reticularis pontis.[16] Neurons in these regions have been shown by means of single unit recording studies to fire selectively during REM sleep (REM-on cells). Other nearby cells are selectively silent during REM sleep (REM-off cells) in the areas of the locus coeruleus and the dorsal raphe. Higher diencephalic and forebrain structures modulate the pontine regions through widespread projections.

Acetylcholine plays an essential role in the neurochemistry of REM sleep, although complete details have not been worked out. Systemic cholinergic agonist administration or localized iontophoresis into selective areas of the tegmentum pontis will facilitate REM sleep. The enzyme choline acetyltransferase is present in these critical areas. REM-on cells appear to be cholinergic while REM-off cells are monoaminergic (responsive to norepinephrine or serotonin). Lesions of the norepinephrine neurons of the locus coeruleus and of serotonergic neurons of the dorsal raphe lead to the appearance of features of REM sleep.

Pharmacologic treatment of narcolepsy facilitates monoaminergic activity. Stimulants enhance synaptic availability of norepinephrine or serotonin and suppress REM sleep. Tricyclic antidepressants inhibit reuptake of monoamines, and fluoxetine directly affects serotonin activity. Those drugs which inhibit monoamine uptake will suppress cataplexy and other REM-associated phenomena. This supports the hypothesis that cholinergic pathways responsible for REM atonia and cataplexy can be inhibited by enhancing norepinephrine activity of the locus coeruleus or serotonin activity of the dorsal raphe.

Clinical and Laboratory Features

The syndrome of narcolepsy in the prepubertal child has been incompletely characterized except in comparison to adult clinical criteria. Therefore, it is unclear whether prepubertal "adult-like" narcolepsy represents the same condition as does excessive sleepiness in children who neither demonstrate cataplexy nor show the expected abnormalities on the MSLT. It is possible that these sleepy children have an early stage or a forme fruste of narcolepsy, but it may also represent an overlapping syndrome or some other condition entirely.

It is likely that narcolepsy either evolves slowly or presents explosively in previously mildly symptomatic individuals. Even when narcolepsy is not diagnosed until adulthood, a history of severe long-standing sleepiness dating back to the teenage years and often into childhood is commonly found. More than 50% of narcoleptic adults report being abnormally sleepy before 15 years of age, and more than 33% had been evaluated for this problem by age 13.[17] In addition, the presence of early-onset narcolepsy can be suggested by the existence of an excessive subjective sleep requirement. In a retrospective analysis of a large group of narcoleptic patients at Stanford University, the majority of adults reported sleeping more than 10 hours per night in the first years of elementary school; 30% were still sleeping this long at age 10 years.[18] Regular daytime naps, extremely uncommon in children of school age, were still present in 30% of those later diagnosed with narcolepsy.

Despite these considerations, it is unusual to be able to make a definitive diagnosis of narcolepsy in the young child. In an early large review of narcolepsy, only 4% were diagnosed before 16 years of age.[19] Recognition of narcolepsy can be delayed because even severely sleepy children often do not develop pathognomonic cataplexy and associated REM phenomena until much later and because pediatric practitioners are not typically knowledgeable about issues of sleep in children.[20] Not infrequently, pathologic sleepiness is overlooked until the onset of REM intrusions. Occurrences of abrupt loss of muscle tone (usually precipitated by strong emotion) may be more dramatic than even longstanding sleepiness, which is often obscured by paradoxical hyperactivity, learning problems, or behavioral disturbances.

There are several small studies of clinically definable narcolepsy in children.[22–23a] Most of the children in these studies, and in the occasional case report, presented suddenly with dramatic daytime sleepiness. They frequently fell asleep whenever sedentary—at school, in the car or school bus, at the dinner table, and while watching television. Some children actually report falling asleep while standing in line or while lying in the bath. Although a number of reported cases of prepubertal onset of narcolepsy did demonstrate definite cataplexy, cataplexy is not essential to the diagnosis. Other REM intrusions, namely sleep paralysis, hypnagogic hallucinations and automatic behavior in which "microsleep" episodes lasting a few seconds interfere with motor performance, concentration, and speech are even less often reported in children with narcolepsy than in adults.

Our current ability to diagnose narcolepsy in children is still based on the same standards of clinical history and laboratory findings established for adults. At all ages, it is essential to exclude other causes of excessive sleepiness including insufficient sleep, schedule disorders, obstructive sleep apnea, obesity-hypoventilation syndrome, underlying medical disorders, psychiatric syndromes, side effects of medications, drug abuse or withdrawal, sleep-related epilepsy, and nocturnal myoclonus (periodic leg movements of sleep).

In addition to a complete medical and psychiatric history, evaluation of a sleep diary, and physical examination, laboratory studies should include overnight PSG and MSLT to establish a diagnosis of narcolepsy. Other investigative studies depend on the specific clinical setting and may include complete blood count, sedimentation rate, thyroid profile, iron studies, Lyme titer, EEG, peak and trough medication levels, drug screen, and CT scan or MRI. It is generally accepted that laboratory confirmation of narcolepsy requires overnight PSG excluding other causes of sleepiness while showing satisfactory REM sleep, followed by an MSLT with short sleep latencies and two or more sleep-onset REM periods (SOREMPs). Some investigators have suggested that narcoleptic individuals show an increased percentage of total REM sleep compared to control subjects. A short mean sleep latency, under 7 minutes, in prepubertal narcoleptic children is similar to MSLT findings in affected adults. Guilleminault reported that SOREMPs are unusual in young narcoleptic children, but most other workers use abnormal SOREMPs on the nocturnal and daytime sleep studies as a major criterion for the diagnosis.[18]

HLA testing may be considered. Since the specificity of a positive (DR2, DQw1) result is low, tissue typing alone cannot establish the diagnosis. However, because there is high sensitivity, a negative test makes the diagnosis very unlikely. This may be very helpful in the evaluation of a sleepy child without definite cataplexy and with ambiguous MSLT results. Still, there are patients who are HLA negative yet fulfill all of the clinical and laboratory criteria for narcolepsy. Some investigators have questioned whether narcoleptic patients negative for DR2 may actually have another disease.

Laboratory testing by itself cannot prove or disprove the diagnosis of narcolepsy.[24] At the Stanford Sleep Disorders Center, records of over 300 adult and pediatric patients with excessive daytime somnolence were reviewed. Cataplexy was compared to the finding of two or more SOREMPs after eliminating definable causes of excessive sleepiness other than narcolepsy (i.e., sleep apnea, restless leg syndrome, schedule disorders.) The subgroup with cataplexy was most homogeneous in clinical and polygraphic features, but only 83% of these patients had two or more SOREMPs on one MSLT. The subgroup defined by two or more SOREMPs mainly included individuals without cataplexy, especially a large number of older women with periodic leg movements. Those with both cataplexy and two or more SOREMPs were most likely to be HLA positive.

Treatment

Treatment of narcolepsy and cataplexy in children reflects the clinical experience with older adult patients. While medication is often necessary to optimize daytime performance, the pediatric emphasis should be on successful education, good sleep hygiene, and appropriate behavior at school and at home. Narcolepsy is a lifelong condition, and it is important for child and family to adjust to, and learn to live with, its associated problems. A carefully structured sleep schedule, judicious naps during the school day, and academic courses timed to the periods of greatest alertness are extremely valuable. While difficult to achieve in many instances, such nonpharmacologic interventions can sometimes avoid or limit drug treatment at least in mild cases. It is equally important to prevent the psychologic consequences of perceived hyperactivity, laziness, disinterest, or unsocial behavior. In one case in the authors' experience, an uninformed and cruel group of elementary school classmates repetitively scared a child into a point of cataplectic status to enjoy the sight of him falling to the ground.

Stimulants are the drugs of choice to treat daytime sleepiness that interferes with normal activities and academic success. A few carefully controlled studies have been carried out to assess the safety and efficacy of stimulants in adult narcolepsy.[25] None have been performed in children. However, there is wide experience with these medications in other clinical conditions, such as attention deficit disorder, which can be extrapolated to narcolepsy.[26–28] Pemoline and methylphenidate are the most widely prescribed stimulants by sleep specialists, although amphetamines are also effective. Personal clinical experience has demonstrated that most affected children benefit from a single dose of pemoline in the morning without unacceptable side effects. When side effects limit the usefulness of pemoline, it is possible to divide the total daily dose with the maximally tolerated amount in the morning supplemented by a small increment at school several hours later. However, this raises the risk of sleep-onset insomnia, since this relatively long-acting medication has a half-life of at least 8 to 12 hours. The starting dose of pemoline is usually 18.75 mg with weekly increases as necessary. Fully grown adolescents may require up to 112.5 mg. Common side effects include tachycardia, irritability, nervousness, nausea, anorexia, and headaches. These are all dose-related problems that usually respond to reduction in total daily amount or a divided schedule. Many specialists in sleep medicine prefer pemoline as a longer acting and less tightly controlled alternative to the other stimulants.

Methylphenidate is the most widely prescribed stimulant in the pediatric population (mostly for attention deficit disorder) and accounts for over 90% of prescriptions. It is usually taken two or three times per day (e.g., 8 AM, noon, and an optional dose at 4 PM for homework or after-school activities). The amount of each dose is approximately 0.3 mg/kg, although doses as high as 1 mg/kg may be successfully tolerated. Although some authors have recommended limiting the total daily dosage to 20 mg, this amount is usually insufficient to treat hypersomnolence in all but the youngest children.[18] Larger doses have been associated with the same side effects as for pemoline as well as growth retardation. Methylphenidate is also available in a sustained release preparation. However, comparison studies in children with attention deficit disorder showed that the regular tablet was generally superior in efficacy.[28] Beyond the sustained release preparation's slower onset of action and lower peak levels, there was a higher incidence of side effects compared to the standard tablet.

Dextroamphetamine is available in a single dose time-release spansule given in the morning and tablets that require a 4-hour dosing schedule similar to methylphenidate. There is a newly released preparation (Adderall®) that combines four different amphetamine salts with varying pharmacokinetic properties to provide a long-acting tablet with an effective single morning-dosing schedule. Total daily dosage of dextroamphetamine ranges from 10 to 30 mg. Most physicians avoid amphetamines in children and adolescents. In addition to a high perceived risk for abuse, amphetamines are more likely to produce tachyphylaxis with increasing dose requirements for sustained effect.

Tricyclic antidepressants are the mainstay for treatment of cataplexy in children as in adults. There is clinical experience with many of the available compounds, but the greatest experience is with imipramine and protriptyline. Imipramine had been widely used to treat enuresis in children, although it is no longer commonly prescribed. Since imipramine often has a sedating effect all, or at least most, of the daily dose (usually 25 to 75 mg) is given at bedtime. At the higher doses, administration of part of the total amount in the morning may avoid anticholinergic side effects. Protriptyline is also effective against cataplexy and other REM intrusions. It has been reported to have activating properties but these have not been confirmed with PSG. Protriptyline is usually prescribed in doses of 5 to 30 mg with the largest dose given in the morning and a small supplement at noon. More recently developed drugs such as fluoxetine and clomipramine have been used successfully in adults with narcolepsy and in children with certain psychiatric disorders. These newer agents are potentially valuable in the treatment of pediatric narcolepsy, although there remain some concerns about excessive sedation (sometimes agitated drowsiness), jerky limb movements, and other side effects. Early anectodal experience has demonstrated the powerful effects and relative safety of these drugs. Furthermore, all tricyclics and selective serotonin reuptake inhibitors can produce anticholinergic side effects of blurred vision, dry mouth, constipation, urinary hesitancy, and sexual dysfunction. In childhood narcolepsy, treatment of cataplexy is not always indicated since symptoms are often mild.

Even when the symptoms of narcolepsy are not disabling, the diagnosis of narcolepsy can lead to emotional consequences and have a profound effect on a child's self-esteem. The loss of control engendered by irresistible napping at inappropriate times, and sudden collapse typically under emotional circumstances, can prove devastating to a child. In most states narcolepsy is grouped with epilepsy as a potentially severe neurologic condition, which requires medical clearance before permission to apply for a driver's license. Even when a teenager with narcolepsy is well-controlled, there is increased concern about his inexperience and possibility of falling asleep at the wheel. One 17-year-old, for example, was sued after being involved in a serious head-on collision after school one day after a normal examination at the regional sleep disorders center, even though there was no evidence that he had fallen asleep and police records showed absence of skid marks by either teenaged driver.

Allsop has suggested that the narcoleptic child's denial of symptoms and failure to accept the consequences of the diagnosis can lead to management difficulties.[23] He emphasized that an additional barrier to effective treatment can be the coexistence of a subclinical depression with low mood, irritability, and social withdrawal. Supportive care of the child and family, an open dialogue with school officials, and pharmacologic intervention can usually produce positive results.

Kleine-Levin Syndrome

Kleine,[29] Lewis,[30] and Levin[31] were the first to describe cases of adolescent boys with recurring episodes of excessive somnolence, abnormal behavior (including overeating and sexual disinhibition), and mental disturbances. Critchley and Hoffman[32] gave this condition the eponymic term *Kleine-Levin Syndrome.* Critchley emphasized additional clinical features: males are principally affected; onset is during adolescence; the syndrome eventually spontaneously disappears; and the overeating is possibly of the compulsive rather than the bulimic type.[33]

Epidemiology

More than 100 typical case reports have been published, with a 3:1 male:female ratio. The median age of onset is during adolescence, earlier in males than in females. At the onset of the first episode specific circumstances are found in approximately half the cases. They consist of a flulike syndrome, upper airway infection, or less frequently, acute drunkenness, seasickness, or a physical blow resulting in loss of consciousness.

Clinical Picture

Excessive somnolence may develop abruptly or gradually. The subject retires to bed and almost refuses to leave it. Sleep is either calm or agitated. Vivid dreams are sometimes reported. Urinary incontinence does not occur. Abnormal behavior—overeating and sexual disinhibition—is generally compulsive. Patients eat all foodstuffs within sight, even if of poor quality, frequently resulting in an increase of weight by the end of the episode. Manifestations of hypersexuality (indiscriminate advances regardless of age and sex, overt masturbation, and public display of sexual fantasy) are reported in approximately one third of the males and less often in females. Mental disturbances vary. Irritability is the most frequent symptom, followed by a feeling of unreality, as if people and things were abnormally distant, and as confusion, and visual or auditory hallucinations. The duration of episodic hypersomnolence varies from 12 hours to 3 to 4 weeks, and their recurrence is at intervals ranging from several weeks to several months. Physical examination may show nonspecific features, such as excessive or depressed deep tendon reflexes, nystagmus, and dysarthria, as well as dysautonomia, congestion of the face, and profuse sweating. After a variable number of days (4 to 7 on the average, 30 at most), symptoms subside. However, a short reaction phase with elation, sleeplessness, or depression, sometimes with suicidal ideation, may occur. Between episodes, physical examination is normal. There is no significant personality disorder.

According to Critchley, attacks gradually decrease in frequency and eventually cease. However, case reports indicate that in numerous instances abnormal episodes are still occurring at the time of the last follow-up visit, as well as cases in which symptoms have been seen after 20 years.

Laboratory Investigations

Electrophysiologic Studies

Routine EEG obtained during attacks show general slowing of the background activity and often paroxysmal bursts of theta activity at 4 to 6 Hz. Twenty-four hour polygraphic recordings show an increased quantity of total sleep time. Short REM sleep latency, increased wakefulness after sleep onset, and diminished NREM sleep stages 3 and 4 have been reported.[33a]

Roentgenographic Studies

Findings on CT or MRI are either normal or remarkable by a relative enlargement of one or both lateral ventricles. Comparative studies performed both during and out of hypersomniac episodes are lacking.

Endocrine Studies

Schematically, two types of laboratory tests have been performed: measures of basal hormonal levels before and after stimulation tests and control of 24-hour or overnight hormonal secretory patterns based on periodic blood sampling.

Basal levels of the main anterior pituitary hormones—growth hormone (GH), prolactin (PRL), thyrotropin-stimulating hormone (TSH), luteinizing hormone (LH), follicle stimulating hormone (FSH), testosterone, and cortisol—have been found to be within the normal limits. The same applied to the levels obtained after stimulation tests with the exception of a paradoxical response of GH to thyro-

tropin-releasing hormone (TRH),[33b] a low or absent response of cortisol to insulin-induced hypoglycemia,[34a, 35] and an abolished response of TSH to TRH.[35]

Different abnormalities have been found in 24-hour or overnight hormonal secretory patterns: increased overnight PRL secretion,[33b, 35] absent nocturnal increased TSH and cortisol secretions, and diminished GH secretion.[35] According to Chesson and associates[34] GH, PRL, and TSH variations during symptomatic periods would favor a reduction of the dopaminergic tone.

Monoamine Assays

Cerebrospinal fluid levels of 5-hydroxyindoleacetic acid (5-HIAA) and homovanillic acid (HVA) have been reported to be normal before administration of probenecid and significantly increased after probenecid.[35a] This finding is in favor of an increased turnover of 5-HIAA and HVA, and hence of serotonin and dopamine.

These results may be disputed. The syndrome is rare and the number of subjects submitted to laboratory investigations during both normal and symptomatic periods is extremely limited. Moreover, a number of results reported in the literature have been obtained in a single subject.

Clinical Variants

Incomplete forms of the Kleine-Levin syndrome are likely to be more numerous than typical cases. They are characterized by recurring episodes of abnormal somnolence without overeating and/or mental disturbances. Natural history and results of laboratory investigations do not differ from those of typical cases. Menstrual-associated periodic hypersomnia is a rare condition. Apparently, the prognosis of this type of recurring hypersomnia does not differ from that of the Kleine-Levin syndrome.

Although most authors report normal behavior between attacks, a recent report described a series of cases with Asperger's syndrome (high functioning pervasive developmental disorder with autistic features).[35b] This raises the possibility that underlying defects of brain organization or neuronal migration may produce or predispose to the Kleine-Levin syndrome.

Pathophysiology

The following group of findings indicates a functional dysregulation of the mesencephalo-hypothalamo-limbic system: abnormal somnolence, overeating, sexual disinhibition, and sometimes heavy sweating and congestion of the face; intermittent occurrence; and lack of abnormality between two episodes.

The frequent occurrence of a flulike syndrome or upper airway infection a few days before the onset of the first episode suggests the role of a virus. Supportive of this hypothesis are the pathologic data reported by Takrani and Cronin[36] and by Carpenter and colleagues[37] on inflammatory lesions—lymphocytic cuffing of small vessels in either the hypothalamus or the thalamus—in favor of a localized encephalitis.

Other features are the similarity of sleep in affective disorders and in some cases of the Kleine-Levin syndrome, pointed out by Reynolds and associates,[38] and the sudden shift from hypersomnia to a provisional state of either elation or depression, sometimes recorded at the end of hypersomniac episodes, reminiscent of the switch process in bipolar depression.

Differential Diagnosis

Recurring hypersomnia may result from an organic insult to the central nervous system (CNS), such as an intraventricular tumor arising from the third ventricle, encephalitis, head trauma, or a cerebrovascular accident.

In contrast, recurring hypersomnia may also stem from affective disorders: major depressions of the recurrent type, bipolar depressions, or neurosis mainly of the hysterical type.

Treatment

Treatment of the Kleine-Levin syndrome and of clinical variants rests on symptomatic and preventive measures. The hypersomniac episodes are treated with stimulant medications, such as the amphetamines, methylphenidate, and pemoline. Generally, the effectiveness of these treatments does not exceed a few hours or so. Preventative therapy is not yet well defined. Some promising results have been obtained, however. Lithium carbonate has been proposed because of the previously men-

tioned similarities between the Kleine-Levin syndrome and affective disorders.[38a] In the case of menstruation-linked hypersomnia, administration of an ovulatory inhibitor has been successful in a few well-documented cases.[39]

Menstrual-Associated Periodic Hypersomnia

Menstrual-associated periodic hypersomnia occurs within the first years after menarche. Episodes generally last 1 to 2 weeks with rapid resolution of each attack at the time of menses.[39] Hormonal imbalance is likely since oral contraceptives will usually lead to prolonged remission, although discontinuation of birth control pills may result in relapse. There is spontaneous resolution within several years of onset or after pregnancy.

Idiopathic Central Nervous System Hypersomnia

CNS hypersomnia is an unusual diagnosis, particularly in childhood. The diagnosis is based on chronic, excessive daytime sleepiness in the absence of medical, toxic, or psychiatric factors; the major disorder to be considered in the differential diagnosis is narcolepsy.[40] In a large retrospective review from Stanford University, no children were found in a series of 74 cases of idiopathic CNS hypersomnia, although there were prepubertal children and adolescents represented in a comparison group of 257 narcoleptics.[40] When HLA DR2 was examined in idiopathic CNS hypersomnia, no increase in frequency of the haplotype was found.[41] Indeed, none of 10 patients carried the allele compared with 22% of normal controls and 100% of 36 narcoleptic patients. These results support the hypothesis that narcolepsy, as currently defined by clinical and laboratory studies, is a different entity from CNS hypersomnia.

The differential diagnosis can be extensive. One neurologic cause of CNS hypersomnia to be excluded in children is hydrocephalus since increased intracranial pressure may lead to marked somnolence without other signs. Excessive sleepiness may also follow acute illnesses with an encephalitic component including Lyme disease, infectious mononucleosis, Guillain-Barré syndrome, and other viral or parainfectious illnesses. There is also significant overlap with the chronic fatigue syndrome (CFS), which is characterized by persistent or recurrent symptoms of decreased alertness, low grade fever, headache, myalgia, depression, memory difficulties, confusion, inability to concentrate, lymphadenopathy, and sore throat in addition to disturbed sleep.[42, 43] Indeed, hypersomnia was found in a majority of adolescents with chronic fatigue whether or not they had symptoms of depression.[44] However, it remains uncertain whether chronic fatigue in childhood actually represents prodromal depression, a discrete psychosomatic illness, an infectious disease, or an immunologic disorder. The absence of systemic complaints, memory problems, and myalgias distinguishes idiopathic CNS hypersomnia from CFS. However, both are poorly defined conditions without any clear pathophysiology, and they remain diagnoses of exclusion.

References

1. Carskadon MA, Dement WC: Sleepiness in the normal adolescent. *In* Guilleminault C (ed): Sleep and Its Disorders in Children. New York, Raven Press, 1987, pp 53–66.
2. Carskadon MA, Keenan S, Dement WC: Nighttime sleep and daytime sleep tendency in preadolescents. *In* Guilleminault C (ed): Sleep and Its Disorders in Children. New York, Raven Press, 1987, pp 43–52.
3. Coble PA, Kupfer DJ, Taska LS, et al: EEG sleep of normal healthy children. Part I. Findings using standard measurement methods. Sleep 7:289, 1984.
4. Carskadon MA: Patterns of sleep and sleepiness in adolescents. Pediatrician 17:5, 1992.
5. Zarcone V: Narcolepsy. N Engl J Med 388:1156, 1973.
6. Mitler MM, Hajdukovich R, Erman M, et al: Narcolepsy. J Clin Neurophysiol 7:93, 1990.
7. Honda Y, Asaka A, Tanaka Y, et al: Discrimination of narcoleptic patients by using genetic markers and HLA. Sleep Res 12:254, 1983.
8. Passouant P, Billiard M: The evolution of narcolepsy with age. *In* Guilleminault C, Dement WC, Passouant P (eds): Narcolepsy. New York, Spectrum, 1976, pp 179–196.
9. Dement WC, Zarcone V, Varner V, et al: The prevalence of narcolepsy. Sleep Res 1:148, 1972.
10. Dement WC, Carskadon M, Ley R: The prevalence of narcolepsy. II. Sleep Res 2:147, 1973.
11. Honda Y, Matsuki K: Genetic aspects of narcolepsy. *In* Thorpy MJ (ed): Handbook of Sleep Disorders. New York, Marcel Dekker, 1990, pp 217–234.
12. Confavreux C, Gebuhrer L, Betuel H, et al: HLA-DR2 negative narcolepsy. J Neurol Neurosurg Psychiatry 50:635, 1987.
13. Roushdy J, Sentot S, Kalb R, et al: A deletion in the second exon of an HLA-DRB1 allele found in a DR2-negative narcolepsy patient. Hum Immunol 37:1, 1993.
13a. Bodmer JG, Marsh SGE, Albert ED, et al: Nomenclature for factors of the HLA system, 1994. Hum Immunol 41:1, 1994.
13b. Matsuki K, Grumet FC, Lin X, Gelb M: DQ (rather than DR) gene marks susceptibility to narcolepsy [letter]. Lancet 339:1052, 1992.
13c. Mignot E, Lin X, Kalil J, et al: DQB1-0602 (DQw1) is not present in most non-DR2 Caucasian narcoleptics. Sleep 15:415, 1992.
13d. Neely S, Rosenberg R, Spire JP, et al: HLA antigens in narcolepsy. Neurology 37:1858, 1987.
13e. Kramer RE, Dinner DS, Braun WE, et al: HLA-DR2 and narcolepsy. Arch Neurol 44:853, 1987.
14. Rechstaffen A, Wolpert W, Dement W, et al: Nocturnal sleep of narcoleptics. Electroencephalogr Clin Neurophysiol 15:599, 1963.
15. Pollak C: Narcolepsy. Third International Symposium, San Diego, June 1988. Unpublished presentation.
16. Aldrich MS: The neurobiology of narcolepsy. Trends Neurosci 14:235, 1991.
17. Merlotti L, Roehrs T, Young D, et al: Symptom patterns of narcolepsy patients: a questionnaire study. Sleep Res 16:391, 1987.
18. Guilleminault C: Narcolepsy and its differential diagnosis. *In* Guilleminault C (ed): Sleep and Its Disorders in Children. New York, Raven Press, 1987, pp 181–194.
19. Yoss RE, Daly DD: Narcolepsy in children. Pediatrics 25:1025, 1960.
20. Mindell JA, Moline ML, Zendell SM, et al: Pediatricians and sleep disorders: training and practice. Pediatrics 94:194, 1994.
21. Young D, Zorick F, Wittig R, et al: Narcolepsy in a pediatric population. Am J Dis Child 142:210, 1988.
22. Kotagal S, Hartse KM, Walsh JK: Characteristics of narcolepsy in preteenaged children. Pediatrics 85:205, 1990.
23. Allsop MR, Zwaiwalla Z: Narcolepsy. Arch Dis Child 67:302, 1992.
23a. Dahl RE, Hohum J, Trubnick L: A clinical picture of childhood and adolescent narcolepsy. J Am Acad Child Adolesc Psychiatry 33:834, 1994.
24. Moscovitch A, Partinen M, Guilleminault C: The positive diagnosis of narcolepsy and narcolepsy's borderland. Neurology 43:55, 1993.
25. Mitler MM, Shafor R, Hajdukovich R, et al: Treatment of narcolepsy: objective studies on methylphenidate, pemoline, and protriptyline. Sleep 9:260, 1986.
26. Conners CK, Taylor E: Pemoline, methylphenidate, and placebo in children with minimal brain dysfunction. Arch Gen Psychiatry 37:922, 1980.
27. Gittleman R, Kanner A: Psychopharmacotherapy. *In* Quay H, Werry J (eds): Psychopathological Disorders of Childhood, 3rd ed. New York, John Wiley & Sons, 1986, pp 455–494.
28. Pelham WE, Jr, Greenslade KE, Vodde-Hamilton, et al: Relative efficacy of long-active stimulants on children with attention deficit-hyperactivity disorder: a comparison of standard methylphenidate, sustained-release methylphenidate, sustained-release dextroamphetamine, and pemoline. Pediatrics 86:226, 1990.
29. Kleine: Periodische schlafsucht. Monatsschr Psychiatr Neurol 57:285, 1925.
30. Lewis NDC: The psychoanalytic approach to the problem of children under twelve years of age. Psychoanal Rev 13:424, 1926.
31. Levin M: Narcolepsy and other varieties of morbid somnolence. Arch Neurol Psychiatry 22:1172, 1929.

32. Critchley M, Hoffman HL: The syndrome of periodic somnolence and morbid hunger (Kleine-Levin syndrome). Br Med J 1:137, 1942.

33. Critchley M: Periodic hypersomnia and megaphagia in adolescent males. Brain 85:627, 1962.

33a. Reynolds CF III, Kupfer DJ, Christiansen CL, et al: Multiple sleep latency test findings in Kleine-Levin syndrome. J Nerv Ment Dis 172:41, 1984.

33b. Gadoth N, Dickerman S, Bechar M, et al: Episodic hormone secretion during sleep in Kleine-Levin syndrome: evidence for hypothalamus dysfunction. Brain Dev 9:309, 1987.

34. Chesson AL, Levine SN, Kong LS, et al: Neuroendocrine evaluation in Kleine-Levin syndrome: evidence of reduced dopaminergic tone during periods of hypersomnolence. Sleep 14:226, 1991.

34a. Koerber RK, Torkelson R, Haven G, et al: Increased cerebrospinal fluid 5-hydroxytryptamine and 5-hydroxyindoleacetic acid in Kleine-Levin syndrome. Neurology 34:1597, 1984.

35. Fernandez JM, Lara I, Gila LK, et al: Disturbed hypothalamic-pituitary axis in idiopathic recurring hypersomnia syndrome. Acta Neurol Scand 82:361, 1990.

35a. Livrea P, Punca FM, Barnaba A, et al: Abnormal central monoamine metabolism in humans with "True hypersomnia" and "subwakefulness." Eur Neurol 15:71. 1977.

35b. Berthier ML, Santamaria J, Encabo DH, et al: Recurrent hypersomnia in two adolescent males with Asperger's syndrome. J Am Acad Child Adolesc Psychiatry 31:735, 1992.

36. Takrani LB, Cronin D: Kleine-Levin syndrome in a female patient. Can Psychiatr Assoc J 21:315, 1976.

37. Carpenter S, Yassa R, Ochs R: A pathological basis for Kleine-Levin syndrome. Arch Neurol 39:25, 1982.

38. Reynolds CF, Black RS, Coble P, et al: Similarities in EEG sleep findings for Kleine-Levin syndrome and unipolar depression. Am J Psychiatry 137:116, 1980.

38a. Goldberg MA: The treatment of Klein-Levin syndrome with lithium. Can J Psychiatry 28:491, 1983.

39. Billiard M, Guilleminault C, Dement WC: A menstruation-linked periodic hypersomnia, Kleine-Levin syndrome or a new clinical entity? Neurology 25:436, 1975.

40. Baker TL, Guilleminault C, Nino-Murcia G, et al: Comparative polysomnographic study of narcolepsy and idiopathic central nervous system hypersomnia. Sleep 9:232, 1986.

41. Poirier G, Montplaisir J, Decary F, et al: ALA antigens in narcolepsy and idiopathic central nervous system hypersomnolence. Sleep 9:153, 1986.

42. Komaroff AL, Buchwald D: Symptoms and signs of chronic fatigue syndrome. Rev Infect Dis 13(Suppl 1): S8, 1991.

43. Katz BZ, Andiman WA: Chronic fatigue syndrome (editorial). J Pediatr 113:944, 1988.

44. Smith MS, Mitchell J, Corey L, et al: Chronic fatigue in adolescents. Pediatrics 88:195, 1991.

CHAPTER

15

Sleep in Children with Neurologic Problems

LAWRENCE W. BROWN, PAUL MAISTROS,
and CHRISTIAN GUILLEMINAULT

While relatively little is known about the developmental aspects of the physiology or anatomic basis of sleep in normal individuals, virtually no information exists on the development of sleep in handicapped or mentally impaired children. The establishment of circadian rhythmicity is determined by many factors including genetic controls of brain differentiation, and it can be affected by exposure of the developing CNS to prenatal, intrapartum, and postnatal environmental influences. Adverse effects from any brain lesion or metabolic perturbation, whether congenital or acquired, can interfere with the development or maintenance of a normal sleep-wake cycle.[1-3] Prematurity, chromosomal disorders, congenital blindness, systemic or primary CNS infection, pervasive developmental disorder (autism), and lead poisoning are among many potential causes that can lead to abnormal sleep and disturbed wakefulness.

Clinical experience has shown that developmentally delayed infants and mentally retarded children often have difficulty acquiring or maintaining a normal sleep-wake schedule. Parents often complain that their handicapped child has his "days and nights reversed." It is common for a severely involved child to have difficulty falling asleep, frequent nocturnal awakenings, or significantly altered total sleep time (see Chapter 9). Blind children understandably may have free-running circadian rhythms as the basis for their apparent schedule problems, but this has not been systematically examined in other handicapping conditions. Although the interrelationship between sleep and epilepsy will not be

addressed here, it is important to note that seizure control is sometimes improved dramatically once there is consolidation of nocturnal sleep; conversely, sleep deprivation has been shown to increase EEG abnormalities as well as to aggravate seizures (see Chapter 13 and Kryger MH, et al: Principles and Practice of Sleep Medicine, 2nd ed, Chapter 77).

Even when there has been no direct adverse effect on the development of normal circadian rhythms, neurologic illness may have other negative influences on normal sleep (see Chapter 9). For example, the anatomic distortions of the upper airway associated with Down Syndrome and Prader-Willi Syndrome often leads to obstructive sleep apnea syndrome (OSAS) (see Chapters 18 and 19), while those associated with myelodysplasia can produce central and/or obstructive events. It is well to consider the potential influence of inadequate sleep regulation or sleep disorders in all handicapped children whose limitations already predispose them to academic, social, and behavioral problems. The toddler with cerebral palsy will not fully respond to physical therapy if he naps through the session, and the excessively sleepy retarded child will not benefit maximally even from a carefully designed individual educational plan.

Blindness

The majority of blind individuals have sleep complaints including difficulty achieving sleep at the desired time, frequent nocturnal arousals, daytime fatigue, and frequent naps. While

135

there are no studies which specifically address these problems in blind children, a survey found that 75% of blind adults had sleep-wake disturbances,[1] and several anecdotal reports have documented these problems in blind children. Okawa and associates studied four congenitally blind children and found free-running circadian rhythms.[2] Palm and associates carefully documented a similar chronobiologic disturbance in a severely retarded child with blindness from congenital toxoplasmosis.[3] Although some blind individuals will respond to a program of rigid day-night routine and others will improve with chloral hydrate or benzodiazepines, this child was resistant. However administration of oral melatonin allowed for entrainment to an appropriate daily schedule.

Only recently has the relationship been explored between the circadian timing system and a daily schedule in a blind person.[4] A congenitally unsighted adult kept meticulous sleep diaries over many years which suggested free-running rhythms; in addition, he underwent extensive chronobiologic studies over an extended period. For 3 months he maintained a constant 24-hour schedule while his endogenous circadian pacemaker (measured by core body temperature, plasma cortisol peaks, and urinary excretion) followed a cycle that was slightly longer. Social cues were insufficient in this case to entrain his endogenous pacemaker. His cyclically recurrent sleep problems related directly to his free-running rhythm; sleep architecture and severity of sleep disruption correlated to lack of synchrony with his circadian phase.

Mental Retardation

Sleep disturbances can be produced by any developmental or acquired structural damage to the critical diencephalic or brainstem nuclei involved in the regulation of wakefulness, alternation between NREM and REM sleep, and normal chronobiologic rhythms. However, the establishment of circadian rhythm requires not only the development of the supra-chiasmatic nucleus of the hypothalamus and its connections, but also perception of environmental cues (zeitgebers). Disturbed sleep can also derive from inadequate visual perception of the light-dark alternation, lack of a regular feeding schedule, or the inability to interpret social interactions.

The abnormal development of circadian rhythms have been examined in severely brain damaged infants. They often lack any identifiable sleep architecture, and it may even be difficult to distinguish between sleep and wakefulness.[5] Okawa and Sasaki also described how abnormal perception and impaired social relationships could lead to free-running circadian rhythms and the appearance of cyclical sleep-wake disorders. Abnormalities of EEG features of sleep have been found in mentally retarded children. (For example, absence of or nearly continuous spindles have been reported in severely retarded children.)[6]

Based on the anecdotal success of melatonin to regulate circadian rhythms in blind adults, a clinical study was undertaken in multiply disabled children with chronic sleep disorders.[6a] While the report lacked careful controls and there was no objective PSG data, the results were strongly encouraging. Neurologically impaired children with and without visual impairment responded to 2 to 10 mg of melatonin given at bedtime. Fragmented sleep, delayed sleep onset, and nonspecific sleep disturbances all improved without adverse effects. Reported benefits included improved mood, reduced irritability, fewer temper tantrums, greater sociability, better appetite, and fewer seizures. The results were so encouraging that further clinical and laboratory investigations are indicated.

In a recent attempt to understand the basis for disturbed sleep-wake activity cycles in severely retarded children, infants with hydranencephaly, a congenital condition in which the cerebral hemispheres are absent but the brainstem and cerebellum are preserved, were examined.[7] Normal circadian activity did not develop in the three cases investigated. Multiple cortisol peaks were seen during the day, growth hormone secretion did not show sleep enhancement, and core body temperature showed inconsistent circadian rhythmicity. These results suggested that rostral brain structures are important in the development of normal sleep-wake cycle even when the midbrain and pons are structurally intact.

Several surveys of mentally handicapped children documenting the frequency of sleep disturbances were reviewed by Stores.[8] One observational study of institutionalized, profoundly retarded, nonambulatory children had irregular and fragmented sleep throughout the day and night; these children spent up to 21 hours per day either in sleep or low level activity without stimulation.[9] Another British examination of 200 severely retarded children living at home found that half had difficulties in falling asleep and two-thirds had frequent nocturnal arousals.[10] Three years later the parents of the majority of affected children still described the same sleep disturbances.

Treatment of schedule disorders in retarded children have not been addressed with rigidly controlled scientific methodology. Many pediatricians provide hypnotic sedatives such as chloral hydrate and diphenhydramine in uncontrolled trials; others have been known to throw up their hands in despair. Recently, behavioral units addressing the needs of mentally retarded children have begun to provide new insights. An interesting single case study using the child as his own control described a model for a combined pharmacologic and behavioral approach for severe sleep-wake schedule disorder in the retarded child.[11] Summers and associates treated a 6-year-old child with Angelman syndrome, a chromosomal deletion syndrome leading to severe mental retardation, microcephaly, seizures, and jerky limb movements. Initial PSG excluded primary sleep disorders including apnea. During a prolonged hospitalization on a specialized behavioral unit, treatment focused on elimination of daytime naps, reduced evening fluids, strict bedtime, and effective hypnotic medication at night. Markedly increased nocturnal sleep (from a baseline of 1.9 hours to 8.3 hours during the treatment phase) and reduced daytime naps (from 1.3 hours to 0.08 hours) were maintained during a trial using placebo instead of diphenhydramine. The improved sleep-wake schedule persisted during an extended home observation period. This single report may encourage professionals and parents to be optimistic that appropriate intervention can reverse chronic schedule disorders in the neurologically impaired child.

Down Syndrome

There has been a recent awareness that children with Down syndrome are at increased risk for sleep disorders, especially for the obstructive sleep apnea syndrome. Many factors predispose these individuals to airway obstruction, which will be discussed in detail in Chapters 18 and 19.

Prader-Willi Syndrome

Prader-Willi syndrome is a congenital disorder usually associated with deletion of part of the long arm of chromosome 15. The syndrome includes dysmorphic features with mild hypotelorism, almond-shaped eyes, down-turned mouth, and high-arched palate.[12] Severe hypotonia and slow weight gain are frequently present in infancy. As the child grows, early failure to thrive is replaced by hyperphagia and marked obesity. During the second year of life there is usually a crossing of the growth parameters with decreased linear growth and rapid weight gain. Mental retardation, hypogonadism, and short stature complete the clinical syndrome.

Excessive daytime sleepiness is a nearly universal feature of the Prader-Willi syndrome, although recent review articles devoted to the condition have overlooked this symptom.[12–14] Even the consensus diagnostic criteria list sleep disturbances and obstructive apnea only as minor criteria.[15] Somnolence is most severe in the morbidly obese patients with sleep apnea and obesity-hypoventilation syndrome. Personal clinical experience suggests that adenotonsillectomy usually improves daytime alertness, but positive results are often incomplete and temporary. The frequent presence of SOREMPs has led to speculation of a possible form of symptomatic, or secondary, narcolepsy, but the effects of sleep disruption and obesity-hypoventilation (pickwickian) syndrome are more likely explanations. Yet another possible basis for abnormal sleep-wake patterns is disturbed hypothalamic function in the Prader-Willi syndrome. When a young adult with Prader-Willi syndrome and SOREMPs in addition to snoring, obstructive sleep apnea (OSA), and daytime sleepiness was given a trial of nasal continuous positive airway pressure, all abnormalities improved except for the SOREMPs.[16]

Developmental changes and gender differences were examined in a large group of children and adults with Prader-Willi syndrome.[17] Surprisingly, only 2 of 24 individuals, both children with enlarged tonsils and adenoids, showed severe OSA; both improved following surgery. Most of the remainder of the group had only mild apnea. However, REM-related oxygen desaturation was very common, and its severity correlated with the degree of obesity. In this study population, REM abnormalities (shortened, fragmented, and multiple REM sleep periods) were seen even in patients without apnea or REM-associated hypoxemia. Although several individuals had at least two SOREMPs on the MSLT, there were no signs of narcolepsy beyond excessive daytime sleepiness. The authors suggested that the pattern of abnormalities supported the hypothesis of underlying hypothalamic dysfunction characteristic of Prader-Willi syndrome.

Rett Syndrome

Rett syndrome is an unusual disorder of unknown etiology characterized by mental retardation, microcephaly, pervasive developmental disorder with autistic features, apnea and hyperventilation in the waking state, and a peculiar motor apraxia leading to the pathognomonic hand wringing. An associated sleep-wake disturbance is so common that it is also considered to be one of the diagnostic behavioral features.[18–20] However, despite parental observations that three quarters of affected girls suffer from frequent night waking, little is known about specific sleep abnormalities in this disorder (Table 15–1).[21]

Rett syndrome is identified by its phenotypic expression and clinical presentation rather than by the presence of a biologic marker. The disorder only (or almost only) affects females.[22] Estimated prevalence is at least 1 in 10,000 girls.[23, 24] Neuropathologic studies show gross cortical atrophy and microcephaly, underpigmentation of the substantia nigra, and evidence of axonal neuropathy.[25, 26] Chromosomal studies are inconclusive. Fragile sites at the Xp22 region have been described by some[27] but negated by others.[28] No cytogenetic abnormalities have been detected. Less than 2% of cases are familial. Since basically all patients are female, the disorder could be X-linked, in which case it would be lethal to males (however, patients' mothers do not report increased miscarriages). Other hypotheses have been proposed.[29] There is usually no history of prenatal problems, and the infants appear normal at birth and for at least the first 6 months of life. Head circumference is normal initially but falls off between 3 months and 4 years. From 9 months to 2 1/2 years there is loss of purposeful hand skills, and there is psychomotor regression with social withdrawal, mental retardation, and communicative dysfunction with loss of speech. Typical, stereotypic "hand washing/wringing" or "tapping/clapping" appear after 1 to 3 years of age. Dyspraxic gait and posture become apparent at 2 to 4 years of age. Other typical features included a characteristic breathing dysfunction, EEG abnormalities, seizures, spasticity,

Table 15–1. THE FOUR CLINICAL STAGES OF CLASSIC RETT SYNDROME

I. Early Onset Stagnation Stage

Duration: months; age: ½ to 1½ years
Developmental arrest—stagnation
Changed communicability? Eye contact?
Unspecified personal deviation?
Diminishing play interest
Hand waving—unspecific? episodic?
Decelerating skull growth

II. Rapid Destructive Stage

Duration: weeks–months; age: 1–4
Developmental deterioration
"Pseudotoxic" at times
Rett stereotypes—autistic manifestations
Severe dementia—quite out
Loss of hand skill/hand use
"Gross motor" better preserved
Mobile—clumsy/apraxic/ataxic
Breathing irregular—hyperventilation
Fits are now problematic

III. Pseudostationary Stage

Duration: years; age: preschool–early school years
Less "out"—some stabilization
Mentally retarded—emotional contact
Autism not a major problem
Gross motor dysfunction
Gait apraxia prominent
Jerky truncal ataxia prominent
Epileptic symptomatology common

IV. Late Motor Deterioration Stage

Duration: decades; age: 5–15–25 years
Decreasing mobility—wheelchair bound
Severe multihandicap syndrome
Para to tetraparetic signs take over
Increasing lower motor neuron signs take over (scoliosis and trophic foot deformity)
Emotional contact improving
Epilepsy less problematic
Cachexia often develops
Growth retardation but normal puberty
Staring unfathomable gaze

Reproduced with permission from Hagberg B, Witt-Engerström I: Rett syndrome: a suggested staging system for describing impairment profile with increasing age towards adolescence. Am J Med Genet 24(Suppl 1):47, 1986.

peripheral vasomotor disturbances, scoliosis, and growth retardation (Table 15–2).

Respiratory abnormalities occur in waking and consist of periodic breathing, intermittent hyperventilation, breath-holding spells, and forced expulsion of air or saliva. Disorganized breathing with elements of obstructive, central, and mixed apnea have been described.[30] The voluntary/behavioral control of breathing is impaired. Breathing is normal in sleep. Dysfunction can occur as early as 10 months of age.[31] Long apneas may be accompanied by cyanosis and fainting.[31]

Table 15–2. RETT SYNDROME: CLINICAL CHARACTERISTICS AND DIFFERENTIAL DIAGNOSIS BY STAGE

Stages	Clinical Characteristics	Differential Diagnosis
Stage I Onset: 6–18 mo Duration: months	Developmental stagnation Deceleration of head/brain growth Disinterest in play activity and environment Hypotonia EEG background: normal or minimal slowing of posterior rhythm	Benign congenital hypotonia Prader-Willi syndrome Cerebral palsy
Stage II Onset: 1–3 yr Duration: weeks to months	Rapid developmental regression with irritability Loss of hand use Seizures Hand stereotypes: wringing, clapping, tapping, mouthing Autistic manifestations Loss of expressive language Insomnia Self-abusive behavior (e.g., chewing fingers, slapping face) EEG: background slowing and gradual loss of normal sleep activity; focal or multifocal spike and wave	Autism Psychosis Hearing or visual disturbance Encephalitis Epileptic encephalopathy Neurocutaneous syndromes Neurodegenerative disorders Various disorders of organic acid and amino acid metabolism
Stage III Onset: 2–10 yr Duration: months to years	Severe mental retardation/apparent dementia Amelioration of autistic features Seizures Typical hand stereotypes: wringing, tapping, mouthing Prominent ataxia and apraxia Hyperreflexia and progressive rigidity Hyperventilation, breath-holding, aerophagia during walking Weight loss with excellent appetite Early scoliosis Bruxism EEG: gradual disappearance of posterior rhythm, generalized slowing, absent vertex and spindle activity, epileptiform abnormalities activated during sleep	Spastic ataxic cerebral palsy Spinocerebellar degeneration Leukodystrophies or other storage disorders Neuroaxonal dystrophy Lennox-Gastaut syndrome Angelman's syndrome
Stage IV	Progressive scoliosis, muscle wasting, and rigidity Decreasing mobility, wheelchair bound Growth retardation Improved eye contact Virtual absence of expressive and receptive language Trophic disturbance of feet Reduced seizure frequency EEG: poor background organization with marked slowing and multifocal spikes and slow spike and wave pattern activated by sleep	Unknown degeneration disorder

Reproduced by permission of Hagberg B, and Witt-Engerström I: Clinical characteristics and differential diagnosis by stage. J Child Neurol 3(Suppl):513, 1988.

The EEG is normal until 1 1/2 to 2 years of age. Then there is gradual slowing of the background with increasing disorganization with age.[32] Focal or multifocal spike and wave complexes develop. A characteristic 3 to 5 hertz slowing appears.[33] After age 6 a monotonous theta rhythm may predominate. In sleep, background activity becomes slow and monotonous with high amplitude multifocal spike and wave discharges followed by brief periods of background activity attenuation.[34] By age 4, k-complexes and spindles disappear. These abnormalities suggest dysfunction in the pontine structures that control sleep cycle generation[30] or in the caudal portion of the locus coeruleus.[35]

Seizures develop in 70 to 80% of patients and usually begin after 2 years of age. They may be localized or generalized, myoclonic or mixed.

Overall sleep architecture and stage distribution may be altered. Changes in amounts of NREM stages are minimal, and both increased[35] and decreased[30] REM sleep have been reported. Decreased total sleep has also been described, at least after age 5 (Table 15–3).[30]

Treatment is unsatisfactory. Intermittent positive pressure breathing (IPPB) may be helpful to control disordered breathing in waking. Other treatment efforts include seizure control, physical and occupational therapy, orthopedic management, and family support. Treatment of sleeplessness remains symptomatic and may require the use of sedation.

Metabolic and Degenerative Disorders

Other specific congenital metabolic or degenerative syndromes have been sporadically and incompletely studied with regards to sleep function. There has been special interest in _phenylketonuria_ (PKU) because catecholamine and serotonin metabolism important in sleep regulation are disturbed in this condition. In the sparse literature addressing the relationship of sleep to PKU in children, sleep architecture has been unaffected.[36] The only unusual PSG findings were premature development of spindles in untreated infants and enhanced spindle activity in those already under dietary treatment.

Trichopoliodystrophy (Menkes's or kinky hair syndrome) is another metabolic condition of interest. The primary disturbance is in copper metabolism. This affects the catecholamine system through its effect on dopamine beta-hydroxylase, a copper dependent enzyme. One carefully studied child showed abnormal sleep architecture and an immature sleep/wake rhythm, neither of which improved after treatment.[1]

Sleep abnormalities have been examined in individual cases with other metabolic or degenerative diseases, but reports are all anecdotal. For example, an adolescent with _Hunter's syndrome_ (type 2 mucopolysaccharidosis) was investigated because his short neck and noisy breathing suggested obstructive apnea.[37] PSG showed both obstructive and central sleep apnea, presumably caused by dysfunction of central chemosensitivity receptors or direct involvement of medullary respiratory centers. _Leigh's syndrome_, a metabolic-degenerative disorder associated with lactic acidosis, can lead to acquired central hypoventilation from bilateral impairment of vital medullary centers.[38] _Familial dysautonomia_ (Riley-Day syndrome) is a severe hereditary sensorimotor neuropathy associated with frequent pulmonary infections, autonomic instability, mild mental retardation, and an ataxic form of cere-

Table 15–3. SLEEP CHARACTERISTICS IN RETT SYNDROME PATIENTS COMPARED WITH AGE-MATCHED CONTROLS

Subjects	Percent Sleep Time*	Stage 1(%)	Stage 2 (%)	Stage 3 (%)	REM (%)	Sleep Latency Minutes	REM Latency Minutes
RS patients 2–5 yr (n–4)	87.8	4.0	50.8†	33.0	14.2†	4.4†	127.0
Control subjects	86.8	8.0	37.7	30.3	22.8	24.6	60.5
RS patients 5–15 yr (n–7)	79.8†	4.9	49.3	34.3	12.4†	19.5	184.8
Control subjects	91.8	4.7	45.2	31.6	21.7	26.2	143.8

*Percent of time asleep during 12 hours total bedtime (20:00–08:00)
†p < 0.01
From Glaze DG, Frost JD, Zoghbi HY, Percy AK: Characterization of respiratory patterns and sleep. Ann Neurol 21:377, 1987.

bral palsy. Children often demonstrate sleep disturbances early in the course. Hypoventilation in NREM sleep, hypercarbia, and mixed apneas can be severe; sleep-disordered breathing worsens with frequent pulmonary infections.[39]

Tourette's Syndrome

Tourette's syndrome is a familial neurobehavioral disorder beginning in childhood. It is characterized by chronic multiple motor and phonic tics, often in association with obsessive-compulsive behavior and attention deficit hyperactivity disorder (ADHD). There is increasing evidence that Tourette's syndrome is an autosomal dominant genetic disorder with variable expressivity and penetrance. Sleep disturbances have been described and several descriptive studies have specifically addressed sleep abnormalities (see Chapter 16).[40–42] Parasomnias (somnambulism and sleep terrors) are increased in children with Tourette's syndrome compared with children with epilepsy or learning disabilities. PSG performed on untreated children with Tourette's syndrome has shown increased slow wave sleep, decreased REM sleep, and an increased frequency of nocturnal arousals, compared with normal age-matched controls.[41] Tics were observed in sleep, in all stages, despite typical parental reports to the contrary. It has been suggested that parasomnias are related more to the attention deficit component than to Tourette's syndrome.[43]

Attention Deficit Hyperactivity Disorder

Attention deficit hyperactivity disorder (ADHD) is a neurobehavioral condition defined by symptoms of inattention, overarousal, hyperactivity, impulsivity, and difficulty in delaying gratification. Although the Diagnostic and Statistical Manual (DSM III-R) has dropped sleep disturbances as a diagnostic criteria, complaints of sleep onset and maintenance are common, and these problems are frequently cited by parents as major concerns (see Chapter 16). They include difficulty in falling asleep, restless sleep, and early morning arousals. The Conner's parent questionnaire asks about each of these problems, and children with ADHD score significantly higher than controls in each of these areas.

Recent studies support the notion that parents perceive children with ADHD as poor sleepers.[44, 45] Preschoolers with the condition showed significantly more difficulty in falling asleep, more night arousals, more crying during the night, and more early morning awakenings compared with normal controls. However, the same researchers were unable to document any differences in total sleep time or sleep latency when using sleep diaries.

Elementary school age children with ADHD have been evaluated with full PSG. Although the methodologic problem of a small sample constrains analysis, there was no difference in sleep architecture between normal children and untreated ADHD.[46] Only chronic treatment with methylphenidate was associated with delayed sleep onset, longer total sleep time, and minor changes in REM variables. These findings were recently confirmed in a drug-placebo crossover, double blinded study performed at home using wrist actigraphy.[47] The authors suggested that longer sleep duration during the baseline and placebo periods in children with ADHD could be attributed to hypoarousal or increased fatigue from hyperactivity during the day. They further implied that the decreased sleep duration during the methylphenidate trial might reflect reversal of a subarousal state underlying the disorder.

There is no doubt that the effects of insufficient or disturbed sleep on daytime function can mimic ADHD or further contribute to the severity of pre-existing attention disorder.[48] Sleep schedule disorders can also contribute to the problem.[49]

It is well known that fatigue in children often leads to paradoxic overactivity and irritability; parents typically recognize that a disturbed schedule can be followed by a day in which the child cannot concentrate, acts wildly, and refuses to cooperate. Any disturbance of sleep can lead to aberrant daytime function. One of the daytime features of OSA of childhood, for example, can be hyperactivity, impulsivity, and behavioral deterioration. These features often resolve when apnea is corrected by appropriate intervention, such as tonsillectomy. Other sleep disorders including narcolepsy can cause similar poor attention and hyperactivity. Periodic leg movements, schedule disorders, and insufficient sleep can impair alertness with resultant hyperactivity.

A novel approach to one group of children with inattentiveness, daydreaming, restlessness, and excessive sleepiness has led to the conclusion that these youngsters have a primary disorder of vigilance.[50] Weinberg and Brumback distinguished this disorder from ADHD, primary affective disorders, narcolepsy, and other conditions.[51] Support for this concept has come from a careful study of preadolescents with ADHD and normal controls employing serial ambulatory PSG and laboratory MSLT.[52] Despite the lack of any major disturbances of nocturnal sleep, 30% of affected children had increased sleepiness by MSLT.

Neuromuscular Diseases

Sleep disorders may occur in patients with neuromuscular disorders associated with respiratory muscle weakness. In terms of actual numbers, this is a more likely consideration than narcolepsy in children. Certainly, in the presence of known muscle weakness, sleep apnea and hypoventilation should be suspected as the most likely cause of disturbed sleep as well as the possible basis for poor school performance or behavior problems (see Chapters 18 and 19).

Respiratory failure has been recognized as a frequent complication and an important cause of death in _Duchenne's muscular dystrophy._[53] Even in affected adolescents and young adults without any complaints of sleep disturbances, morning headaches, or daytime hypersomnolence, periods of hypopnea and apnea were observed in all patients studied.[54] Significant oxygen desaturations were noted, especially during REM sleep. This group did not have abnormal waking arterial blood gases. The severity of daytime pulmonary function studies did not predict the degree of central events during sleep. In a slightly younger group of adolescent boys with Duchenne's dystrophy without any evidence of nocturnal oxygen desaturations, there was still evidence for significant sleep fragmentation, recurrent hypoventilation, and reduced REM sleep.[55] The authors speculated that even these minor disturbances could aggravate existing behavioral and learning problems. Furthermore, the disease could be worsened by an increased risk for aspiration, which is known to occur with experimental sleep fragmentation.[56] Repeated aspiration is an important cause of progressive respiratory insufficiency in chronic neuromuscular disease. Other important considerations include chronic lung infections, scoliosis, chest wall deformities, and intercostal muscle weakness in addition to abnormal control of ventilation.[57]

Myotonic dystrophy is another important muscle disease that presents with early sleep disturbances. Guilleminault has suggested that myotonic dystrophy may be the most common undiagnosed cause of excessive daytime sleepiness in children.[58] This condition has multiple organ involvement including heart, brain, eye, and other organs. The etiology of somnolence in myotonic dystrophy is occasionally obscure. Respiratory failure from alveolar hypoventilation can be found in the presence of only mild respiratory muscle weakness; in these cases impaired neural control of ventilation has been implicated. One recent study of ambulatory patients without chronic lung disease showed hypoxic ventilatory responses which were significantly reduced, while hypercapnic ventilatory responses were only irregularly affected.[59] In addition to central apnea, probably from direct weakness of intercostal and accessory muscles of respiration as well as diaphragmatic involvement, some patients also show typical obstructive apnea. Although it is tempting to attribute cognitive deficit to disturbed sleep, another study demonstrated no correlation between fragmented sleep or apnea with daytime dysfunction.[60] These authors proposed that the neuropsychologic deficits in myotonic dystrophy probably represent a direct effect of CNS lesions rather than disturbed sleep function.

There have been fewer investigations in other neuromuscular diseases, but case reports have implicated several nonprogressive, slowly progressive, and infectious conditions such as _nemaline myopathy, congenital muscular dystrophy, spinal muscular atrophy, transverse myelitis and poliomyelitis._[61-63] Affected individuals were chronically symptomatic with morning headaches and excessive sleepiness or acutely ill with ventilatory failure and cor pulmonale. A recent large series has confirmed the frequency of respiratory involvement across the entire spectrum of primary muscle diseases.[64] Although respiratory failure often paralleled the severity of the muscle weakness, some patients developed pulmonary problems at an earlier stage of their disease, often in association with intercurrent illness. Respiratory involvement was relatively early particularly in inflammatory muscle disorders and acid maltase deficiency.

In most instances, the identification of symptomatic sleep problems heralds end-stage disease. Under these circumstances, treatment of respiratory failure is sometimes not instituted, although aggressive management can be associated with successful weaning from mechanical ventilation if precipitated by acute illness.[65] When early diagnosis prior to respiratory failure is made, there are a variety of successful treatment options. Nocturnal endotracheal intubation now can usually be replaced by negative pressure ventilation or positive pressure ventilation through a nose mask.[66–68] Other preventative strategies which can ameliorate respiratory compromise include early treatment of scoliosis, weight control, and improved sleep positioning.

Another less obvious presentation of disturbed respiration in neuromuscular disease can be *nocturnal seizures*.[69] Presumably this occurs on a hypoxic rather than an epileptic basis. Treatment of a young adult with congenital muscular dystrophy by nocturnal ventilatory support led to resolution of nocturnal seizures as well as resolution of all sleep-disordered breathing and normalization of blood gases.

Myelodysplasia, Hydrocephalus, and Other Structural Lesions

Infants and children with structural brain lesions may demonstrate clinically significant sleep disorders. Myelodysplasia (spina bifida) is frequently associated with apnea and hypoventilation. The presence of vocal cord paralysis presenting with stridor and swallowing incoordination strongly points toward the brainstem involvement due to mechanical disturbance of nuclei and pathways involved in the control of respiration. Anatomic distortion of important structures can be caused by the effects of hydrocephalus and the Chiari II malformation which typically occur in association with spina bifida. Likely mechanisms are direct compression or traction of the medulla or vascular compromise. The range of clinical presentation varies widely, but some infants are so severely affected that they are ventilator dependent. Although large scale studies are unavailable, even apparently asymptomatic infants with myelodysplasia have a high incidence of abnormalities when studied with screening home pneumograms.[70] Apnea, cyanosis, and irregular breathing during sleep have also been seen in adolescents with this condition.[71] This population showed blunted hypercapnic ventilatory responses indicating disturbed central chemosensitivity.

Treatment options include tracheostomy and surgical decompression with cervical laminectomy.[72] However, the long-term outcome remains poor for these symptomatic children with severe respiratory problems. An alternative nonsurgical approach was recently suggested by Milerad and associates who treated two affected infants with acetazolamide.[73] These authors argued that the increased ventilatory drive from pharmacologic stimulation of peripheral and central chemoreceptors markedly reduced the frequency of hypoventilation and hypoxemia by recruitment of chest wall muscles and increased upper airway patency. Interestingly, the beneficial effects of a 3-month course of acetazolamide were maintained after discontinuation.

There are several reports of sleep abnormalities in syringobulbia and syringomyelia which add support to the concept of an anatomic disruption of midline medullary nuclei and pathways as the basis for central and obstructive apnea.[74–76] Central and mixed apnea was a frequent finding even in asymptomatic patients with syringomyelia, and obstructive apnea was present in all patients with syringobulbia who demonstrated dysphagia. Patients with advanced syringomyelia and syringobulbia are at high risk for life-threatening respiratory events during sleep. A high level of clinical concern should incorporate periodic pulmonary function studies and PSG in order to anticipate the need for ventilatory support in those patients at increased risk of sudden death.

References

1. Miles LEM, Wilson MA: High incidence of cyclic sleep/wake disorders in the blind. Sleep Res 6:192, 1977.
2. Okawa M, Nanami T, Wada S, et al: Four congenitally blind children with circadian sleep-wake rhythm disorder. Sleep 10:101, 1987.
3. Palm L, Blennow G, Wetterberg L: Correction of non-24 hour sleep/wake cycle by melatonin in a blind retarded boy. Ann Neurol 29:336, 1991.
4. Klein T, Martens H, Dijk DJ, et al: Circadian sleep regulation in the absence of light perception: chronic non-24-hour circadian rhythm sleep disorder in a blind man with a regular 24-hour sleep-wake schedule. Sleep 16:333, 1993.
5. Okawa M, Sasaki H: Sleep disorders in mentally retarded and brain-impaired children. *In* Guilleminault C (ed): Sleep and Its Disorders in Children. New York, Raven Press, 1987, pp 269–290.
6. Shibagaki M, Keyono S, Takeuchi T: Nocturnal sleep in infants with congenital cerebral malformations. Clin Electroencephalogr 17:92, 1986.
6a. Jan JE, Espeze LH, Appleton RE: The treatment of sleep disorders with melatonin. Dev Med Child Neurol 36:97, 1994.

7. Hashimoto T, Fukuda K, Endo S, et al: Circadian rhythm in patients with hydranencephaly. J Child Neurol 7:188, 1992.

8. Stores G: (Annotation) Sleep studies in children with a mental handicap. J Child Psychol Psychiatry 33:1303, 1992.

9. Landesman-Dwyer S, Sackett GP: Behavioral changes in nonambulatory, profoundly mentally retarded individuals. Monogr Am J Ment Defic 3:44, 1978.

10. Quine L: Sleep problems in children with mental handicap. J Ment Defic Res 35:269, 1991.

11. Summers JA, Lynch PS, Harris JC, et al: A combined behavioral/pharmacological treatment of sleep-wake schedule disorder in Angelman Syndrome. J Dev Behav Pediatr 13:284, 1992.

12. Cassidy SB: Prader-Willi syndrome. Curr Prob Pediatr 14:1, 1984.

13. Bray GA, Dahms WT, Swerdloff RS, et al: The Prader-Willi syndrome: a study of 40 patients and a review of the literature. Medicine 62:59, 1983.

14. Cassidy SB, Ledbetter DH: Prader-Willi syndrome. Neurol Clin 7:37, 1989.

15. Holm VA, Cassidy SB, Butler MG, et al: Prader-Willi syndrome: consensus diagnostic criteria. Pediatrics 91:398, 1993.

16. Sforza R, Krieger J, Geiser J, et al: Sleep and breathing abnormalities in a case of Prader-Willi syndrome. Acta Paediatr Scand 80:80, 1991.

17. Hertz G, Cataletto M, Feinsilver SH, et al: Sleep and breathing patterns in patients with Prader-Willi syndrome (PWS): effects of age and gender. Sleep 16:366, 1993.

18. Hagberg B, Aicardi J, Dias K, et al: A progressive syndrome of autism, dementia, ataxia and loss of purposeful hand use in girls: Rett's syndrome: report of 35 cases. Ann Neurol 14:471, 1983.

19. Hagberg BA: Rett syndrome: clinical peculiarities, diagnostic approach, and possible cause. Pediatr Neurol 5:75, 1989.

20. Naidu S, Murphy M, Moser HW: Rett syndrome—natural history in 70 cases, Am J Med Genet 24:61, 1983.

21. Coleman M, Brubaker J, Hunter K, et al: Rett syndrome: a survey of North American patients. J Ment Defic Res 32:117, 1983.

22. Goutieres F, Aicardi J: Atypical forms of Rett syndrome. Am J Med Genet 24:183, 1986.

23. Hagberg B: Swedish approach to analysis of prevalence and cause. Brain Dev 7:277, 1985.

24. Kerr AAM, Stephenson JBP: Rett's syndrome in the West of Scotland. Brit Med J 291:579, 1985.

25. Jellinger K, Seitelberger F: Neuropathology of Rett's syndrome. Am J Med Gen 24:259, 1986.

26. Haas R, Love S: Peripheral nerve findings in Rett's syndrome. J Clin Neurol 3 Suppl:S25, 1988.

27. Moore JW, Tucker-Miller CM, Murphy M, et al: Chromosome studies in 10 patients with Rett's syndrome. Am J Med Genet 24:345, 1986.

28. Romeo G, Archidiacono N, Ferlini A, et al: Rett's syndrome: lack of association with fragile site Xp22 and strategy for genetic mapping of X-linked new mutations. Am J Med Genet 24(Suppl 1):355, 1986.

29. Zoghbi HY: Genetic aspects of Rett's syndrome. J Child Neurol 3(Suppl):S76, 1988.

30. Glaze DG, Frost JD, Zoghbi HY, Percy AK. Characterization of respiratory patterns and sleep. Ann Neurol 21:377, 1987.

31. Lugaresi E, Cirignotta F, Montagna P: Abnormal breathing in the Rett syndrome. Brain Dev 7:329, 1985.

32. Robb SA, Harden A, Boud SG: Rett's syndrome: an EEG study in 52 girls. Neuropediatrics 20:192, 1989.

33. Ishizaki A, Inoue Y, Sasaki H, et al: Longitudinal observations of EEG in the Rett's syndrome. Brain Dev 11:407, 1989.

34. Trauner A, Haas RH: Electroencephalographic abnormalities in Rett's syndrome. Pediatr Neurol 3:331, 1987.

35. Nomura Y, Segawa M, Hasegawa M: Rett's syndrome clinical studies and pathophysiological considerations. Brain Dev 6:475, 1986.

36. Schulte JJ, Kaiser HJ, Engelbart S: Sleep patterns in hyperphenylalaninemia: a lesson on serotonin to be learned from phenylketonuria. Pediatr Res 7:588, 1973.

37. Kurihara M, Kumagai K, Goto K, et al: Severe type Hunter's syndrome. Polysomnographic and neuropathological study. Neuropaediatrie 23:248, 1992.

38. Cummiskey J, Guilleminault C, Davis R, et al: Automatic respiratory failure: sleep studies and Leigh's disease (case report). Neurology 37:1876, 1987.

39. Guilleminault C, Stoohs R, Quera-Salva MA: Sleep-related obstructive and nonobstructive apneas and neurologic disorders. Neurology 42 (Suppl 6):53, 1992.

40. Barabas G, Matthews WS, Ferrari M: Disorders of arousal in Gilles de la Tourette's syndrome. Neurology 34:815, 1984.

41. Glaze DG, Frost JD, Jankovic J: Sleep in Gilles de la Tourette's syndrome: disorders of arousal. Neurology 33:586, 1983.

42. Barabas G, Matthews WS, Ferrari M: Somnambulism in children with Tourette syndrome. Devel Med Child Neurol 26:457, 1984.

43. Allen RP, Singer HS, Brown JE, et al: Sleep disorders in Tourette syndrome: a primary or unrelated problem? Pediatr Neurol 8:275, 1992.

44. Salzarulo P, Chevalier A: Sleep problems in children and their relationship with early disturbances of the waking-sleeping rhythms. Sleep 6:47, 1983.

45. Kaplan BJ, McNicol RD, Conte RA, et al: Sleep disturbance in preschool-aged hyperactive and nonhyperactive children. Pediatrics 80:839, 1987.

46. Greenhill L, Puig-Antich J, Goetz R, et al: Sleep architecture and REM sleep measures in prepubertal children with attention deficit disorder with hyperactivity. Sleep 6:91, 1982.

47. Tirosh E, Sadeh A, Munvez MA, et al: Effects of methylphenidate on sleep in children with attention-deficit hyperactivity disorder: an activity monitor study. Am J Dis Child 147:1313, 1993.

48. Weinberg WA, Emslie GJ: Attention deficit hyperactivity disorder: the differential diagnosis. J Child Neurol 6(suppl):S21, 1991.

49. Dahl RE, Puig-Antich JP: Sleep disturbances in child and adolescent psychiatric disorders. Pediatrician 17:32, 1990.

50. Weinberg WA, Harper CR: Vigilance and its disorders. Neurol Clin 11:59, 1993.

51. Weinberg WA, Brumback RA: Primary disorder of vigilance: a novel explanation of inattentiveness, daydreaming, boredom, restlessness, and sleepiness. J Pediatr 116:720, 1990.

52. Palm L, Persson E, Bjerre I: Sleep and wakefulness in preadolescent children with deficits in attention, motor control and perception. Acta Paediatr 81:618, 1992.

53. Inkley SR, Oldenburg FC, Vignos PJ: Pulmonary function in Duchenne muscular dystrophy related to stage of disease. Am J Med 56:297, 1974.

54. Smith PEM, Calverley PMA, Edwards RHT: Hypox-

emia during sleep in Duchenne muscular dystrophy. Am Rev Respir Dis 137:884, 1988.

55. Redding GJ, Okamato GA, Guthrie RD, et al: Sleep patterns in nonambulatory boys with Duchenne muscular dystrophy. Arch Phys Med Rehab 66:878, 1985.

56. Bowes G, Woolf GM, Sullivan CE, et al: Effect of sleep fragmentation on ventilatory and arousal responses of sleeping dogs to respiratory stimuli. Am Rev Respir Dis 122:899, 1980.

57. Begin R, Bureau MA, Lupien L, et al: Control of breathing in Duchenne muscular dystrophy. Am J Med 69:227, 1980.

58. Guilleminault C: Sleep disorders of children. *In* Berg BO (ed): Neurological Aspects of Pediatrics. Boston, Butterworth Heinemann, 1992, pp 617–626.

59. Carroll JE, Zwillich CW, Weil JV: Ventilatory response in myotonic dystrophy. Neurology 27:1125, 1977.

60. Broughton R, Stuss D, Kates M, et al: Neuropsychological deficits and sleep in myotonic dystrophy. Can J Neurol Sci 17:410, 1990.

61. Heckmatt JE, Loh L, Dubowitz V: Nocturnal hypoventilation in children with non-progressive neuromuscular disease. Pediatrics 83:250, 1989.

62. Maayan C, Springer C, Armon Y, et al: Nemaline myopathy as a cause of sleep hypoventilation. Pediatrics 77:390, 1986.

63. Thorpy MJ, Schmidt-Nowara WW, Pollak CP, et al: Sleep-induced nonobstructive hypoventilation associated with diaphragmatic paralysis. Ann Neurol 12:308, 1982.

64. Howard RS, Wiles CM, Hirsch NP, et al: Respiratory involvement in primary muscle disorders: assessment and management. Q J Med 86:175, 1993.

65. O'Donohue WJ, Baker JP, Bell GM, et al: Respiratory failure in neuromuscular disease: management in a respiratory intensive care unit. JAMA 235:733, 1976.

66. Braun SR, Sufit RL, Giovanni BA, et al: Intermittent negative pressure ventilation in the treatment of respiratory failure in progressive neuromuscular disease. Neurology 37:1874, 1987.

67. Ellis ER, Bye PTP, Bruderer JW, et al: Treatment of respiratory failure during sleep in patients with neuromuscular disease. Am Rev Respir Dis 135:148, 1987.

68. Gilgoff IS, Kahlstrom E, MacLaughlin E, et al: Long-term ventilatory support in spinal muscular atrophy. J Pediatr 115:904, 1989.

69. Kryger MH, Steljes DG, Woon-Chee Y, et al: Central sleep apnoea in congenital muscular dystrophy. J Neurol Neurosurg Psychiatry 54:710, 1991.

70. Davidson-Ward SL, Jacobs RA, Gates EP, et al: Abnormal ventilatory patterns during sleep in infants with myelomeningocele. Pediatr 109:631, 1986.

71. Swaminathan S, Paton JY, Ward SL, et al: Abnormal control of ventilation in adolescents with myelodysplasia. J Pediatr 115:898, 1989.

72. Charney EB, Rorke LB, Sutton LN, et al: Management of Chiari II complications in infants with myelomeningocele. Pediatrics 80:231, 1987.

73. Milerad J, Lagercrantz H, Johnson P: Obstructive sleep apnea in Arnold-Chiari malformation treated with acetazolamide. Acta Paediatr 81:609, 1992.

74. Encabo H, Gene R, Nogues MA: Polysomnographic findings in syringomyelia and syringobulbia. Sleep Res 16:474, 1987.

75. Nogues MA, Gene R, Encabo H: Risk of sudden death during sleep in syringomyelia and syringobulbia. J Neurol Neurosurg Psychiatry 55:585, 1992.

76. Adelman S, Dinner DS, Goren H, et al: Obstructive sleep apnea in association with posterior fossa neurologic disease. Arch Neurol 41:509, 1984.

16

Sleep in Behavioral and Emotional Disorders

RONALD E. DAHL

Child and adolescent psychopathology is a problem of enormous magnitude. Estimates from a recent report from the Institute of Medicine indicate that greater than 15% of American youth have significant behavioral or emotional problems.[1] These problems appear to be increasing and represent serious disorders. For example, completed suicides among adolescents have tripled over the past three decades, and suicide is now the second leading cause of mortality in this age group.[2]

The regulation of sleep appears to have a close relationship with behavioral and emotional disorders. Sleep complaints and sleep disturbances occur frequently with these disorders, the medications used to treat the disorders often affect sleep, and sleep loss can exacerbate mood and behavioral symptoms. There are also numerous examples of primary sleep disorders masquerading as psychiatric disorders (and vice versa). Although sleep, mood, and behavior are closely related in this age group, the details of the relationships are poorly understood. The limited information available comes from two perspectives: (1) measures of sleep disturbances within the context of specific psychiatric disorders and (2) measures of behavioral and emotional disturbances within the context of specific sleep disorders. Each perspective will be presented in this chapter.

Specific Psychiatric Disorders

Child and Adolescent Affective Disorders

Major depressive disorder (MDD) is a common problem, with prevalence estimates rang-ing from 2 to 5% in the child and adolescent age range.[3, 4] Recent evidence supports the continuity between early onset MDD and adult depression, indicating that these problems in children and adolescents may represent the beginning of a lifetime of problems.[5-7]

Subjective sleep complaints are very common in children and adolescents with MDD. These include insomnia in approximately 75% of cases and hypersomnia in 25% of cases.[8] Hypersomnia symptoms become much more prevalent after puberty.[9] Approximately 30 to 40% of depressed children and adolescents complain of severe insomnia, often describing extreme difficulty falling asleep or a subjective sense of having not slept deeply all night. Early morning awakening is less common in young depressed subjects than in adult MDD. There is also an overlap with late sleep-wake schedule disorders and depression in adolescence. That is, depressed adolescents frequently have difficulty falling asleep, are unable to get up on time for school, sleep in very late during the day, and have extreme daytime fatigue (and over time, shift to very delayed sleep-wake schedules (see Chapter 10)). It is often quite difficult to sort out the components of these problems with respect to decreased motivation, delayed circadian phase, and the depressive symptomatology. From a clinical perspective, the possibility of a MDD should be assessed when a child or adolescent presents with significant and persistent sleep complaints. Consideration of depression should include an assessment for other symptoms of major depression (Table 16–1). In addition, a positive family history for affective disorders also warrants more careful assessment of chil-

Table 16–1. MDD CRITERIA SYMPTOMS (5 REQUIRED)

Depressed or irritable mood
Diminished interest or pleasure
Appetite or weight change
Insomnia or hypersomnia
Psychomotor agitation or retardation
Fatigue or loss of energy
Worthlessness or excessive guilt
Diminished concentration
Thoughts of death, suicidal ideation, or plan, or suicide attempt

dren with sleep complaints because of the strong evidence for increased familial loading in cases of early onset affective disorders.[6, 7] Once a diagnosis of MDD is made, treatment should focus on the depression as the primary illness, as evidence supports improved sleep following recovery. Following rules for good general sleep hygiene with regular sleep-wake schedules also makes good sense within the overall treatment for depression.

In contrast to the convergence of evidence for *subjective* sleep complaints associated with early onset depression, EEG studies of sleep in depressed children and adolescents have not reliably revealed the same objective abnormalities that have been well-described in *adult* patients with MDD.[10–17] Although a few controlled studies have found significant differences in sleep latency,[10, 16] mildly increased sleep continuity disturbances,[11, 13] and reduced REM latency,[15, 16] these abnormalities have not been seen consistently across studies in this age group. Furthermore, there have been no documented abnormalities in delta sleep.

There are at least three interpretations to the discrepancies between subjective and objective studies in child and adolescent depression. One possibility is that MDD is associated with a change in the perception of sleep rather than physiologic changes as measured by EEG studies. A second alternative is that the sleep disruptions associated with MDD in younger subjects are masked by maturational effects on sleep. A third interpretation is that age and depression may interact in producing the psychobiologic changes associated with depression, including the pattern of sleep changes.[18]

Another clinical presentation of sleep disturbances related to affective disorders is seen in adolescents with a bipolar affective disorder who present with a dramatically decreased need for sleep. During manic episodes, these adolescents can show a drastically reduced sleep requirement with increased energy, elation, grandiosity, and other signs of mania.

There is a general need for better assessment in children and adolescents for both mood- and sleep-related disturbances. Frequently, adolescents are reluctant to voice complaints and parents can often be unaware of their children's sleep problems. Many people tend to attribute mood changes and significant sleep changes to normal adolescent turbulence. However, when there is a deterioration in school and/or social functioning in children and adolescents, it is important to carefully assess for sleep and mood symptoms. The early identification and treatment of sleep and mood problems may significantly reduce the morbidity and mortality of these disorders. There is also evidence from adult studies that sleep disturbances may *precede* the development of depression in MDD.[19]

Attention Deficit Hyperactivity Disorder (ADHD)

Inattentiveness, impulsivity, restlessness, hyperactivity, and disruptive behavior are common sources of complaints by parents and teachers. Within this clinical entity of attention-related problems, sleep complaints are also frequently reported (see Chapter 15). Difficulties falling asleep, restless sleep, night waking, and early morning waking are reported more frequently by the parents of children with attention deficit hyperactivity disorder (ADHD) than age-matched controls.[20–22]

In addition, there is evidence that inadequate sleep can at least exacerbate, if not cause, ADHD-like symptoms in some children. Specifically, sleep loss in children frequently results in symptoms of inattention, irritability, distractibility, and impulsivity. Dahl and associates[23] recently reported the case of a 10-year-old girl with ADHD and longstanding sleep difficulties (delayed sleep phase insomnia), who demonstrated significant improvement of ADHD and learning disability symptoms (as determined by blind raters in a controlled research setting) following treatment of her sleep problems. Children with obstructive sleep apnea (OSA) syndrome also may show improvement or resolution of ADHD symptoms following treatment of the sleep-disordered breathing.[24] Despite this evidence implicating sleep as having an important role in ADHD, objective EEG studies of sleep in a controlled setting generally have not revealed significant sleep disturbances.[25, 26] Some non-specific sleep changes have been reported in children with ADHD, including reduced REM sleep,[27] signs of sleepiness by pupillometry,[28] and decreased threshold of arousal to sounds during sleep.[29]

From a clinical perspective, it is prudent to carefully assess children with ADHD symptoms for sleep problems. When sleep disturbances are identified, treatment should address both behavioral and physiologic components of the sleep problem. Adequate or optimal sleep is not well-defined in children. There is a wide range of individual variation in sleep requirements and many children seem to "adapt" to getting by on little sleep. However, some of these children may show an improvement in daytime behavioral symptoms with increased sleep. Thus, if inadequate sleep or sleep disturbances are suspected in children with ADHD-type symptoms, one prudent approach is to attempt to increase or improve the sleep and evaluate for signs of improved daytime functioning.

Another important aspect of the relationship between sleep and ADHD is the sleep effects of the stimulants often used to treat ADHD. Some of these children receive late doses of stimulants or long-acting preparations that can prolong sleep latency. However, there are families who report significant *improvement* in their child's sleep when the child is placed on stimulants, even on a late dose. This improvement may result from better organized behavior around bedtime, compliance with going to bed, and earlier sleep onset. Thus, sleep effects with stimulants in ADHD appear to be highly individualized. EEG sleep studies of children on stimulant medication have revealed (overall) small delays of 15 to 20 minutes in sleep onset during medication condition compared to nonmedication condition.[30-32]

Conduct Disorder

Conduct disorder is the general term used to describe a group of disorders in children characterized by a persistent pattern of conduct violating the rights of others (at least 6 months of major violations of age appropriate rules or norms). Families of children with conduct disorder often present sleep-related complaints similar to children with ADHD. With respect to objective abnormalities, a study by Coble and associates,[33] utilizing automated analyses of subtypes of EEG waves in children with psychopathology, identified a group of prepubertal children with conduct disorder with increased counts of delta waves in the first half of the night compared with age-matched normal controls. The group also exhibited less total sleep, increased arousals, and more stage 1 sleep compared with the rest of the group. Although there is not a specific clinical conclusion to these findings, the authors interpret them as encouraging in the application of automated techniques in detecting subtle sleep changes associated with child psychopathology, which may not be evident with routine EEG sleep studies. It is also possible that these children may have adapted to getting less sleep and more arousals by deeper delta sleep in the first half of the night. From a clinical perspective, one should ensure that these children are obtaining adequate amounts of undisturbed sleep. Behavioral treatments targeting bedtime and other sleep-related, limit-setting policies can help to improve the amount of sleep in some oppositional children who may have relative sleep deprivation because of an inadequate number of hours in bed.

Tourette's Syndrome

Gilles de la Tourette's syndrome is a child-onset disorder of multiple motor and/or vocal tics. In approximately 50 to 75% of cases there is a positive family history of Tourette's or simple tics, and about 10% overlap with familial obsessive-compulsive disorder.[34] Sleep disturbances are reported in over 50% of subjects with Tourette's syndrome and occur more frequently in family members of individuals with Tourette's syndrome (see Chapter 15).[34, 35] In addition, Tourette's syndrome represents one of the few movement disorders in which movements can continue through all stages of sleep.[34, 36-39] Patients with Tourette's syndrome also have increased partial arousals from deep stage 4 sleep (night terrors, sleep walking) and more frequent enuresis.[36-39] Treatment of Tourette's syndrome improves tics as well as decreasing partial arousals from sleep.[37]

At Western Psychiatric Institute, a number of children with Tourette's syndrome have been studied who have frequent sudden arousals through all stages of sleep and frequent partial arousals from stage 4. It is also evident that many of these same children have significant daytime difficulties with irritability, inattentiveness, and impulsivity. (There is a well-documented overlap of ADHD-like symptoms in Tourette's.[35] Adding a dose of medication such as clonidine or clonazepam near bedtime has resulted in significant decrease in EEG arousals from sleep and an improvement in daytime irritability and tiredness, which may have been a result of chronically disturbed sleep. Behavioral treatments targeting adequate amounts of nighttime sleep can also be essential adjuncts to treatment.

Behavioral Treatment of Inadequate Sleep

In a number of these disorders (ADHD, conduct disorder, and Tourette's), there has been a general recommendation toward "optimizing" nighttime sleep. This process can be broken down into three components:

1. Eliminating identifiable causes of sleep disturbance (e.g., sleep apnea, environmental disturbances).
2. Teaching good general sleep hygiene.
3. Behavioral treatments focused on *target behaviors* that are interfering with sleep (e.g., late night television, oppositional behaviors at bedtime, erratic schedules).

The first step in these interventions is to correctly identify the causes of inadequate sleep. The second step is to help the family understand the consequences of inadequate sleep in the child (exacerbation of emotional and behavioral symptoms in the daytime). Third, a specific behavioral contract should be drawn up with the family specifying the changes in target behaviors (for example, in bed with lights and television out by 9:00 PM) and subsequent rewards or consequences for successes and failures. The emphasis should be on a positive, helpful approach (*helping the child and family make desired changes*). Relaxation therapy (with positive imagery) can also be an important adjunct for children who have trouble "unwinding," unless they are completely exhausted.

Specific Sleep Disorders

Narcolepsy

Early onset narcolepsy can be difficult to diagnose and can be confused with early behavioral or psychiatric disorders (see Chapter 14). Although the typical age of diagnosis for narcolepsy is reported to be late adolescence to early adulthood, many patients describe the onset of symptoms during school age and early adolescence. Documented clearcut cases of narcolepsy have been reported as early as 6 to 8 years of age.[40–42] The diagnosis can be very difficult to make in early cases, even when a full assessment is being performed by clinicians experienced with narcolepsy.[43] In addition, behavioral and emotional symptoms are frequently significantly concomitant with early narcolepsy.[43] Thus, early cases may be misdiagnosed as behavioral or psychiatric disorders.[44] Two cases were seen at the Western Psychiatric Institute of undiagnosed narcolepsy in adolescents admitted to a psychiatric hospital with a diagnosis of psychotic depression. In each case, the adolescents had shown social withdrawal, pervasively depressed mood, fatigue, increased sleep, and a variety of "unusual" behaviors (cataplexy and hypnagogic hallucinations) that were misinterpreted as psychotic symptoms. A recent description of consecutive cases of early onset narcolepsy in a psychiatric setting has been reported emphasizing the complexity and overlap of symptoms.[45] In many cases involving children and younger adolescents, even when narcolepsy is suspected, history alone is not adequate in distinguishing narcolepsy from other causes of sleepiness and mood disturbances. (Symptoms of weakness with laughter or seeing things before falling asleep can be nonspecific in children.) Therefore, when children and adolescents present with persistent hypersomnia and mood or behavioral problems, the possibility of narcolepsy must remain high on the list of differential diagnoses.

Obstructive Sleep Apnea Syndrome

Many children with mild to moderate OSAS present with a constellation of daytime symptoms consistent with chronically disturbed nighttime sleep (see Chapters 18 and 19). This includes irritability, emotional lability, difficulty with concentration, and inattentiveness. Many young children may not show frank somnolence with chronically disturbed sleep, only the irritability and inattentiveness. As reported by others,[24] the author has also seen a number of these children carrying the diagnosis of ADHD and being treated with stimulant medication. Positive therapeutic response to stimulants does not rule out OSAS, as stimulant medication will improve daytime symptoms of chronically disturbed sleep. In a number of these cases, the apnea index and size of the tonsils and adenoids were otherwise felt to be "borderline" (apnea index 2 to 5) and not clearly indicative of treatment by tonsillectomy and adenoidectomy. In some of these cases, we strongly recommended treatment for the apnea because of the behavioral-emotional symptoms, which can have such a negative impact on school and social function.

Parasomnias

There appears to be a higher rate of significant parasomnias, especially night terrors and agitated partial arousals, in children with concurrent psychopathology (see Chapter 11). There are at least three possible components to this relationship: (1) abnormal physiologic arousal patterns related to psychopathology; (2) abnormal sleep patterns related to psychopathology; (3) psychologic factors. Each will be discussed briefly.

1. There is a subgroup of children with abnormal, sudden arousals throughout the night, similar to the Tourette's patients. PSG studies of these children show brief periodic paroxysmal arousals throughout the night. The author has observed this pattern primarily in children with severe psychopathology, in children with Tourette's syndrome, and in two children with obsessive-compulsive disorder. When these arousals coincide with stage 4 sleep, night terrors and agitated partial arousals often occur. In some of these cases, the parasomnia events are very frequent and severe and require aggressive treatment with medications to suppress the arousals.

2. Many children with significant behavioral and emotional problems develop erratic sleep-wake schedules with frequent bedtime struggles and late night bedtimes. Although the children may seem to "adapt" to getting by on less sleep than one would predict for age, this "adaptation" usually results in high-intensity stage sleep early in the night and may predispose to more frequent partial arousals. In these children, behavioral treatment and increasing the total amount of sleep are usually effective in eliminating the parasomnias.

3. Psychologic factors may also be important in the relationship between psychopathology and parasomnias. Klackenberg,[46] and Ferber,[47] have commented on the role of "repressed anxiety and aggression." In many cases, these children are quiet and well behaved but seem to have a great deal of unexpressed tension. We have observed that some of these children focus on anxious thoughts and worries at bedtime and have difficulty falling asleep, which may be a variant of sleep loss/parasomnias. For some of these children, addressing the sources of their fears and anxieties and helping them express these in healthy ways while awake may also contribute to improvements in parasomnias.[46]

General Points

1. There is a strong relationship between the control of sleep and the regulation of emotion and behavior in children and adolescents. Children with significant behavioral and emotional problems should be assessed for sleep disorders. The possibility of a primary psychiatric disorder must be considered in patients with sleep disorders and vice versa. In addition, it is likely that a subgroup of children with behavioral-emotional problems may show clinical improvement in behaviors after optimization of sleep (quantity and quality). Behavioral methods to optimize sleep include good sleep hygiene with regular bedtime hours (including weekends), avoidance of caffeine and other stimulants in the diet, and relaxation techniques and positive imagery at bedtime (for children with difficulty falling asleep).

2. Effective management of sleep difficulties is a central pragmatic issue for clinicians dealing with a wide range of child and adolescent psychiatric disorders. Sleep-related problems in children with behavioral and emotional problems often affect the entire family. Struggles to get children into bed at night and battles to wake adolescents up in the morning for school can become a source of major conflict for families. Middle of the night arousals in young children usually disturb the parents' sleep as well. In severe cases, such as with severe mental retardation or children with multiple handicaps, the pragmatic issues of dealing with problem behaviors at night can tip the balance toward the need for institutional care. Thus, effective management of sleep related problems is a major issue for clinicians working with child and adolescent psychiatric populations.

3. Our current knowledge of these complex relationships between sleep, development, and psychiatric well-being is at an embryonic state. Both sleep problems and emotional problems

are common among our youth. There is a clear need for improved understanding of these relationships along with better diagnosis and more effective treatments.

References

1. Institute of Medicine Report of Research on Child and Adolescents with Mental, Behavioral and Developmental Disorders. National Institute of Mental Health, U.S. Department of Health and Human Services. Public Health Service On Alcohol, Drug Abuse and Mental Health Administration. DHHS Pub. #(ADM90-1659), 1990.
2. Centers For Disease Control: Suicide Surveillance 1970–1980. Atlanta, U.S. Department of Health and Human Services, Public Health Service, Violent Epidemiology Branch, Center for Health Promotion and Education, 1985.
3. Kashani JH, Sherman DD: Childhood depression: epidemiology, etiological models, and treatment implications. Integr Psychiatry 6:1, 1988.
4. Bird HR, Canino G, Rubio-Stipec M, et al: Estimates of the prevalence of childhood maladjustment in a community survey in Puerto Rico. Arch Gen Psychiatry 42:689, 1985.
5. Strober M, Morrell W, Burroughs J, et al: A family study of bipolar I disorder in adolescence: early onset symptoms linked to increased family loading and lithium resistance. J Affect Dis 15:255, 1988.
6. Weissman MM, Gammon GD, John K, et al: Children of depressed parents. Increased psychopathology and early onset of major depression. Arch Gen Psychiatry 44:847, 1987.
7. Puig-Antich J, Goetz D, Davies M, et al: A controlled family history study of prepubertal major depressive disorder. Arch Gen Psychiatry 46:406, 1989.
8. Ryan ND, Puig-Antich J, Rabinovich H, et al: The clinical picture of major depression in children and adolescents. Arch Gen Psychiatry 44:854, 1987.
9. Williamson DE, Dahl RE, Ryan ND: Subjective sleep disturbances in children and adolescents with major depressive disorder. Sleep Res 20:193, 1991.
10. Dahl RE, Puig-Antich J, Ryan ND, et al: EEG sleep in adolescents with major depression: the role of suicidality and inpatient status. J Affect Dis 19:63, 1990.
11. Goetz R, Puig-Antich J, Ryan ND, et al: Electroencephalographic sleep of adolescents with major depression and normal controls. Arch Gen Psychiatry 44:61, 1987.
12. Young W, Knowles JB, MacLean AW, et al: The sleep of childhood depressives: comparison with age-matched controls. Biol Psychiatry 17:1163, 1982.
13. Appleboom-Fondu J, Kerkhofs M, Mendlewicz J: Depression in adolescents and young adults—polysomnographic and neuroendocrine aspects. J Affect Dis 14:35, 1988.
14. Puig-Antich J, Goetz R, Hanlon C, et al: Sleep architecture and REM sleep measures in prepubertal major depressives during an episode. Arch Gen Psychiatry 39:932, 1982.
15. Lahmeyer HW, Poznanski EO, Bellur SN: EEG sleep in depressed adolescents. Am J Psychiatry 140:1150, 1983.
16. Emslie GJ, Rush AJ, Weinberg WA, et al: Children with major depression show reduced rapid eye movement latencies. Arch Gen Psychiatry 47:119, 1990.
17. Kahn AU, Todd S: Polysomnographic findings in ado-

18. Reynolds CF, Kupfer DJ: State-of-the-art review: sleep research in affective illness: state of the art circa 1987. Sleep 10:199, 1987.
19. Ford DE, Kamerow DB: Epidemiological studies of sleep disturbances and psychiatric disorders: an opportunity for prevention? JAMA 262:1479, 1989.
20. Kaplan BJ, McNicol J, Conte RA, et al: Sleep disturbance in preschool-aged hyperactive and nonhyperactive children. Pediatrics 80:839, 1987.
21. Salzarulo P, Chevalier A: Sleep problems in children and their relationship with early disturbances of the waking-sleeping rhythms. Sleep 6:47, 1983.
22. Ross DM, Ross SA: Hyperactivity: Current Issues, Research and Theory, ed 2. New York, John Wiley & Sons, 1982.
23. Dahl RE, Pelham WE, Wierson M: The role of sleep disturbances in attention deficit disorder symptoms: a case study. J Pediatr Psychol 16:229, 1991.
24. Guilleminault C, Winkle R, Korobkin R, et al: Children and nocturnal snoring: evaluation of the effects of sleep related respiratory resistive and daytime functioning. Eur J Pediatr 139:165, 1982.
25. Greenhill L, Puig-Antich J, Goetz R, et al: Sleep architecture and REM sleep measures in prepubertal children with attention deficit disorder with hyperactivity. Sleep 6:91, 1983.
26. Busby K, Firestone P, Pivik RT: Sleep patterns in hyperkinetic and normal children. Pediatrics 4:366, 1981.
27. Kahn AU: Sleep REM latency in hyperkinetic boys. Am J Psychiatry 139:1358, 1982.
28. Knopp W, Arnold LE, Andras RL, et al: Predicting amphetamine response in hyperkinetic children by electronic pupillography. Pharmacopsychiatry 6:158, 1973.
29. Busby K, Pivik RT: Auditory arousal thresholds during sleep in hyperkinetic children. Sleep 8:332, 1985.
30. Chatoor I, Wells KC, Conners KC, et al: The effects of nocturnal behavior in hyperactive children. J Am Acad Child Adolesc Psychiatry 22:337, 1983.
31. Haig JR, Schroeder CS, Schroeder SR, et al: Effects of methylphenidate on hyperactive children's sleep. Psychopharmacologia 37:185, 1974.
32. Small A, Hibi S, Feinberg I: Effects of dextroamphetamine sulfate on EEG sleep patterns of hyperactive children. Arch Gen Psychiatry 25:369, 1971.
33. Coble PA, Taska LS, Kupfer DJ, et al: EEG sleep 'abnormalities' in preadolescent boys with a diagnosis of conduct disorder. J Am Acad Child Adolesc Psychiatry 23:438, 1984.
34. Jankovic J, Rohaidy H: Motor, behavioral, and pharmacologic findings in Tourette's syndrome. J Can Sci Neurol 14:3(suppl):541, 1987.
35. Nee LE, Caine ED, Polinsky RJ, et al: Gilles de la Tourette syndrome. Clinical and family study of 50 cases. Ann Neurol 7:41, 1980.
36. Glaze DG, Frost JD, Jankovic J: Sleep in Gilles de la Tourette's syndrome. Disorder of arousal. Neurology 33:586, 1983.
37. Jankovic J, Glaze DG, Frost JD: Effect of tetrabenazine on tics and sleep of Gilles de la Tourette's syndrome. Neurology 34:688, 1984.
38. Burd L, Kerbeshian J: Nocturnal coprolalia and phonic tics. Am J Psychiatry 145:132, 1988.
39. Barabas G, Matthews WS, Ferrari M: Disorders of arousal in Gilles de la Tourette's syndrome. Neurology 34:815, 1984.

lescents with major depression. Psychiatry Res 33:313, 1991.

40. Chisholm RC, Brook CJ, Harrison GF, et al: Prepubescent narcolepsy in a six year old girl. Sleep Res 15:113, 1985.
41. Young D, Zorick F, Wittig R, et al: Narcolepsy in a pediatric population. Am J Dis Child 142:210, 1988.
42. Wittig R, Zorick F, Roehrs T, et al: Narcolepsy in a 7 year old child. J Pediatr 102:725, 1983.
43. Kotagal S, Hartse KM, Walsh JK: Characteristics of narcolepsy in preteenaged children. Pediatrics 85:205, 1990.
44. Mahowald M, Rosen G: Verbal communications, 1990.
45. Dahl RE, Holttum J, Trubnick L: A clinical picture of child and adolescent narcolepsy. J Am Acad Child Adolesc Psychiatry 33:834, 1994.
46. Klackenburg G: Incidence of parasomnias in children in a general population. *In* Guilleminault C (ed): Sleep and Its Disorders In Children. New York, Raven Press, 1987, pp 99–113.
47. Ferber RA: Sleepwalking, confusional arousals, and sleep terrors in the child. *In* Kryger MH, Roth T, Dement WC (eds): Principles and Practices of Sleep Medicine. Philadelphia, WB Saunders, 1989, pp 640–642.

Primary Snoring in Children

JOHN L. CARROLL and GERALD M. LOUGHLIN

Approximately 1 in 10 children exhibit habitual snoring, that is, snoring during sleep every night or "most nights."[1–3] Although, at any point in time, there are millions of children with habitual snoring, it is believed in most cases to be a benign condition that does not need treatment. Snoring in children would not be a problem were it not for the fact that snoring is also a major presenting symptom of childhood obstructive sleep apnea syndrome (OSAS). Childhood OSAS, unlike primary or benign snoring, is associated with significant nighttime symptoms, daytime symptoms, and serious complications. Childhood OSAS is also discussed in Chapters 18 (clinical features and pathophysiology) and 19 (diagnosis and management).

Since the mid 1970s, when childhood OSAS was brought to the attention of pediatricians by Guilleminault and others,[4] increasing attention has been focused on snoring and breathing during sleep in children. More and more, physicians and parents recognize snoring in a child as a marker for a potentially serious disorder and children are now frequently referred for evaluation. The difficult challenge for the sleep disorders specialist is to determine whether a snoring child suffers from childhood OSAS or only primary snoring (PS).

Unlike adults, in whom the main presenting symptom of OSAS is excessive daytime somnolence (EDS), children are brought to the doctor because of snoring or difficult breathing during sleep. Thus, the main differential diagnosis of childhood snoring is between primary snoring (PS) and childhood OSAS, which are defined as follows:

PS in children is characterized by snoring during sleep without associated apnea, hypoventilation, hypoxemia, or hypercarbia. There is no associated sleep disturbance and no associated daytime symptoms other than those directly related to adenotonsillar hypertrophy.

Childhood OSAS is characterized by episodes of partial or complete upper airway obstruction during sleep, usually associated with a reduction in oxyhemoglobin saturation and/or hypercarbia. Nighttime and daytime symptoms and findings are present.

Classification into benign or primary snoring versus harmful snoring or OSAS appears to be a clinically useful separation. PS is a diagnosis of exclusion based on the assumption that snoring is benign when it is not associated with hypoxemia, hypercarbia, sleep disruption, or daytime symptoms. The usefulness of this clinical distinction is based on the assumption that PS does not require treatment, whereas OSAS does. As our knowledge of childhood OSAS increases, the present classification system may be displaced by one more consistent with the physiology of sleep-associated airway obstruction.

Much of the diagnostic evaluation for OSAS aims to distinguish between childhood OSAS and PS. PS is discussed as a separate clinical entity even though there is significant overlap between the symptoms of PS and OSAS. Indeed, it is this overlap that makes diagnosis problematic. In the absence of complications, PS is difficult to distinguish from childhood OSAS by history alone.

Predominant Symptoms and Main Features

Snoring is a vibratory sound produced in the upper airway, usually during the inspiratory phase of breathing, and almost always occurring during sleep. It can be distinguished by ear or by sophisticated computerized sound analysis from stridor—a sound with different characteristics, occurring during wakefulness as well as sleep, and originating from different anatomic sites in the airway.[5, 6] Some authors use the term "snoring" to refer to inspiratory sounds with specific characteristics,[5, 6] although to others it means *any* inspiratory breathing noise produced during sleep. Most studies of snoring or OSAS in children have avoided any attempt to precisely define the term. There is very little published information on PS in children. Although there is a great deal of literature on the general subject of snoring, studies do not distinguish between PS and OSAS and there have been no large studies on the clinical features of children with proven PS. Studies on patterns of snoring in children with PS are also lacking. Table 17–1 summarizes the clinical features of primary snoring, based on available literature and experience with over 4000 children referred to the Johns Hopkins Pediatric Sleep and Breathing Center for evaluation of snoring between 1985 and 1995.

Experience indicates that the snoring in a child with PS may be loud or soft, continuous or intermittent. Even when continuous (i.e., without apparent apneic interruptions), such snoring is not diagnostic of PS. The same pattern may also be heard in children with continuous partial upper airway obstruction (obstructive hypoventilation). Daytime symptoms should be absent, except those related to adenotonsillar hypertrophy such as mouth breathing, dry mouth, speech defects, swallowing difficulties, nasal stuffiness, and halitosis.[7, 8]

Course

The course of PS in children is not known. It is believed that some children with PS are at risk to develop OSAS. Guilleminault and associates reported five infants who initially presented with "near miss for SIDS," then gradually developed snoring during sleep, and finally by age four developed childhood OSAS.[9] Although this could be interpreted as showing the progression of PS to OSAS, these cases may not be representative of otherwise normal children.

Since the prevalence of habitual snoring appears to be at least four- to fivefold greater than the prevalence of OSAS, and since not all snoring children undergo adenotonsillectomy, it can at least be said that some proportion of snoring children do not develop OSAS. Some cases of PS must represent an early stage

Table 17–1. SYMPTOMS OF PRIMARY SNORING VERSUS CHILDHOOD OSAS

Primary Snoring	OSAS
Common features:	
May be loud	
May disturb others in house	
Worse in supine position	
Often present for months or years	
Worse during upper respiratory infection	
Worsened by obesity	
Worsened by sedatives or alcohol	
Continuous pattern usually	
May be intermittent	
Both may be associated with:	
Mouth breathing	
Nasal stuffiness	
Frequent otitis media	
Frequent sore throats	
Halitosis	
PS not usually associated with:	**OSAS may be associated with:**
Frequent arousals from sleep	Snoring or gasping
Disturbed sleep	Frequent arousals
Significant retraction*	Disturbed sleep
Unusual sleeping position	Significant retractions
Daytime sleepiness	Unusual body positions
Morning headache	Morning headache
School problems	Excessive daytime sleepiness
Behavior problems	School and behavior problems

*Paradoxical inward rib cage motion (retractions) can be normal in REM sleep in infants and children <2 years of age.

that will progress to childhood OSAS. But which ones? Is there any way to predict which snoring children are at risk to develop OSAS? Longitudinal studies of children with PS are needed to answer this important question.

Predisposing Factors

Enlarged adenoids predispose to snoring in children.[10, 11] Obesity predisposes to snoring in adults and is widely believed to do so in children. However, although obese children are considered to be at high risk for sleep-associated breathing disorders,[12] the prevalence of PS and OSAS in an unselected sample of obese children is not known. Snoring has been reported to be associated with numerous specific craniofacial abnormalities and inherited syndromes, including retrognathia, mandibular hypoplasia, macroglossia, nasal polyps, upper respiratory tract infection, and other causes of partial nasal or nasopharyngeal obstruction (Table 17–2), but no studies have investigated the precise role of these factors in producing snoring in children. Clinical experience suggests that snoring is more common in children with nearly any cause of neurologic impairment (such as cerebral palsy), but again no studies have reported the prevalence or course in an unselected sample. Snoring in children aged 6 to 13 is associated with parental cigarette smoking and is significantly related to the "dosage" of passive smoke.[3] Snoring in adults is also associated with cigarette smoking.[13]

Prevalence

The term "habitual snoring" has been used to refer to snoring that occurs frequently or constantly, often, or on most nights. Despite the lack of a standard definition of snoring, prevalence figures from 3 different countries are similar. Brouillette and associates reported the prevalence of frequent or constant snoring in normal children aged 1 to 10 years to be 9%.[1] A recent study from Italy, using questionnaires to evaluate 1615 school children aged 6 to 13 years, found that 8.5% reported snoring apart from when they had colds and 7.3%

Table 17–2. PREDISPOSING FACTORS FOR PRIMARY SNORING AND CHILDHOOD OSAS

Airway Narrowing or Dysfunction:	*Suppression of Airway Control:*
Airway muscle dysfunction	Alcohol
Airway tissue infiltration	Anesthesia
Allergic rhinitis	Chloral hydrate
Familial (?)	Narcotics
Hypothyroidism	Sedatives
Lingual tonsil hypertrophy	
Macroglossia	*Syndromes:*
Micrognathia	Achondroplasia
Nasal polyps (other nasal obstruction)	Apert's syndrome
Nasopharyngeal foreign body	Arthrogryposis multiplex congenita
Neurofibroma (laryngeal)	Beckwith-Wiedemann syndrome
Obesity	Conradi-Hünermann syndrome
Oropharyngeal papillomatosis	Crouzon syndrome
Previous airway surgery	Down syndrome
Post-transplant lymphoproliferative disorder	Facioauriculovertebral sequence
Repaired cleft palate	Fragile X syndrome
Retrognathia	Hallermann-Streiff syndrome
Sarcoidosis of the tonsils/adenoids	Hemifacial microsomia (mandibular hypoplasia)
Sleep deprivation	Hunter's syndrome
Smoking in home	Hurler's syndrome
	Klippel-Feil syndrome
Neurologic:	Kleeblattschädel deformity
Arnold-Chiari malformation	Larsen's syndrome
Hydrocephalus	Marfan's syndrome
Meningomyelocele	Mucopolysaccharidosis type VI
Myotonic dystrophy	Pfeiffer's syndrome
Syringobulbia-myelia	Pierre-Robin syndrome
Temporal lobe astrocytoma	Rubinstein-Taybi syndrome
	Stickler syndrome
	6q deletion syndrome
	Treacher Collins syndrome
	Velocardiofacial syndrome

reported habitual snoring (defined as snoring often).[3] Similar results have been found in England, where 8.7% of 4- to 5-year-old children were reported to snore on most nights.[2]

Census figures for 1988 for the United States indicated that there were about 32 million children 1 through 9 years old.[14] If the prevalence of habitual snoring is 7 to 9% as suggested by the above data, then there should be about 2 million children in the United States who snore most nights. Since the prevalence of OSAS in children is thought to be about 1.5 to 2%, about 1 in 5 children who snore most nights would be expected to have OSAS. It would then follow that most patients referred to otolaryngologists and pediatric sleep clinics for a complaint of loud snoring should have only primary snoring, not childhood-type OSAS. At present, lacking data on referral patterns of snoring children or the epidemiology of snoring in large unselected populations, these speculations cannot be confirmed.

Gender and Age

Corbo and associates[3] demonstrated that the prevalence of habitual snoring was the same in girls and boys. They also demonstrated that within the 6- to 13-year-age range the prevalence of snoring decreased with age. In contrast, the prevalence of habitual snoring (often, every night) in adults is about 13 to 17% and its prevalence increases with age.[13] This suggests that the prevalence of habitual snoring decreases during childhood, reaches a nadir at some (as yet undefined) age, and then begins to increase with age. Nothing is known about the prevalence of snoring in adolescents or the mechanisms underlying changes with age.

Genetics

Little is known about the role of inheritance in primary snoring. Snoring has been described in families,[15, 16] but the role of inheritance of specific determinants of snoring versus nonspecific predisposing factors (obesity) and environmental factors (pollution, pollen) is not known.

Pathophysiology

There is much speculation about the mechanisms of snoring but little data on this subject in children. Although past literature discusses mechanisms of heavy snoring in children,[17, 18] most of these children would now be classified as having obstructive hypoventilation (see Chapter 18). Snoring is assumed to result from oropharyngeal tissue vibrations caused by inspiratory airflow and to necessarily involve some degree of partial upper airway obstruction. Neuromuscular, mechanical, and structural determinants of snoring in children are not known.

Complications

Most complications of snoring reported in the literature are actually complications of chronic obstructive hypoventilation, or OSAS. Little or nothing is known about the complications of PS per se. It is well known that chronic upper airway obstruction (childhood-type OSAS) leads to ventricular dysfunction and cor pulmonale.[19–22] Since snoring involves some degree of partial upper airway obstruction, it would be expected that children with primary snoring have negative inspiratory pressures outside of the normal range. We have measured inspiratory pressures during PS as low as -40 cm H_2O (normal $= -2$ to -15 cm H_2O). Whether years of such a breathing pattern during sleep could adversely affect a child is not known.

PS may be a significant social handicap in some children or adolescents, for example, when sharing the same room with other youngsters at camp or in a dormitory.

Diagnosis

The clinician must differentiate between PS and other conditions associated with snoring in children (such as OSAS). Clinical history should elicit information about sleep, breathing during sleep, daytime symptoms, complications, and previous airway surgery. Specific information should be sought concerning the nature and quality of the snoring and parental observations of cyanosis, apnea, inspiratory struggles, retractions, the need to shake the child (to make him/her breathe) or to watch the child sleep (for fear that he/she might stop breathing).

Can PS be diagnosed by history alone? This question was recently investigated at the Hopkins Center. Patients were evaluated in clinic and a questionnaire was used to inquire about the parents' observations of their sleeping child. Questions related to cyanosis, observed apnea, difficult breathing during sleep, watching in fear, and shaking the child. PSG was used to classify patients as PS or OSAS. Using logistic regression analysis, it was found that observed apnea, shaking the child, or watching in fear were significant risk factors for OSAS. However, all other historic factors (including snoring) were not significantly different between the two groups, and no model using any combination of symptoms was found to be predictive.[23] A history of snoring is particularly of little value since, at least in the Johns Hopkins clinic, nearly all children (PS or OSAS) are reported to snore loudly on most nights. Leach and associates also evaluated the usefulness of clinical history in 93 children referred to otolaryngology for symptoms of sleep-related airway obstruction. They found no difference in historic features between children with and without OSA on PSG.[24] Others in an otolaryngology setting have reported that snoring in referred children is universal and therefore valueless as a distinguishing feature.[25] Thus, evidence to date indicates that PS cannot be distinguished from OSAS on the basis of history alone.

Several studies have suggested that a clinical score[1] or history combined with screening tests, such as pulse oximetry,[25] can accurately diagnose childhood-type OSAS and obviate the need for PSG in selected children. The problem with these studies is that control groups that contained nonsnorers were used to derive an algorithm for using history to identify OSAS. Pediatric pulmonary subspecialty, sleep, and otolaryngology clinic referral populations consist almost entirely of children who snore. In these settings, it has not been demonstrated that PS can be distinguished from OSAS without PSG. This fact is important since roughly 80% of children with habitual snoring do not have OSAS and thus would not necessarily need surgical intervention for snoring (although some will undergo adenotonsillectomy or surgery for other indications). Since parental pressure and the emotional needs of the parents are no longer acceptable indications for adenotonsillectomy, it is crucial to make the correct diagnosis of PS or OSAS before subjecting a child to potentially unnecessary surgery.[26]

Additional studies of measurement techniques, complications, course, and the natural history of PS are needed. In one study of children with snoring and OSAS, adenotonsillectomy was delayed up to 24 months to determine if spontaneous improvement would occur. Eight patients (8.6%), two of whom had OSAS, showed spontaneous improvement and surgery was unnecessary.[27] Avoidance of unnecessary risk is only one issue requiring further study. Future investigations must balance the costs of laboratory evaluation (PSG) against savings gained by avoiding unnecessary hospital stays, anesthesia, and surgery.

Diagnostic Criteria

There are no standard diagnostic criteria for PS that apply specifically to children. Therefore, we use diagnostic criteria that are *modeled after* the primary snoring criteria published in the International Classification of Sleep Disorders: Diagnostic and Coding Manual (ICSD), but modified so that they apply to children (Table 17–3).[28] A provisional diagnosis can be made if A plus B (snoring without daytime symptoms or sleep disruption) are present. Confirmation of the diagnosis, and the ruling out of OSAS or other causes of noisy breathing

Table 17–3. DIAGNOSTIC CRITERIA FOR CHILDHOOD PRIMARY SNORING

Diagnostic Criteria

A. Complaint of snoring by an observer.
B. No evidence of daytime symptoms or sleep disruption resulting from the snoring.
C. Polysomnography demonstrates:
  1. Snoring (usually inspiratory) often occurring for prolonged periods during sleep.
  2. No associated arousals, disturbed sleep, oxyhemoglobin desaturation, hypercarbia, or arrhythmias.
  3. Normal sleep pattern for age.
  4. Normal respiratory pattern for age during sleep.
D. Does NOT meet diagnostic criteria for other sleep disorders, e.g., OSAS, central alveolar hypoventilation syndrome, sleep-related laryngospasm.

Severity Criteria

Mild:	Snoring does not occur every night and is not disturbing to others.
Moderate:	Snoring occurs nightly, occasionally disturbs others.
Severe:	Snoring occurs every night, usually disturbs others. Siblings may have to sleep in another room because of loudness of snoring. Adolescents often not able to sleep in the same room with others (i.e., in a dormitory).

Modified for children. Format of criteria *modeled after* International Classification of Sleep Disorders: Diagnostic and Coding Manual criteria for adult OSAS.[28]

during sleep, requires further evaluation. At the present time, the best method available for confirmation is overnight PSG. If PSG is unavailable, hospital admission for direct observation of the child during sleep may be an alternative. Home videotaping of what is perceived by the parents to be their child's worst snoring may also be a useful screening test but has never been evaluated by scientific study. No method of testing in the patient's home has been validated as being useful in children.

Severity Criteria

Because data concerning adverse outcome in children with PS are lacking, severity criteria are arbitrary. Since PS may be quite loud, severity criteria include disturbing other family members and snoring as a social handicap. The criteria listed in Table 17–3 were adapted from those proposed in the ICSD[28] and modified for children based largely on clinical experience. Future studies must determine markers for adverse outcome and relate these to features of PS.

Duration Criteria

Some children snore only during an upper respiratory infection and during these episodes could be said to have acute PS. In the absence of better information, the presently proposed duration criteria[28] should be viewed as completely arbitrary.

Polysomnographic Features

Children with PS demonstrate snoring during the inspiratory phase of breathing. Because snoring reflects a mild degree of partial upper airway obstruction, signs of increased work of breathing or respiratory effort will often be evident. Rib cage distortion will be especially pronounced during REM sleep. In children with PS alone, there will be no findings of abnormal oxyhemoglobin desaturation, hypercarbia, or sleep disturbance.

Differential Diagnosis

The differential diagnosis for PS overlaps that of childhood-type OSAS. There is no evidence that reported snoring characteristics help to differentiate the diagnoses under consideration. Snoring must be differentiated from stridor, which is also an inspiratory noise but is not sleep dependent. Children with stridor, from laryngomalacia, have noisy breathing that is also present on waking and worsens with agitation.

Treatment

Does true PS require treatment? There is little or no information concerning this question. If, by definition, PS is not causing symptoms, then what could be the indications for treatment? It may be that symptoms or physiologic changes are present but unrecognized. Because PS may be associated with abnormally large intrathoracic pressure swings and increased left ventricular afterload, it is possible that adverse effects on cardiac function may occur over years. However, there are no data to answer this question at the present time. In adolescents whose PS is causing significant social dysfunction, therapy should be considered. Parents and siblings may decide that separate rooms or closed doors are preferable to surgical intervention.

Significant changes in a snoring child's behavior may be noted after adenotonsillectomy, even if OSAS could not be documented preoperatively.[25, 27] The authors' experience, and that of others (R. Ferber, personal communication), is that in some cases parents note remarkable improvement in their child's behavior only in retrospect, after adenotonsillectomy. Therefore, in children with severe PS, especially if there are ill-defined behavioral features that may be related to the adenotonsillar hypertrophy and snoring, surgical treatment may still be indicated even if PSG does not demonstrate OSAS. The mechanism of postoperative improvement in such children is unknown. Large adenoids, chronic tonsillitis, and partial nasal obstruction cause difficulties with breathing, swallowing, and eating as well as other direct sequelae of chronic adenotonsillar infection. It is conceivable that adenotonsillectomy could result in behavior changes that have nothing to do with the associated snoring. On the other hand, snoring always involves some degree of upper airway obstruction, the effects of which may be subtle. Indications for treating childhood PS will have to be revised as our knowledge of snoring in children increases.

Besides adenoidectomy and/or tonsillectomy, treatment choices for snoring children are limited. A variety of mechanical devices and intraoral appliances are commercially available for the treatment of snoring in adults. There is no information at the present time to indicate whether such devices are appropriate for snoring children. Even if these devices are appropriate for children, PSG is required to rule out OSAS before prescribing an intraoral appliance. Uvulopalatopharyngoplasty and other surgical procedures aimed at reducing snoring have not been systematically evaluated in children.

References

1. Brouillette R, Hanson D, David R, et al: A diagnostic approach to suspected obstructive sleep apnea in children. J Pediatr 105:10, 1984.
2. Ali NJ, Pitson D, Stradling JR: The prevalence of snoring, sleep disturbance and sleep related breathing disorders and their relation to daytime sleepiness in 4-5 year old children. Am Rev Respir Dis 143:A381 (abstract), 1991.
3. Corbo GM, Fuciarelli F, Foresi A, et al: Snoring in children: association with respiratory symptoms and passive smoking. Br Med J 299:1491, 1989.
4. Guilleminault C, Eldrige F, Simmons FB, et al: Sleep apnea in eight children. Pediatrics 58:23, 1976.
5. Leiberman A, Cohen A, Tal A: Digital signal processing of stridor and snoring in children. Int J Pediatr Otorhinolaryngol 12:173, 1986.
6. Schafer J, Pirsig W: Digital signal analysis of snoring sounds in children. Int J Pediatr Otorhinolaryngol 20:193, 1990.
7. Hibbert J: The occurrence of adenoidal signs and symptoms in normal children. Clin Otolaryngol 6:97, 1981.
8. Potsic WP, Pasquariello PS, Baranak CC, et al: Relief of upper airway obstruction by adenotonsillectomy. Otolaryngol Head Neck Surg 94:476, 1986.
9. Guilleminault C, Souquet M, Ariagno RL, et al: Five cases of near-miss sudden infant death syndrome and development of obstructive sleep apnea syndrome. Pediatrics 73:71, 1984.
10. Sorensen H, Solow B, Greve E: Assessment of the nasopharyngeal airway. A rhinomanometric and radiographic study in children with adenoids. Acta Otolaryngol (Stockh) 89:227, 1980.
11. Fukuda K, Matsune S, Ushikai M, et al: A study on the relationship between adenoid vegetation and rhinosinusitis. Am J Otolaryngol 10:214, 1989.
12. Mallory GB, Jr, Fiser DH, Jackson R: Sleep-associated breathing disorders in morbidly obese children and adolescents. J Pediatr 115:892, 1989.
13. Stradling JR, Crosby JH: Predictors and prevalence of obstructive sleep apnea and snoring in 1001 middle aged men. Thorax 46:85, 1991.
14. U.S. Bureau of the Census: Statistical Abstract of the United States: 1991. Washington, DC, U.S. Government Printing Office, 1991.
15. el-Bayadi S, Millman RP, Tishler PV, et al: A family study of sleep apnea. Anatomic and physiologic interactions. Chest 98:554, 1990.
16. Strohl KP, Saunders NA, Feldman NT, et al: Obstructive sleep apnea in family members. N Engl J Med 299:969, 1978.
17. Guilleminault C, Winkle R, Korobkin R, et al: Children and nocturnal snoring: evaluation of the effects of sleep related respiratory resistive load and daytime functioning. Eur J Pediatr 139:165, 1982.
18. Guilleminault C, Stoohs R: Chronic snoring and obstructive sleep apnea syndrome in children. Lung 168 (Suppl):912, 1990.
19. Tal A, Leiberman A, Margulis G, et al: Ventricular dysfunction in children with obstructive sleep apnea: radionuclide assessment. Pediatr Pulmonol 4:139, 1988.
20. Nussbaum E, Hirschfeld SS, Wood RE, et al: Echocardiographic changes in children with pulmonary hypertension secondary to upper airway obstruction. J Pediatr 93:931, 1978.
21. Brown OE, Manning SC, Ridenour B: Cor pulmonale secondary to tonsillar and adenoidal hypertrophy: management considerations. Int J Pediatr Otorhinolaryngol 16:131, 1988.
22. Wilkinson AR, McCormick MS, Freeland AP, et al: Electrocardiographic signs of pulmonary hypertension in children who snore. Br Med J 282:579, 1981.
23. Carroll JL, McColley SA, Marcus CL, et al: Can childhood obstructive sleep apnea syndrome (OSA) be diagnosed by a clinical symptom score? Am Rev Respir Dis 145(Part 2):A179, 1992.
24. Leach J, Olson J, Hermann J, et al: Polysomnographic and clinical findings in children with obstructive sleep apnea. Arch Otolaryngol Head Neck Surg 118:741, 1992.
25. van Someren VH, Hibbert J, Stothers JK, et al: Identification of hypoxaemia in children having tonsillectomy and adenoidectomy. Clin Otolaryngol 15:263, 1990.
26. Furman R: Handling parental pressure for the T and A. J Pediatr 54:195, 1959.
27. Ahlqvist-Rastad J, Hultcrantz E, Svanholm H: Children with tonsillar obstruction: indications for and efficacy of tonsillectomy. Acta Paediatr Scand 77:831, 1988.
28. Diagnostic Classification Steering Committee, Thorpy MJC (Chairman): International Classification of Sleep Disorders: Diagnostic and Coding Manual. Rochester, MI, American Association of Sleep Disorders Associations, 1990.

Obstructive Sleep Apnea Syndrome in Infants and Children: Clinical Features and Pathophysiology

JOHN L. CARROLL and GERALD M. LOUGHLIN

Infants and children with chronic sleep-related upper airway obstruction may develop a characteristic clinical syndrome, defined as follows:

Childhood obstructive sleep apnea syndrome (OSAS) is characterized by episodes of partial or complete upper airway obstruction that occur during sleep, usually associated with a reduction in oxyhemoglobin saturation and/or hypercarbia. Nighttime symptoms include snoring, paradoxical chest-abdomen motion, retractions, observed apnea, observed difficulty breathing during sleep, cyanosis during sleep, or disturbed sleep. Daytime symptoms include nasal obstruction, mouth breathing and other symptoms of adenotonsillar hypertrophy, behavior problems, or excessive daytime sleepiness. Severe forms may be associated with cor pulmonale, developmental delay, failure-to-thrive, or death.

This chapter reviews the clinical features and pathophysiology of childhood OSAS. Primary snoring (PS) in children was discussed in Chapter 17. Diagnosis and management of childhood OSAS is discussed in Chapter 19.

The first series of patients with childhood-type OSAS was reported in 1976 by Guilleminault and associates.[1] Much has changed in the 16 years since that landmark publication. Awareness has now increased to the point that children with OSAS are referred for evaluation much earlier in the course of the disease than was the case 10 to 15 years ago. As a result, the literature before 1983 describes the most severe forms of OSAS, those with the highest incidence of complications. In addition, definitions of OSAS in children have been constantly changing since 1976, and there has never been agreement on the definitions of obstructive apnea, obstructive hypopnea or hypoventilation, mixed apnea, sleep disturbance, and arousal in childhood OSAS. Children with OSAS may be seen by various specialists: pediatricians, psychiatrists or psychologists, neurologists, otolaryngologists, and pediatric pulmonologists, and the referrals may be for different reasons. Pediatricians may see patients for failure-to-thrive, neurologists for sleepiness, otolaryngologists for adenotonsillar hypertrophy, psychiatrists or psychologists for behavior problems, and pulmonologists for snoring and difficulty breathing. These factors lead to further difficulties interpreting the literature.

Terminology. Sleep-related obstructive breathing disorders in children have come to be called "obstructive sleep apnea syndrome" even when there is absence of apnea per se. Thus, the terms "childhood OSAS" or "childhood-type OSAS" will be used to refer to all symptomatic sleep-related upper airway obstruction in children. Furthermore, most terms relating to disordered breathing during sleep can be defined from a clinical, physiologic, or polysomnographic (PSG) viewpoint. Clinical definitions are listed in Table 18–1, and PSG definitions are listed in Chapter 19, Table 19–4.

Historic Perspective

William Osler described childhood OSA in his 1892 textbook of medicine[2]; a century

Table 18–1. DEFINITIONS—GENERAL*

Snoring. A vibratory sound produced in the nasopharynx during the inspiratory phase of breathing. Snoring may be a low frequency sound produced by vibration of the soft palate and the pillars of the oropharyngeal inlet[30] (usual in adults). With adenotonsillar enlargement the movement of the soft palate is impeded and snoring may be higher pitched (usual in children). In children the frequency content of snoring is variable.

Primary Snoring (PS). In children PS is characterized by snoring during sleep without associated apnea, hypoventilation, hypoxemia or hypercarbia, sleep disturbance, or daytime symptoms other than those directly related to adenotonsillar hypertrophy (e.g., nasal obstruction, mouth breathing, nasal congestion, frequent otitis media, frequent sore throats, and halitosis).

Childhood Obstructive Apnea Syndrome. OSAS is characterized by episodes of partial or complete upper airway obstruction that occur during sleep, usually associated with a reduction in oxyhemoglobin saturation and/or hypercarbia. Nighttime symptoms include snoring, paradoxical chest and abdomen motion, retractions, observed apnea, observed difficulty breathing during sleep, cyanosis during sleep, or disturbed sleep. Daytime symptoms include nasal obstruction, mouth breathing and other symptoms of adenotonsillar hypertrophy, behavior problems, or excessive daytime sleepiness. Severe forms may be associated with cor pulmonale, developmental delay, failure-to-thrive, or death.

Apnea. Absence of air flow at the nose or mouth. In *central apnea* airflow is absent due to the absence of respiratory efforts. In *obstructive apnea* airflow is absent, in spite of continuing respiratory efforts, due to collapse of the upper airway. In *mixed apnea* central and obstructive apnea occur sequentially with no normal breathing between the two events.

Hypoventilation. A decrease in pulmonary ventilation below the minimum level necessary to maintain normoxia or normocapnia. In *nonobstructive hypoventilation* ventilation is inadequate due to decreased central nervous system respiratory drive, neuromuscular abnormalities, or pulmonary restrictive abnormalities. *Obstructive hypoventilation* is characterized by partial upper airway obstruction leading inadequate pulmonary ventilation; overall respiratory drive is normal or increased.

*See Table 19–4 for PSG definitions.

later, modern texts have not improved upon Osler's superb description. Sixty-four years passed before Spector and Bautista alerted the medical community (again) to the possibility that adenotonsillitis could cause upper airway obstruction and respiratory distress in children.[3] Nine years later, in 1965, Noonan described reversible cor pulmonale in children with adenotonsillar hypertrophy.[4] By 1975 OSA in children was still described in the medical literature only when associated with cardiac failure. In 1976, Goodman and associ-

ates asked "Is there a *forme fruste* of the syndrome?"[5]; then quotes Jaffee from 1974: "it is my feeling that many youngsters seen in consultation have less severe manifestations of these severe obstructive conditions. This is probably the reason that following adenotonsillectomy in selective cases there occurs a period of rapid growth and development."[6] We now know that Jaffee and Goodman were correct. Following Guilleminault's description of eight children with OSAS in 1976,[1] larger series were reported in the early 1980s,[7, 8] and the first controlled study on the clinical features only appeared in 1984.[9]

In 1995, the clinical "syndrome" of childhood-type OSAS is still not clearly defined and there is no true consensus concerning its diagnosis or treatment. Information on fundamental aspects such as natural history, prevalence, pathophysiology, diagnosis, appropriate management, and markers of adverse outcome is scant or missing. "In spite of the thorough ventilation of this subject by specialists" wrote Dr. Osler in 1892, "practitioners do not appear to have grasped as yet the full importance of this disease."[2] One hundred years later the importance of childhood-type OSAS is still not fully appreciated. A 1988 article states that OSAS is a "rare condition in childhood."[10]

Essential Features

Childhood OSAS is not adult OSAS in little people. Several of the essential clinical features differ markedly from the adult syndrome (Table 18–2). An important feature of childhood OSAS is the variety of possible manifestations of the clinical syndrome. In children, the spectrum runs from obstructive hypoventilation without *any* complete obstructive apnea, through a mixture of obstructive apnea and obstructive hypoventilation, to pure obstructive apnea without obstructive hypoventilation. Some children will exhibit excessive daytime sleepiness (EDS), but most will not. Some are obese, but most are not. Some show suboptimal growth or failure-to-thrive, but most do not. Some children with severe breathing disturbance have small tonsils and adenoids, while some with enormous adenoids or tonsils have only mild OSAS (or are completely asymptomatic).

Nighttime Symptoms

"At night the child's sleep is greatly disturbed; the respirations are loud and snoring, and there are

Table 18–2. FEATURES OF ADULT VS CHILDHOOD OSAS

	Adult	**Child**
Snoring	Usually alternating with pauses	Often continuous
Excessive daytime sleepiness	Main presenting symptom	Minority of patients
Associated obesity	Majority of patients	Minority of patients
Underweight or failure-to-thrive	No	Minority of patients but not rare
Daytime mouth breathing	No	Common
Gender	M:F = 8–10:1	M:F = 1:1
Differential diagnosis	Other causes of excessive sleepiness or sleep disruption	Other causes of snoring or breathing difficulty during sleep
Enlarged tonsils and adenoids	Uncommon	Most common
Predominant obstructive pattern	Obstructive apnea	Obstructive hypoventilation
Arousal on apnea termination	Nearly always	Usually not
Sleep pattern disruption	Nearly always	Sleep stages (%) often normal
Complications	Mainly cardiopulmonary and complications of EDS	Cardiopulmonary, growth, behavior, developmental, perioperative
Surgical correction	Only in selected cases (minority)	Successful in most cases (adenotonsillectomy)
CPAP*	Most common treatment	Only in selected cases (minority)
Mortality	Sudden death during sleep or from cardiovascular complications	Usually perioperative

*Continuous positive airway pressure.

sometimes prolonged pauses, followed by deep, noisy inspirations."

WILLIAM OSLER, 1892

Snoring

In the 100 years since Osler described OSAS in children, there have been no large studies of the most common symptom of childhood-type OSAS, snoring. Except for studies of the acoustical characteristics of snoring,[11, 12] most studies do not define what is meant by the term "snoring." Nearly all children with OSA snore and most are perceived to snore loudly. Many parents report that their child's snoring disturbs them or others in the home. However, significant OSAS can occur without snoring or with only high-pitched grunting noises during sleep. In one clinic, 97% of parents of children with proven OSAS report loud snoring on "most nights of the week" but so do 87% of parents of children with primary snoring.[13] Many investigators have reported anecdotally that snoring is exacerbated by upper respiratory tract infection.[7, 8]

In children with OSAS, patterns of either OSA or sleep-associated obstructive hypoventilation may predominate. For this reason, children exhibit two major patterns of snoring: fairly continuous snoring[14] and snoring punctuated by episodes of silence, which are usually terminated by a loud gasp or snort.[7, 15, 16] There is little or no scientific information on the relationship between specific snoring and breathing patterns and nothing is known about how these patterns vary within or across nights, or how diurnal snoring characteristics compare with snoring during daytime naps.

Increased Respiratory Effort

Increased respiratory effort is evident in nearly all children with OSAS. Esophageal pressures in the range of −50 to −70 cm H_2O have been documented in children with sleep-related airway obstruction.[17, 18] The increased effort required during obstructed breathing is manifested as intercostal, sternal, suprasternal, and supraclavicular retractions; costal margin flaring; visibly detectable use of accessory muscles of respiration; and paradoxical inward rib cage motion (PIRCM) during inspiration. Normally the chest and abdominal wall move outwardly together during the inspiratory phase of breathing. During obstructed breathing, the downward motion of the diaphragm causes the abdomen to move outwardly but the markedly negative intrathoracic pressures cause "paradoxical" inward movement of the rib cage. PIRCM is normal in newborns and in infants and older children during REM sleep. There have been no formal studies of the signs of increased respiratory effort in childhood-type OSAS.

Parents of children who snore loudly not only notice the increased breathing effort, but they are often terrified by the look and sound of their child's breathing during sleep. Frank and associates reported on parents staying up watching their children sleep, and waking them if obstructive apnea was not resolving spontaneously.[7] Carroll and associates investigated this question in 31 children with PS and 34 children with OSAS, and found that watching children sleep for fear that they would "stop breathing" was reported by 94% of OSAS parents and 71% of PS parents.[13] Shaking the child during sleep "to make him or her breathe" was reported by 56% of OSAS parents and by 23% of PS parents. Observed obstructive apnea was reported by 74% of parents of OSAS and by 39% of PS children.[13] All of these were significantly more likely to be observed by parents of children with OSAS but none was predictive. Loud snoring is often frightening to parents, regardless of whether the child simply has loud PS or OSAS.

Patterns of Obstruction

Konno and associates clearly described two patterns of sleep-associated airway obstruction in children: continuous partial obstruction and obstructive apnea.[14] The former was associated with loud continuous snoring but a stable oxygen saturation, stable EEG, and less sleep disruption.[14] The second or "periodic" pattern was associated with periodic complete obstruction, large periodic variations in intrathoracic pressure, regular rapid oxygen desaturation episodes, and EEG arousal following each obstruction.[14] Although both patterns of obstruction were shown to occur in children, the prevalence of each type is not known. The largest series of the continuous partial obstruction pattern was reported by Guilleminault and associates in 1982 in which 25 children, aged 2 to 14 years, had heavy nighttime snoring and moderate–severe daytime symptoms but none exhibited obstructive apnea; about one third had EDS, one half showed significant behavior problems; and most were underweight.[17] During sleep there was loud snoring, large negative inspiratory intrathoracic pressures, and relatively mild hypoxemia. The authors emphasized that severe obstructive hypoventilation can cause the full daytime "syndrome" in children without *any* obstructive apnea.[17] Brouillette and associates also pointed out that same year that obstructive hypoventilation in children may be just as severe or even worse than OSA.[8]

Obstructive Apnea

There are no large scientific studies on the characteristics of obstructive apnea per se in children, and surprisingly few articles have provided details about obstructive apnea in children, although there have been large series reported of patients undergoing adenotonsillectomy[19, 20] or those with obesity.[21] Guilleminault's 1976 series reported on 8 children who all exhibited very severe OSAS with 78 to 816 obstructive events per night, average obstructive durations of 15 to 32.5 seconds, and complications such as cor pulmonale.[1] Eight years of experience at the Johns Hopkins Pediatric Sleep Center suggests most patients do not exhibit such severe OSAS. In 1983, Frank and associates reported on 32 moderate-to-severely affected children with OSAS, although it is not clear exactly what criteria were used to make this diagnosis.[7] In their study of 2- to 13-year-old children, the average frequency of obstructive events was about 20 per hour, with average durations for obstructive and mixed apneas of 17.3 seconds, and 13.6 seconds for hypopneas.[7] If significant duration is defined as any apnea lasting longer than two breathing cycles, then one finds that average apnea duration is quite variable.[3] Some children, especially older ones, show apnea durations in the range reported above, while others, often young children or infants, exhibit desaturation with obstructions as brief as 3 to 4 seconds. The older studies mentioned provide a picture of the child with severe OSAS, but little is known about children with mild to moderate OSAS, or the characteristics of obstructive apnea if duration is not arbitrarily limited.

Data on the fundamental diagnostic features of the OSAS disorder are lacking. This includes information on the relationship between obstructive event duration and severity, between duration and oxyhemoglobin desaturation (desaturation), between sleep state and duration or desaturation, and between age, size, gender, or other patient characteristics and the various apnea characteristics.

Sleep

Effects on sleep in childhood OSAS are also poorly understood. The observation that EDS is present only in a minority of children with OSAS suggests two possibilities: most children with OSAS get sufficient adequate-quality sleep to avoid EDS or the daytime manifestations of sleep disruption are different in children than adults.[7, 13, 17, 22–24] There is evidence to support both of these possibilities. Several investigators have found that, in contrast to adults, many children with OSAS have normal amounts of delta sleep,[7, 13, 22, 25] and children with continuous partial obstruction during sleep do not show sleep fragmentation.[17] In studies by Frank and associates and Zucconi and associates, sleep stage distribution was normal preoperatively and remained so after adenotonsillectomy.[7, 26] Frank and associates also found that sleep efficiency and arousal rate did not change significantly by 4 to 6 weeks after surgery, in spite of a marked improvement in breathing during sleep.[7] This would imply that sleep was normal to begin with, that sleep disturbance was not related to OSA, that 4 to 6 weeks was not enough time for recovery, or that sleep analysis methods failed to detect significant sleep disruption. It has been suggested that standard sleep scoring, using 20 or 30 second epochs, may fail to detect transient or microarousals and that evaluating miniarousals often gives a better picture of the sleep disturbance than any other sleep score.[27] However, there have been no controlled studies in children linking mini- or microarousals to daytime symptoms, and miniarousals in children with OSAS have never been shown to alter the sleep time, time spent awake after sleep onset, distribution of sleep stages, or overall sleep quality.

Many investigators have described "restless" sleep or "bed thrashing" in children with OSAS.[7, 15, 16, 20, 28, 29] Restlessness during sleep is defined as persistent or recurrent body movements, arousal, and brief awakening in the course of sleep.[30] Unfortunately, we do not know what is normal. One way around this is to study reported sleep quality before and after surgical intervention. In one study, adenotonsillectomy reduced complaints of restless sleep by about 75%.[29] Swift reported that 70% of children with OSAS showed restless sleep preoperatively but none did after surgery.[31] Ahlqvist-Rastad and coworkers found that restless sleep dropped from 55 to 13% after tonsillectomy.[20] There are a few studies comparing symptoms in children with OSAS with those of normal controls. Stradling and associates found that about 75% of children with OSAS were often perceived as restless sleepers compared with about 10% of controls and observations suggested that the restless sleep was associated with upper airway obstruction.[29] In another study, restless sleep in OSAS and controls was 80 and 23%, respectively.[9]

A potential problem with studies comparing OSAS children with normal controls is that these control groups may consist of mostly nonsnorers. However, nonsnoring children are easily identified by clinical history without need of further study. The clinician must differentiate PS from OSAS. Children with large tonsils and adenoids and loud snoring can be restless sleepers whether they have obstructive sleep apnea or not. This is not surprising since large adenoids lead to difficulty breathing through the nose and can be associated with posterior nasal mucus drainage. Large tonsils may be chronically infected and painful. Resulting symptoms could lead to disturbed sleep even if the child does not have OSA. Nasal occlusion in normal adults leads to severe sleep disturbance[32] and adults with allergic rhinitis have 10 times more microarousals than normal controls.[33] On the other hand, surgical removal of tonsils and adenoids may directly result in improved sleep quality by a mechanism not involving OSAS. Improvement in sleep quality may be concomitant with, but not necessarily due to, elimination of sleep-associated airway obstruction.

Sleeping Position

Children with OSAS may sleep in bizarre or unusual positions, often with neck extension.[17, 29] Stradling and associates found that about 65% of OSAS children slept in odd positions compared with almost none in the control group.[29] Children may sleep with their neck hyperextended, in a kneeling knee-chest position or propped up on pillows or sitting upright (usually obese children).[34, 35] Occasionally parents will report intervening by changing the child's head position. The mechanisms underlying spontaneous position changes during sleep to improve airway patency are not known.

Sweating

In a study of 50 children with OSAS, 96% showed profuse sweating during sleep.[15] A later controlled study found that excessive sweating during sleep was present in 50% of OSAS children compared with only 16% of matched controls.[9] Infants with brief upper airway obstructions during sleep also show a significantly higher incidence of profuse sweating (15%) than infants without such obstructions (7%).[36] This finding is noteworthy since one quarter of children dying of sudden infant death syndrome (SIDS) were described by Kahn and associates as exhibiting excessive or profuse sweating during sleep.[37] The prevalence and correlates of excessive sweating in sleep in children remain unknown.

Enuresis

Enuresis or bedwetting is said to be a common feature of childhood-type OSAS.[7, 15, 38] Brouillette and associates found enuresis in 8% of OSAS children but also in 4% of matched controls (no significant difference).[9] Swift found that 3 of 19 (16%) children with OSAS had enuresis preoperatively but that only 1 became dry after surgery.[31] Thus, from these studies it might seem that enuresis is not specifically associated with OSAS. On the other hand, Frank and associates reported enuresis in 33% of children with OSAS over 4 years old, although they did not study a control group.[7] Weider and Hauri reported in 1985 that in 26 of 35 children with nocturnal airway obstruction and enuresis, the enuresis was cured or significantly improved after surgical removal of the tonsils or adenoids.[39] However, the patient group in this study was heterogeneous and the proportion that actually had OSAS is not clear since only four had PSG.[39] Therefore, the role of OSAS per se in producing enuresis in these children was not apparent. A more recent publication from the same group reports 115 children, 3 to 19 years of age, with symptoms of upper airway obstruction and nocturnal enuresis.[22] Upper airway surgery dramatically diminished enuresis in 76% of their patients, leading them to conclude that enuresis should be an indication for adenotonsillectomy or other upper airway surgery.[22] Unfortunately Weider and associates collected these patients over 12 years and did not state the overall incidence of enuresis in their referral population. Furthermore, PSG was performed in only 11 of 115 patients.[22] Although it is stated that all 115 patients were obligate nighttime mouth breathers and had symptoms of upper airway obstruction, the proportion of children with OSAS, the incidence and degree of sleep disturbance, and the severity cannot be known. Again, the role of OSAS per se is not clear. Abnormalities in diurnal secretion of antidiuretic hormone (ADH) in children with enuresis have recently been reported, but there are no reports suggesting such abnormalities are caused by OSAS.[40] Weider and associates speculated that improvement of enuresis after surgery was due to elimination of sleep disruption and the subsequent normalization of arousal mechanisms.[22] However, there are no data to support this contention at the present time.

Daytime Symptoms

"The expression is dull, heavy, and apathetic . . . In long-standing cases the child is very stupid-looking, responds slowly to questions, and may be sullen and cross. Among other symptoms may be mentioned headache, which is by no means uncommon, general listlessness, and an indisposition for physical or mental exertion. The influence upon the mental development is striking."

WILLIAM OSLER—1892

Symptoms on Awakening

Symptoms reported to be present on awakening in the morning include dry mouth, grogginess, disorientation, confusion, and headaches. Potsic and associates, using questionnaires from parents of 100 children with symptoms of airway obstruction, found that children with OSAS were perceived as cranky in the morning and tired during the day.[16] Butt and associates reported morning irritability in 9 of 14 children with OSA, but control data was not provided.[41] These data are hard to interpret without knowing the proportion of normal children that are perceived by parents to be cranky or irritable in the morning.

Brouillette and associates found that 15% of children with OSAS complained of frequent morning headaches but so did 7% of matched controls (difference not significant).[9] Guilleminault also found morning headaches in 16% of children with OSAS, but since the study was not controlled (at least with respect to daytime symptoms), it is not known if this differs compared with children without OSAS.[15] Consistent with the findings of Brouillette and associates, morning headaches are a common and nonspecific complaint in adults with a variety of sleep disorders and sleep-disordered breathing other than OSAS. Headaches show no particular association with OSAS.[42] Even less is known about the prevalence of morning grogginess, confusion, and disorientation. Dry mouth in the morning would be expected in any child with adenotonsillar hypertrophy and nighttime mouth breathing and has not been linked specifically to childhood OSAS.

Excessive Daytime Sleepiness

In the International Classification of Sleep Disorders Diagnostic and Coding Manual, the first diagnostic criterion for OSAS is: "The patient has a complaint of excessive sleepiness or insomnia."[30] However, EDS does not appear to be a major feature of childhood OSAS. In the 1976 series reported by Guilleminault and associates, EDS was a prominent symptom,[1] and a 1981 article from the same group reports EDS as the most common complaint (84%) in 50 children with OSAS.[15] However, in 1981 childhood OSAS was still widely viewed as the adult syndrome in children; therefore, it is not surprising that EDS was the most common reason for referral at that time. Since then, numerous studies have shown that EDS is not a common complaint in children with OSAS. Reports have found the proportion of OSAS children with EDS to be 8%,[28] 15%,[43] 18%,[24] 23%,[8] 27%,[13] 31%,[7] 32%,[17] 33%,[9] 43%,[41] 57%,[18] and 62%.[1] It is unusual for EDS to be the main presenting symptom. Frank and associates reported EDS as a marked problem in only 9%,[7] and Carroll and associates found that only 13% of parents with children with OSAS report EDS as a moderate, considerable, or great problem.[13] The incidence of reported EDS in children with OSAS is not significantly different from non-OSAS controls with only snoring.[13, 24]

Nearly all of the literature on EDS in children with snoring or OSAS deals with hypersomnolence as a subjective symptom rather than an objectively measured finding. Parents' answers to questions about EDS depend very much on how the questions are asked. There has been no standardization of questionnaires, and questions are usually not specified in published studies. Thus, there are significant problems even detecting EDS in children. Children less than 4 to 5 years of age are expected to nap during the day and may not be perceived to have a problem. On the contrary, the ability of children 2 to 5 years old to sleep during the day is often considered a blessing. Children who sleep in school may be labeled as dull or lazy. Even if school-aged children are correctly perceived as excessively sleepy, EDS may not be perceived as a serious medical symptom that warrants attention. Adolescents frequently are sleep deprived and fall asleep when bored. In these cases the significance of EDS can be easily overlooked by parents, teachers, or other caregivers. Thus, the actual prevalence of EDS in children with OSAS remains to be determined. At present it appears that EDS is not a common complaint in children with OSAS.

Daytime Behavior

There is little information on daytime behavior disorders due to OSAS in children. In a small study of eight patients reported by Guilleminault and associates in 1976, there was a high incidence of impaired school performance, hyperactivity, decreased intellectual performance, and emotional problems (50% were receiving counseling).[1] Another study, of 25 children with continuous partial airway obstruction during sleep, reported pathological shyness or withdrawn behavior in 40%, aggressive behavior in 40%, hyperactivity in 48%, and learning problems in 40%.[8] Although others describe hyperactivity and abnormal behavior in children with OSAS, most of these studies have not been controlled (at least with respect to behavior problems). In 1984, Brouillette and associates asked parents of OSAS children about bizarre behavior, discipline problems, hyperactivity, and aggressive behavior.[9] These features were present to varying degrees in 9 to 31% of children with OSAS but were also present in matched controls to a similar degree (no significant differences).[9]

Weissbluth and associates took a different approach to this question. They surveyed the parents of 2076 children and identified 71 as having behavioral, developmental, or academic problems.[44] Five controls were then selected for each problem child and the occurrence of certain features in the two groups was compared. Problem children reported significantly greater snoring, mouth breathing when awake, mouth breathing when asleep, and difficulty breathing when asleep.[44] When the authors culled out a subgroup whose parents described academic problems or hyperactivity-attention deficit disorder (ADD) the same relationships were found; markers of disturbed sleep and breathing during sleep were significantly more common in the problem group.[44] The authors point out that these findings should be interpreted with caution. Children in this study were not studied by PSG, and it is not known what proportion actually had OSAS or significant sleep disturbances.[44]

There are numerous case reports of developmental delay in children with OSAS; however, there have been no controlled studies. Developmental delay in a child with severe OSAS has been reported to improve within days of tracheostomy and, over time, to resolve completely.[8] Significant developmental delay may be overlooked in children with Down syndrome and other genetic disorders because they are expected to be mentally retarded and developmentally delayed. Several children with achondroplasia, severe OSAS, failure-to-thrive, and developmental delay have been seen at the Johns Hopkins Pediatric Sleep Center. In other genetic syndromes, it is also possible that the mental retardation and developmental delay accepted as part of the phenotype are actually due, in part, to unrecognized OSAS.

Older studies of children with OSAS characterized the most severely affected patients. In the 1990s, children are referred earlier with the result that obvious developmental and behavioral problems appear less commonly than originally reported. No large, well-controlled study has shown that daytime behavior problems are common in childhood-type OSAS or specifically related to any particular feature of OSAS. No behavioral problem has been shown to be of value in differentiating between OSAS and other diagnoses. Still, behavioral problems and developmental delay do occur in certain children with OSAS and may be severe. It is also possible that OSAS leads to subtle, currently unrecognized, developmental impairment.

Bedtime Behavior Problems

Several investigators have reported behavior problems in children with OSAS centered around bedtime.[1, 18] Guilleminault described children with OSAS who avoided bed and fought desperately against sleepiness.[1] Miyazaki and associates described 9 of 15 children (60%) with OSAS who fought sleep and had to be "forced" to go to bed (symptoms resolved by 6 months after adenotonsillectomy.)[18] Experience at the Johns Hopkins Pediatric Sleep Center with hundreds of children with OSAS suggests that bedtime-centered behavior problems are not common and that bizarre sleeping postures are rare. Controlled studies are needed.

Daytime Cognitive Function

Effects of OSAS on daytime cognitive function in children are virtually unexplored. Adults with OSAS have been shown to have impaired attention span, concentration, memory, vigilance, and motor skills. Several of these studies have shown correlations between nocturnal hypoxemia and daytime cognitive impairment.[45, 46] Since many children with OSAS suffer moderate-to-severe hypoxemia during sleep, it is likely that their daytime

cognitive function is similarly impaired. The pediatric literature contains mostly anecdotal reports of improved behavior after surgical relief of chronic upper airway obstruction. Lind and Lundell described 14 children with OSAS, growth impairment, and CO_2 retention and state that a great improvement in school results was noted in several children after tonsillectomy.[47] Guilleminault and associates reported on 5 children aged 11 to 14 years with continuous partial airway obstruction during sleep who showed abnormal average sleep latencies (on MSLT testing) and impaired cognitive function on the Wilkinson Addition Test preoperatively, and all returned to normal after tonsillectomy and/or adenoidectomy.[17] Children with OSAS may be impaired at critical times during development, making detection even more essential.

Adenotonsillar Hypertrophy and Mouth Breathing

It appears that most otherwise normal children with OSAS have hypertrophied tonsils and adenoids, although the actual number is not known. OSAS in children is characterized by symptoms and signs that are also seen in children without OSAS but with adenotonsillar hypertrophy. Swift found that 95% of 20 children with OSAS showed mouth breathing and only 5% continued mouth breathing after surgical intervention.[31] Data from questionnaires given to parents of children undergoing adenotonsillectomy for airway obstruction showed daytime mouth breathing in 75%.[16] Brouillette and associates reported that 87% of children with OSAS exhibited mouth breathing while awake compared with only 18% of normal controls (controls in this study were normal children selected from general pediatrics clinics).[9] A more relevant comparison is between children with adenotonsillar hypertrophy with and without OSAS. Carroll and associates found no significant difference in the prevalence of daily daytime mouth breathing in primary snorers (45%) compared with children with OSAS (64%).[13] Hibbert and colleagues compared signs and symptoms of adenotonsillar hypertrophy in children awaiting adenoidectomy with control children who had never consulted an otolaryngologist.[48] They found that nasal obstruction (64% vs 21%), snoring (78% vs 33%), and speech defects (52% vs 10%) were significantly more common in children awaiting adenoidectomy than controls.[48] Mouth breathing tended to be more common in children awaiting adenoidectomy than in controls (38% vs 21%), but the difference was not statistically significant.[48] Therefore, it appears that mouth breathing in children is not even specific for adenotonsillar hypertrophy, much less for OSAS.

In most studies, the term mouth breathing is not precisely defined. As pointed out by Klein,[49] most mouth breathers *can* breathe through their noses at least to some degree. The determinants of habitual mouth breathing in children are not known. Some mouth breathers have no evidence of nasal obstruction. This has led to confusion in the literature concerning the effects of mouth breathing on facial development. Although it is commonly said that mouth breathing is an important factor in the development of the "long-face syndrome" or "adenoid facies," one study of 106 children aged 6 to 13 years found that mouth breathing was correlated with dental malocclusion but not with adenoid facies.[49] Other studies have found mouth breathing to be associated with both abnormal facial development and dental malocclusion.[50, 51] No study has investigated the role that obstructive sleep apnea per se might play in facial development or malocclusion.

Adenoid Facies

It is often stated that adenoid facies is a common feature of children with OSAS. However, Butt and associates reported that only 3 of 20 (15%) children aged 6 months to 3 years with OSAS had adenoid facies, even though the tonsils and adenoids were moderately to grossly enlarged in approximately 90% of patients.[41] The low proportion of patients with adenoid facies in this study may be attributable to the young age of the study group (median age 14 months).[41]

Speech, Eating, and Swallowing

Many studies have reported speech defects, eating and swallowing difficulties, and halitosis in children with OSAS. Although 27% of the 122 children with tonsillar obstruction reported by Ahlqvist-Rastad and associates had swallowing difficulties, interference with swallowing was one of their patient selection criteria.[20] Of the 20 children with OSAS reported by Swift, 65% reported noisy eating, which was virtually eliminated after surgical removal of tonsils and/or adenoids.[31] Potsic and associates reported slow eating in 60%, dry mouth

in 42%, and trouble swallowing in 37 children undergoing adenotonsillectomy for airway obstruction.[16] Brouillette and associates found that a variety of symptoms were significantly more common in OSAS than in normal children: nausea and vomiting (30% vs 2%), difficulty swallowing (26% vs 2%), and poor appetite (30% vs 9%).[9] Monoson and Fox found that 8 of 13 adults with OSAS had disordered speech compared with 1 of 13 controls.[52] Ahlqvist-Rastad and associates reported that the majority of children with symptoms of tonsillar obstruction showed phoniatric signs (however, speech impairment was one of the criteria for patient selection in that study).[20] Although it is often mentioned in correction with childhood-type OSAS, there have been no studies of disordered speech in children with OSAS.

Associated Features

Associated features are those features that are often but not invariably present in or appear as complications due directly to OSAS.[30] These features are not always the same as those listed in the adult classification. Obesity, for example, is often but not invariably present in adults with OSAS, but most children with OSAS are not obese. Therefore, in childhood-type OSAS, obesity is discussed under predisposing factors, not associated features. Other associated features of adult OSAS are discussed only when they differ markedly from childhood OSAS.

Growth Impairment

One of the main associated features of childhood-type OSAS is impaired somatic growth. Most early case reports of childhood OSAS, from 1956 to 1976, described impaired growth.[3–5, 53–71] Because earlier series described more severely affected patients, the reported prevalence of growth impairment was higher than one would expect to find now. Five of the eight OSAS patients (62%) reported by Guilleminault in 1976,[1] 56% of the 50 children reported by Guilleminault and associates in 1981,[15] 27% of the children reported by Brouillette and associates in 1982,[8] and 69% of patients reported by Butt and associates in 1985[41] showed growth impairment. Guilleminault and associates reported in 1982 that 76% of children with obstructive hypoventilation (loud snoring, partial upper airway obstruction, no complete obstructive apnea, minimal or no hypoxemia, minimal sleep fragmentation, daytime symptoms) were underweight.[17] Individual case reports of OSAS causing failure-to-thrive were still appearing in the literature as recently as 1987.[72, 73] Bate and associates in 1984 described a 4-year-old girl with OSAS, short stature (height less than the third percentile), and a rapid growth spurt following tonsillectomy.[74]

Children labeled as failure-to-thrive show obvious growth impairment including low weight for age. In the early 1980s it was discovered that OSAS could affect growth without causing full-blown failure-to-thrive. Lind and Lundell described 14 children with OSAS whose height and weight gain velocity increased after surgical intervention even though 13 of 14 were within 2 standard deviations of mean height or weight for age.[47] Stradling and associates reported 61 snoring children undergoing adenotonsillectomy for recurrent tonsillitis, 61% of whom exhibited hypoxemia due to sleep-related upper airway obstruction.[29] Although most of these patients were within the normal range for height, they were significantly shorter than matched controls, and growth velocity increased significantly after adenotonsillectomy.[29] Stradling and associates did not perform PSG and did not correlate disordered breathing during sleep with the magnitude of the postoperative growth spurt.[29] Williams and associates recently described 37 children, aged 6 to 36 months, who underwent inpatient adenotonsillectomy or adenoidectomy for symptoms of sleep-related airway obstruction.[75] Although the severity of OSAS was not known, 46% of patients were at or below the fifth percentile for weight, and most patients (65%) showed at least a 15% increase in percentile after surgery.[75] The high incidence of growth failure reported by Williams and associates may reflect the young age group studied, the fact that 32% had additional medical problems, or underdiagnosis of milder cases of OSAS.

Many questions about childhood OSAS and somatic growth remain unanswered, especially regarding the relationship between age and growth impairment, the relationship between growth impairment and the severity of OSAS, the role of adenotonsillar hypertrophy per se (which possibly interferes with eating or appetite), and the relative roles of sleep disruption, hypoxemia, hypercarbia, and increased work of breathing. Because growth hormone (GH) release occurs during sleep, and sleep frag-mentation has been shown to impair GH release in a child with OSAS,[76] deficient GH release has been proposed as the cause of suboptimal growth in childhood-type OSAS. However, children with OSAS often have normal amounts of delta sleep (when GH is released) and minimal sleep fragmentation. Furthermore, Bate and associates described normal GH release during sleep in a 4-year-old with short stature due to OSAS,[74] and otherwise normal children with mild or moderate OSAS have not shown abnormal GH release. Bate and associates suggested that CO_2 retention and acidosis may impair end organ response to growth factors, but CO_2 retention or acidemia in children with OSAS have never been shown to correlate with growth impairment.[74] Chronic adenotonsillar hypertrophy may lead to poor appetite, difficulty swallowing, and eating or feeding difficulties. Thus, enlarged tonsils and adenoids could interfere with caloric intake and impair growth whether or not the child has OSAS. Finally, partial upper airway obstruction leads to marked increases in respiratory effort and presumably work of breathing. Various combinations of poor intake, increased caloric expenditure, hypoxemia, and sleep disturbance could lead to suboptimal growth.

Sudden Awakening

Children may awaken suddenly and cry, scream, moan, or change body position following obstructive events. The International Classification of Sleep Disorders describes "sudden awakenings" with complaints of "chest discomfort, choking, or suffocation that are associated with intense anxiety,"[26] although it is not clear that these features occur in childhood-type OSAS. Frank and associates reported that frequent awakenings seen in 60% of children were a major source of anxiety to the parents.[7] Swift reported that 70% of children with OSAS exhibited episodic choking during sleep, which completely resolved after surgical intervention.[31] At the Johns Hopkins Pediatric Sleep Laboratory, review of videotapes taken during PSG of hundreds of children with snoring and OSAS shows that awakenings in children are quite variable. Some children, especially at the end of a prolonged obstructive event, exhibit sudden awakenings with crying out or moaning, others suddenly sit up or change sleeping position, and many children produce loud snorting and snoring noises. Whether children with OSAS awaken with intense anxiety about their sleep-related airway obstruction is not known.

Gastroesophageal Reflux

Gastroesophageal reflux (GER) is said to occur in adults with OSAS in association with the effort to reestablish breathing.[30] However, analysis of 445 apneas in 7 obese adults showed no relationship between GER and apnea termination.[77] It is attractive to speculate that large negative intrathoracic pressures in patients with OSAS may lead to GER. Buts and associates reported that in children with asthma the percentage of sleep time spent with GER is 40 times greater than in asymptomatic controls.[78] Although this would seem to support the possibility that children with airway obstruction during sleep are predisposed to GER, asthmatic children also have hyperinflation and diaphragm flattening, are usually on medication associated with GER, and in some GER may be the cause of bronchospasm.

Aspiration

Sleep-related upper airway obstruction in children may be linked to aspiration of nasopharyngeal contents or secretions. Konno and associates, studying children 2 to 10 years of age with marked adenotonsillar hypertrophy and snoring, instilled contrast media into the nasopharynx during sleep.[79] They found that 8 of 10 OSAS children showed pulmonary aspiration of the contrast media compared with only 1 of 7 normal control children.[79] Whether aspiration of oropharyngeal secretions in children with OSAS is harmful is not known. Konno proposed that OSAS may predispose children to recurrent lower respiratory tract infection,[79] although there is no evidence that otherwise normal children with OSAS have a higher incidence of lower respiratory disease. The combination of GER and OSAS in one patient could theoretically predispose the child to aspiration of stomach contents.

Hypoxemia

Hypoxemia, usually defined as an arterial oxyhemoglobin saturation of less than 90 or 92%, is present in many children with OSAS. Surprisingly, there is not much quantitative data on hypoxemia during sleep in children with OSAS. It is not even known what proportion of children with OSAS have hypoxemia during sleep or what the relationship is between hypoxemia or hypercarbia and the severity of sleep-related airway obstruction. Some children with severe OSAS have drops in SaO_2 to values below 50%, while others have OSAS with daytime symptoms but no hypoxemia. Children with obstructive apnea usually show a repetitive pattern of desaturation during apnea with recovery of SaO_2 when breathing resumes. In children with continuous partial obstruction SaO_2 may decrease at the start of the event and remain low (and unsteady) for long periods. Brouillette and associates reported transcutaneous pO_2 values as low as 7 mmHg during obstructive hypoventilation in a child who was left with severe neurologic damage.[8] Although the effects of asphyxia are clear in such cases, little is known about how the degree and duration of hypoxia during sleep relates to outcome in children. This is a complex question since the pattern of hypoxemia may also be important. Multiple brief oxyhemoglobin desaturations may not be as harmful as prolonged episodes, even though total hypoxic duration is the same. The link between hypoxia and specific adverse effects is also unknown except in a rough qualitative way. For example, although it is well known that hypoxemia during sleep can cause pulmonary hypertension and cor pulmonale, it is not known how much hypoxemia a child can tolerate before developing cor pulmonale. Finally, the effects of mild hypoxemia and subsequent indications for treatment are unknown.

Hypercarbia

Hypercarbia during sleep is a feature of childhood-type OSAS. Some investigators define obstructive hypopnea or hypoventilation as a reduction in oronasal airflow, while others require a rise in end-tidal CO_2. Most studies do not report measurements of end-tidal CO_2 in a systematic and quantitative fashion. For this reason, the literature is difficult to summarize. In the older literature most children reported had severe OSA and presented in respiratory failure with hypercarbia even while awake.[4, 54–56, 58, 61, 62, 66, 69, 80] Ainger described 6 children, 18 months to 6 years of age, with severe OSAS and cor pulmonale; 5 of 6 had $PaCO_2$ values between 52 and 68 mmHg.[56] About one half of the 22 children reported by Brouillette and associates in 1982 showed hypercarbia (end-tidal CO_2 >45 mmHg) related to OSAS or continuous partial obstruction.[8] There is a general impression that most children presenting with OSAS today do not have daytime hypercarbia. However, the proportion of children with OSAS with some degree of hypercarbia during sleep is unknown.

Neuropsychiatric Disturbances

The International Classification of Sleep Disorders Manual describes depression, irritability, anxiety, and profound despair as commonly associated with OSAS in adults as well as blackouts, disorientation, and periods of automatic behavior with amnesia. It is not known if these symptoms are features of childhood OSAS. In one report of 25 children with continuous partial obstruction, 40% manifested aggressive and rebellious behavior or pathologic shyness and social withdrawal.[17] It is likely that psychologic dysfunction occurs in many other children with OSAS, but this remains to be studied.

Course

Since childhood OSAS has various causes and may occur at any age from infancy to adolescence, a single course is unlikely. It is clear from the large number of case reports between 1956 and 1976 associating adenotonsillar hypertrophy with cor pulmonale, in some children untreated OSAS will progress to pulmonary hypertension and heart failure. Other reports suggest that some children with OSAS develop failure-to-thrive and neurologic and developmental impairments. However, it must also be true that some children with OSAS experience spontaneous resolution over time and do not develop obvious complications. One problem is that the course or natural history of OSAS is likely to be different in mild, moderate, and severe childhood-type OSAS; in infants, young children, older children, and adolescents; in obese children; and in children with craniofacial abnormalities.

Another problem is that physicians often see patients only at a single point along their course. One patient may have severe OSAS with cor pulmonale and failure-to-thrive, whereas another may have only mild obstructive hypoventilation and no daytime symptoms. The determinants of why one child pro-

gresses to a bad outcome and another does not are not known. Nor is it known what adverse outcomes are possible. Mild OSAS, for example, may not lead to cor pulmonale, but there may be subtle effects on behavior and daytime cognitive function. Snoring and mild OSAS may affect development in other ways not yet recognized. Finally, it is not known whether children with OSAS will grow up to be adults with OSAS.

Predisposing Factors and High-Risk Groups

Anything that reduces the caliber, increases the collapsibility, or interferes with the neural control of the nasopharyngeal airway could predispose a child to the development of sleep-related upper airway obstruction. Possibilities include large tonsils or adenoids, macroglossia, abnormalities of the soft palate, micro- or retrognathia, other craniofacial abnormalities, obesity, mucosal swelling, polyps, foreign bodies, tumors, abscesses and other infections, tissue infiltration (storage diseases), and neurologic lesions affecting upper airway dilator muscles (see Table 17–2). Young age and small stature may also be predisposing factors.

Obesity

Although obesity appears to predispose children to OSAS, most children with OSAS are not obese. In 1977, Stool and associates reported on three children aged 5, 6, and 12 years of age with adenotonsillar hypertrophy, obesity, daytime hypersomnolence, hypoxemia, hypercarbia, and OSAS; all were above the 97th percentile for weight and were 150 to 195% of ideal weight for height.[34] One boy, 6 years old, had complete resolution of OSAS symptoms for 1 year after adenotonsillectomy, but symptoms returned when he gained 24 pounds.[34] Mallory and associates reported on 41 children with sleep-related disordered breathing and morbid obesity (>150% of ideal weight).[21] They found no correlation between clinical history and any abnormality on PSG. Fifteen patients (37%) showed mild abnormalities and 2 (5%) showed abnormalities severe enough to warrant surgical intervention.[21] However, this study used "adult" definitions of OSA (apnea index >5, end-tidal CO_2 >50 mmHg for more than 5% of sleeptime,

$SaO_2 < 90\%$ for more than 3% of sleeptime, minimum apnea duration at least 10 sec). The reported patients were referred from 222 patients in a pediatric obesity clinic. If the 181 patients not referred for breathing problems did not have OSAS, then the proportion of obese children with sleep-related breathing abnormalities would be 15/222, or about 7%.[21] This figure of 7% from the Mallory study probably *underestimates* the incidence of sleep-related upper airway obstruction in obese children given the definitions they used.[21] This estimate is still higher than any estimate of childhood-type OSAS prevalence in the general population. The actual prevalence of sleep-related breathing abnormalities in unselected obese children is not known.

It might be expected that OSAS symptoms would correlate with the severity of obesity. Silvestri and associates recently addressed this question using PSG to study 32 obese children referred for assessment of snoring and difficulty breathing during sleep.[81] Although these patients had a high incidence of OSAS symptoms such as difficulty breathing during sleep (59%), apnea (50%), and EDS (59%), individual symptoms did not correlate with the severity of PSG abnormalities and PSG findings did not correlate with the degree of obesity. The only significant finding was that end-tidal CO_2 was higher in patients >200% ideal body weight than in those patients who weighed less. A significant proportion of the obese children reported in this study were hypoxic and hypercarbic while awake.[81]

Infants

Some amount of obstructive apnea is normal in premature infants and full-term newborns. Kahn and associates recently reported that brief obstructive apnea during sleep is associated with symptoms even in normal infants.[36] When normal infants with brief obstructive apneas are compared to infants without such obstructions, they are found to have a higher incidence of reported breathholding spells and fatigue during feeding while awake and profuse sweating, snoring, and noisy breathing while asleep.[36] It is not known if normal brief obstructive apneas are an early sign of childhood OSAS.

The prevalence of OSAS in infants is not known. Leiberman and associates reported on 14 infants, 10 boys and 4 girls, aged 7 to 18 months of age with OSAS diagnosed by adult criteria during PSG or direct observation.[82] Presenting symptoms in all children included snoring or noisy breathing and a history of apnea. Three infants showed failure-to-thrive, two showed developmental delay, and two had craniofacial abnormalities. Snoring was the most common initial symptom, and onset of symptoms occurred between 2 and 6 months of age.[82] Adenotonsillectomy led to marked improvement in 13 infants; the one that did not improve also had micrognathia. Growth charts showed "remarkable catch-up" after surgery.[82]

Down Syndrome

Down syndrome is one of the strongest known risk factors for OSAS in children. Although it was suspected for many years that the incidence of OSAS was high in Down syndrome patients, this was not confirmed until 1991. Marcus and associates, studying 53 Down syndrome subjects (2 weeks to 51 years old) using daytime nap PSG, found that 45% had OSA and 66% showed obstructive hypoventilation during sleep.[83] A subgroup also had overnight PSG, which showed that nap PSG underestimated the presence of abnormalities. Confirming the speculations of Loughlin and associates[84] and Rowland and associates[85] from 10 years earlier, there was no clinical suspicion of OSAS in 68% of the subjects. Age, obesity, and the presence of congenital heart disease were not correlated with OSA, hypoxemia, or hypoventilation during sleep.[83] Although PSG improved in the eight patients who underwent adenotonsillectomy, it did *not* normalize in five subjects (62%).[83] Thus, postoperative PSG in Down syndrome patients should be strongly considered.

The findings that most patients with Down syndrome have sleep-associated upper airway obstruction and about one-third show hypoxemia during sleep may have important implications. Some of the features of Down syndrome such as pulmonary hypertension, behavioral problems, and mental retardation may be due, at least in part, to unrecognized OSAS with its associated hypoxemia, hypercarbia, and sleep disturbance.

Craniofacial Syndromes

Jamieson and associates reported that over 90% of adults with OSAS have abnormal cephalometric landmarks[86]; the corresponding information is not available for children. Children with craniofacial abnormalities (see Table 17–2) would be expected to have a high incidence of OSAS, although actual incidence is still unknown. Midfacial hypoplasia and increased nasal resistance, soft palate abnormalities, macroglossia, mandibular hypoplasia, muscular hypotonia, abnormal neural airway control, and structural defects could all play a role. Infants with Pierre Robin syndrome (micrognathia, glossoptosis, and cleft palate) have been known for years to have upper airway obstruction leading to complications such as cor pulmonale and sudden death.[87–89] Appropriate management during infancy can prevent most of these complications,[89] and micrognathia and airway obstruction slowly resolve or at least improve with age. Spier and associates performed PSG on eight patients between 8 and 22 years of age with Pierre Robin syndrome and found that minor clinically significant sleep disturbance was common but that only one patient had OSAS.[88] However, this was a limited follow-up study of only 8 of 36 consecutive patients with Pierre Robin syndrome.

OSAS has been reported in association with Pierre Robin syndrome,[8, 15, 87–89] Klippel-Fiel syndrome,[15, 90, 91] Hallermann-Streiff syndrome,[92, 93] Treacher Collins syndrome,[15, 94, 95] Apert's syndrome,[96] Pfeiffer's syndrome,[96] Larsen's syndrome and arthrogryposis multiplex congenita,[8] facioauriculovertebral sequence,[95] Crouzon's syndrome,[8, 15, 95] Stickler syndrome, craniosynostosis with arachnodactyly and abdominal hernias, velocardiofacial syndrome, pycnodysostosis,[95] Prader-Willi syndrome,[15] Marfan's syndrome,[97] osteopetrosis,[98] Rubinstein-Taybi syndrome,[99] fragile X syndrome,[100] and deletion of a portion of the long arm of chromosome 6.[101] Sher and associates studied a number of these patients endoscopically and described that the site of airway obstruction was variable, both between and within syndromes.[95] At the Johns Hopkins Sleep Center, OSAS has been diagnosed in children with many of these syndromes and in many patients with what Sher and associates called "provisionally unique syndromes" (one-of-a-kind, multiple anomalies).[95] It should be remembered that many of these children have other airway abnormalities that could lead to obstruction such as completely cartilaginous trachea in Crouzon's syndrome,[102] palatal thickening due to accumulation of mucopolysaccharides in Apert's syndrome,[103] macro-

glossia in Beckwith-Wiedemann syndrome,[104] and laryngomalacia, tracheomalacia, and bronchomalacia in Apert's and Pfeiffer's syndromes.[96] A child in the clinic at Johns Hopkins with deformity of kleeblattschädel, severe OSAS, failure-to-thrive, developmental delay, and congestive heart failure also was found to have asymmetry of the cardiac septal hypertrophy. Although there are no studies of OSAS in children with pre-existing heart disease, there is the clinical impression that children with pre-existing structural cardiac disease are more vulnerable to the complications of OSAS than are normal children.

Achondroplasia

Children with achondroplasia are at risk for several respiratory complications including OSAS. In 1978 Smith and associates diagnosed OSAS using fluoroscopy in a 12-year-old boy with achondroplasia.[105] Stokes and associates in 1983, reported 7 of 85 patients in an achondroplasia clinic at the Johns Hopkins Children's Center with OSAS or loud snoring and hypoxemia (in retrospect, probably obstructive hypoventilation).[106] At the same institution, Reid and associates prospectively evaluated 26 children with achondroplasia and found that 15 (58%) had a history of loud snoring and 9 (35%) had OSA on overnight PSG.[107] Experience during the last 5 years in the same clinic indicates that more than 50% of the patients had evidence of obstructive apnea or hypoventilation on PSG. The rising incidence figure probably represents increased recognition of the disorder, increased referrals of children with achondroplasia for sleep-related breathing problems, and changing definitions of childhood-type OSAS. It should be noted that these figures come from a tertiary referral center with widely known expertise in the area of sleep-disordered breathing in achondroplasia; the incidence of OSAS in a less selected sample is not known.

Nelson and associates prospectively evaluated 32 patients with achondroplasia (mean age, 8.1 years) using nap or overnight PSG.[108] This study is difficult to interpret since they used adult criteria (obstructive events lasting <10 sec, and oxygen desaturations <10%, were not counted) and obstructive events in REM were excluded.[108] Even so, 6 of the 32 patients (19%) showed upper airway obstruction during sleep.

The determinants of upper airway collapse

and predisposing factors for OSAS in these patients are not known. Midfacial hypoplasia, increased nasal resistance, structural abnormalities of the nasopharyngeal airway, and abnormal neural control of upper airway muscle tone are all possible. Abnormalities at the craniocervical junction could affect airway control by cervicomedullary compression, including compression of cranial nerves IX and XII. Five patients who underwent surgical posterior fossa decompression were reported by Nelson and associates to show improvement on postoperative PSG.[108] Also in that study was the finding that a history of apnea was not sufficient to confirm or rule out abnormal breathing during sleep.[108] Achondroplastic patients may present with failure-to-thrive and cor pulmonale and still have their sleep-associated airway obstruction unrecognized. Given current knowledge, PSG evaluation of all patients with achondroplasia seems reasonable.

Mucopolysaccharide Storage Diseases

The mucopolysaccharidosis (MPS) and mucolipidosis (ML) are caused by biochemical defects that result in accumulation of macromolecules, eventually leading to structural changes in tissues, including the respiratory tract.[109] Of the 21 patients (children and adults) with MPS or ML reported by Semenza and Pyeritz, 18 (86%) had upper airway narrowing, 12 (57%) had macroglossia, and 14 (67%) showed adenotonsillar hypertrophy.[109] Nine of twelve patients with symptoms of OSAS underwent PSG, and OSA was found in 8 (89%).[109] Nearly all (20 of 21) patients had chronic pulmonary disease and thus were particularly prone to develop hypoxemia and hypercarbia during sleep if upper airway obstruction is superimposed.

Specific syndromes that have been associated with OSAS include Hurler's syndrome (MPS-IH), Hurler-Scheie syndrome (MPS-IH/S), Hunter's syndrome (MPS-II), Morquio's syndrome (MPS-IV), Sly's syndrome (MPS-VII), and Sanfilippo's syndrome (MPS-III).[18, 109–112] At Johns Hopkins, an 8-year-old boy was seen with OSAS and Maroteaux-Lamy syndrome (MPS-VI). Shapiro and associates described four children with Hurler's and Hunter's syndromes and OSAS.[110] All of these children had purulent rhinitis and chronic nasal congestion that persisted after adenoidectomy or tonsillectomy.[110] Myer described the radiographic features of Hurler's syndrome in

four children 4 months to 4 years old (two with OSA), which included short neck, adenotonsillar hypertrophy, macroglossia, and a high epiglottis.[113] Although adenotonsillar hypertrophy is often present, their removal may not be effective.[110, 113] Tracheostomy relieves the sleep-related upper airway obstruction, but perioperative morbidity due to other tracheobronchial abnormalities in common.[110, 113] Malone and associates reported a 3-year-old girl with Hurler's syndrome and OSAS in whom biopsy showed that more than 50% of tonsil volume was attributable to lysosomal inclusions in macrophages.[111] OSAS resolved in this patient after bone marrow transplantation, and follow-up tonsil biopsy revealed that the lysosomal inclusions were no longer present.[111] MPS patients present very complex airway management problems and even tracheostomy does not insure control of the airway.[110] These children should be referred to centers with otolaryngology and pulmonology expertise in the management of MPS and ML patients.

Neurologic Disorders

In adults there is evidence that central nervous system lesions such as syringobulbia-myelia,[114] lateral medullary syndrome,[115] and posterior fossa tumors[116] can cause OSA. However, neurologic lesions have not been shown to *cause* typical OSAS in children. Syringobulbia has been associated with laryngeal stridor in children.[117] Infants[118] and adolescents[119] with meningomyelocoele, hydrocephalus, and Arnold-Chiari malformation have been shown to have life-threatening central apnea as well as vocal cord paralysis with upper airway obstruction, but OSA due to pharyngeal airway collapse in such cases has not been documented. Prolonged central apnea and obstructive apnea associated with seizures developed in an infant with a left temporal lobe astrocytoma.[120] Although Guilleminault and associates reported on six children with neurologic (Arnold-Chiari malformation, syringomyelobulbia) or neuromuscular (myotonic dystrophy) disease and OSAS,[121] it was not clear if the neurologic disorder per se was a causative factor in the OSAS.

Miscellaneous Predisposing Factors

Anesthesia and sedatives are known to be associated with increased upper airway obstruction in children. Alcohol is likely to predispose children to OSA, as it does adults. Nasal obstruction with mouth breathing and snoring in an 11-year-old boy was found to be caused by Hodgkin's disease of the nasopharynx (this child had no complaints of sleep apnea and no polysomnography).[122] A 12-year-old black girl with adenotonsillar hypertrophy, chronic mouth breathing, and loud snoring was found to have noncaseating granulomas of the tonsils and adenoids consistent with sarcoidosis.[123] Symptoms of behavior disturbances, daytime hypersomnolence, enuresis, and snoring with restless sleep were caused by OSA in a 10-year-old boy with an antral choanal polyp.[124] Polypectomy was unsuccessful owing to regrowth of polypoid mucosa, but after a Caldwell-Luc procedure PSG became normal and symptoms resolved.[124] OSAS in young children can also be caused by cystic hygroma,[125] massive oropharyngeal papillomatosis,[126] and nasopharyngeal foreign body.[127] In one infant, OSAS was associated with congenital hypothyroidism.[15]

OSAS has been linked to lymphoproliferative disorders in adults and children. Fairley and associates reported on three patients, including a 6-year-old girl, who were immunosuppressed following heart-lung transplants.[128] In two of these patients on long-term cyclosporin therapy, massive adenotonsillar enlargement causing OSA was found to be caused by an Epstein-Barr virus (EBV) lymphoproliferative disorder.[128] Transplant-associated lymphoproliferative disorder leading to adenotonsillar enlargement has also been reported to cause OSAS in a 2-year-old child on cyclosporin following liver transplantation.[129]

Prevalence

In 1988 one report stated that, "Obstructive sleep apnea syndrome is a rare condition in childhood."[10] Far from being rare, however, OSAS in childhood is a public health problem of potentially immense proportions. Approximately 7 to 9% of children suffer from habitual snoring,[9, 130, 131] and the prevalence of OSAS is suspected to be about 2%.[130] These data have two major implications. Since most children with habitual snoring do not have OSAS (see Chapter 17), identifying the 20% of habitual snorers who do have OSAS, in a cost-effective manner, is a difficult and important public health goal. Effective screening

tests do not yet exist, and the cost of performing PSG on every snoring child would be prohibitive. Furthermore, since there are approximately 32 million children aged 1 to 9 years in the United States,[132] and even if the prevalence of OSA were only 1%, there would still be 320,000 children with OSAS.

Age of Onset

The clinical syndromes of sleep-associated upper airway obstruction may begin in infancy.[8, 41, 82, 133] Frank and associates studying children 2 to 13 years of age (parental reporting of symptoms subject to recall-bias errors) found that 28% of parents described symptoms (snoring) dating back to the "first few months of life."[7] In the 22 patients reported by Brouillette and associates in 1982, the mean age of onset for OSAS was 14 ± 12 months (the earliest occurrence being in the newborn period).[8] Guilleminault and Stoohs reported 25 full-term infants who presented in infancy with an apparent life-threatening event (ALTE) and developed OSAS by 5 years of age.[133]

Sex Ratio

Estimates based on the current literature suggest that the sex ratio for OSAS in prepubertal children is roughly 1:1. There is a strong clinical impression that OSAS is unusual in postpubertal girls, but this has not been confirmed.

Genetics

Little is known about the role of inheritance in childhood-type OSAS. As with snoring, OSAS has been described in families,[134, 135] but the role of specific inheritable determinants of OSAS versus nonspecific predisposing factors (e.g., obesity) and environmental factors is not known. The recent controlled study by Redline and associates of 272 subjects in 29 families found a familial aggregation of OSAS symptoms suggesting a significant genetic component.[136] Although there were some children identified as having OSAS, this study did not examine childhood OSAS per se. Furthermore, Redline used a questionnaire (filled out by the parents) to identify children with OSAS, which may not accurately identify children with OSAS as opposed to those with primary snoring.[137] In the Guilleminault and Stoohs report, 25 infants presented with an ALTE during infancy and later developed OSAS.[133] These infants were more likely to have a family history of OSAS and snoring, to still have home monitor alarms at 9 months of age, and to have significantly smaller airway dimensions on cephalometric radiographs than matched ALTE controls.[133] These data suggest that genetic influences on airway structure may play a role in the development of childhood OSAS.

Pathophysiology

The mechanisms of OSA in children are not known. Although some data pertaining specifically to children can be found in the literature, studies directly investigating the mechanisms of childhood OSAS are few. Clearly, there is not a single mechanism in all children with OSAS. It is probable that OSAS in children with adenotonsillar hypertrophy differs from OSAS in children with craniofacial or neurologic syndromes. At the very least, it should not be assumed that mechanisms of childhood OSAS are the same as in adults.

The term "upper airway" refers to the tube formed by the nasopharynx, oropharynx, and hypopharynx. Studies in dead infants have shown the following: the oropharynx is the most compliant or collapsible segment of the upper airway; the closing pressure of the airway (without muscle activity) is near atmospheric; once the airway collapses more force is required to open it; and negative pressure inside the airway pulls in the anterior, lateral, and posterior airway walls.[138, 139] Airway patency is ordinarily maintained by muscle activity and by other factors. It would be important to know the determinants of airway collapse and the mechanisms by which obstructive apnea or hypopnea (hypoventilation) are terminated.

Sites of Obstruction

Felman and associates, using fluoroscopy to study children with obstructive sleep apnea, described two patterns of inspiratory obstruction: posterior movement of the soft palate with occlusion of the nasal canal and posterior movement of the tongue plus thickening of the prevertebral tissues leading to hypopharyngeal collapse.[140] Fernbach and associates used

lateral neck radiographs and airway fluoroscopy to study children with OSAS.[141] They found that during obstructed inspiration the pharyngeal airway collapsed and the posterior pharyngeal wall moved forward, which was sometimes associated with posterior movement of the tongue, elongation of the tonsils, and inferior or posterior tonsillar displacement.[141] The soft palate remained unchanged or became apposed to the prevertebral tissues. The airway below the site of obstruction was seen to collapse on inspiration; whereas above the obstruction, dilation was observed.[141] Endoscopic examination in children has revealed pharyngeal collapse at the site of large adenoids and tonsils[142, 144] and at the level of the soft palate.[142, 143]

In children with craniofacial abnormalities, the site of obstruction is also variable. Even without adenotonsillar hypertrophy, such children may show pharyngeal or hypopharyngeal obstruction during inspiration. In Pierre Robin syndrome, a normal-sized tongue was endoscopically observed to move posteriorly and obstruct the airway.[143] In achondroplasia, sleep-associated inspiratory obstruction started at the base of the tongue and extended to the epiglottis.[105] In Down syndrome, obstruction occurred at the tongue base in 4 of 6 patients described by Croft and associates and at the tonsils and adenoids in 2 of 6.[143] A child with Beckwith-Wiedemann syndrome and macroglossia had obstruction due to posterior tongue displacement.[142]

Studies in adults[145] and children[105] show that inspiratory obstruction usually begins in the pharynx and extends downward during the apnea. This has also been demonstrated using power spectral density analysis and acoustical analysis of an estimated cross-sectional area.[11] The acoustical studies show that the site of obstruction moves during inspiration, starting at the nasopharynx and moving down to the supralaryngeal area by the end of inspiration.[11]

In all studies, OSA occurs only during sleep and is usually due to pharyngeal/hypopharyngeal collapse or apposition of the soft palate and adenoids during inspiration. Collapse of the upper airway is a dynamic process that involves interactions between sleep state, pressure-flow mechanics, and respiratory drive. Unfortunately, observing the airway collapsing around and below large tonsils and adenoids does not explain why it does so in some children but not in others (see below). Even less is known about the sites and dynamics of partial airway collapse in children.

Mechanisms of OSAS in Children

Most otherwise normal children with OSAS have enlarged tonsils and/or adenoids and no clinically apparent craniofacial or upper airway structural abnormalities.[8, 16, 31, 140, 145, 146] However, numerous studies have failed to find a relationship between tonsil or adenoid size and sleep-associated upper airway obstruction in children (see below). Several questions remain: Is there a single mechanism, even in normal children? Why do some children without adenotonsillar enlargement have OSAS, while others with severe adenotonsillar hypertrophy do not? Is OSAS in children simply due to mechanical airway obstruction from large tonsils or adenoids, or is it necessary for the child have an underlying abnormality of upper airway control or structure?

It has been proposed that enlarged tonsils and/or adenoids lead to increased upper airway resistance, which combined with decreased upper airway dilator muscle activity at sleep onset leads to upper airway collapse during inspiration.[8, 140] However, children do not show decreased genioglossus muscle or diaphragm activity at the onset of obstructive sleep apnea.[147] Jeffries and associates pointed out that decreased phasic upper airway dilator muscle activity cannot be the *primary cause* of OSA in children since normal children do not have phasic upper airway dilator muscle activity during sleep.[148] It is possible that when the airway is preloaded with large tonsils and adenoids, the increased resistance leads to activation of upper airway dilator muscles which *then* play a significant role in the maintenance of upper airway patency. However, this hypothesis does not explain why some children with huge tonsils and adenoids have minimal or no OSA, while other children with small tonsils and adenoids can have severe OSA. It appears likely that other etiologic factors such as subtle abnormalities of airway configuration, abnormal upper airway dilator muscle control, or abnormal arousal mechanisms are necessary to fully explain childhood OSAS.

Role of Adenotonsillar Hypertrophy

Large adenoids can be shown to correlate with snoring and nasal obstruction.[149, 150] Brodsky and associates compared children with chronic tonsillitis but *no snoring* with OSAS children diagnosed *by history alone*.[146] It is not surprising that subtle differences were found in oropharyngeal soft tissue dimensions; OSAS children had less space between lateral pharyngeal walls compared with nonsnorers.[146, 150] The results of these studies are difficult to interpret since it has not been shown that childhood OSAS can be distinguished from PS by history.[13, 137] Croft and associates reported a significant relationship between sleep apnea or sleep disturbance (sleep grade) and tonsillar size.[19] However, this relationship can be explained by the observation that 50% of the patients in this study did not snore at all. When the analysis is restricted to patients with snoring, there appears to be no relationship between tonsil size and upper airway obstruction.[19] They also reported that the size of the oropharyngeal airway, measured on lateral cephalometry, was an important contributor to sleep apnea and sleep disturbance.[19] Again, when nonsnorers are dropped from the analysis, there appears to be no correlation between airway dimensions and OSA per se.

Tonsil Size

Ahlqvist-Rastad and associates investigated tonsil size in 93 children with symptoms of OSAS, mouth breathing, and swallowing difficulties.[20] They found no correlation between tonsil size and OSAS or swallowing difficulties, suggesting that other factors such as adenoidal hypertrophy were causally related to OSAS or feeding difficulties. Some children with nearly normal tonsil size (+1 on a scale of 0 to +4) showed severe obstructive symptoms.[20] Brodsky and associates found that large tonsils (+3 or +4) may or may not be associated with OSAS in children.[150] After excision, large nonobstructing tonsils and large tonsils from OSAS children weighed nearly the same, but tonsil volume was significantly greater in those from OSAS children.[150] This could imply that there is a difference between tonsillar hypertrophy in obstructed and nonobstructed patients. More importantly, when patients with and without OSAS were matched for tonsil size (+3 or +4), there were no significant differences in oropharyngeal or nasopharyngeal dimensions.[150]

Adenoid Size

Although studies suggest that tonsillar enlargement alone cannot account for OSAS in children, there is little information about the role of adenoidal hypertrophy. Adenoidal hypertrophy has been correlated with snoring[150] but has not been shown to correlate with OSA. Even when nonsnorers were included in the analysis, Croft and associates found that the thickness of the "adenoid pad" on lateral cephalometry did not correlate with OSA.[19]

Effect of Adenoid and/or Tonsil Removal

At the Johns Hopkins Pediatric Sleep Center many patients have been encountered who experience dramatic resolution of OSAS following adenotonsillectomy, only to have symptoms return during an upper respiratory tract infection. This implies that such children are still not completely normal after adenotonsillectomy. In addition, many children continue to snore after adenotonsillectomy and some continue to have OSA. Maw and associates found that 52% of children who snore continue to do so after adenoidectomy and 70% continue mouth breathing.[151] The persistence of snoring postoperatively correlated with adenoid volume but mouth breathing did not.[151] It is not known whether the persistence of snoring and/or OSA after adenotonsillectomy correlates with the tonsil or adenoid volume removed. The observation that most children improve after adenotonsillectomy leads many to assume that adenotonsillar hypertrophy causes OSAS. However, it is possible that adenotonsillar hypertrophy is merely an exacerbating factor that causes snoring in normal children but causes OSAS only in children with abnormal upper airway structure or control.

Keeping in mind that most of the aforementioned studies did not use PSG to diagnose OSA, it would appear that large tonsils and adenoids are a major factor producing snoring, mouth breathing, and nasal obstruction. In addition, the nature of the hypertrophy may be different in obstructing tonsils. However, the observations that large tonsils or adenoids may not be associated with OSAS[150] and that severe OSAS may occur in children with small tonsils[20] strongly suggest that factors *other than adenotonsillar hypertrophy* must be important in the development of obstructive sleep apnea in children.

Underlying Airway Structure

Although Brodsky and associates have found trends toward subtle differences in oropharyngeal dimensions in children with large obstructing as opposed to large nonobstructing tonsils,[150] no study has documented that normal children with OSAS have abnormal underlying upper airway structure.

The Role of Mucosal "Stickiness"

In animals it has been demonstrated that more pressure is required to open the collapsed airway than to close an open airway,[152, 153] a finding thought to be related to adhesive surface forces between the apposed mucosal surfaces. Enlargement of the tonsils and adenoids leads to major changes in airway size and anatomic relationships between mucosal surfaces. It is also possible that the properties of the mucosal surfaces or the mucus itself may be different in children with OSAS from that in normal children (see Other Mechanisms).

Role of Arousal from Sleep in Apnea Termination

Obstructive apnea in adults is usually terminated by central nervous system (CNS) arousal,[154, 155] but the situation is not so clear in children. Several investigators have found that children terminate a significant proportion of obstructive events without the EEG arousal seen in adults.[25, 156] In addition, the occurrence of prolonged periods of obstructive hypoventilation or profound hypoxemia without CNS arousal and the minimal degree of sleep fragmentation seen in many children with OSAS, suggests that arousal mechanisms in children are different from those in adults.

The idea that heart rate or breathing changes occurring in isolation represent CNS arousal has lead to confusion in the literature. Based on known interactions between cardiac and respiratory systems, heart rate would be expected to slow during obstructive apnea and to accelerate immediately upon apnea termination, purely on a reflex basis. This reflex can be demonstrated in decerebrate and anesthetized animals, involves feedback from the pulmonary stretch receptors, and is vagally mediated. Although data are not available for human children, Baker and Fewell have demonstrated in lambs that heart rate changes associated with relief of airway obstruction are related to cardiopulmonary reflexes and not to arousal.[157]

Sleep Deprivation

There is evidence that sleep-deprivation can lead to development of OSA in healthy infants. Canet and associates studied sleep-deprived healthy infants 1 to 6 months of age and found a 12-fold increase in the amount of obstructed breathing during sleep.[158] Therefore, it is possible that OSA, initially caused by an upper respiratory infection, leads to sleep deprivation and worsening of OSA in a vicious circle.

Other Mechanisms

Is there something different about the adenotonsillar hypertrophy in children who develop OSAS? Pransky and associates compared adenoid and tonsil histology in children with obstructive adenotonsillar hypertrophy with children with recurrent tonsillitis without obstructive symptoms.[159] They found that 18% of all patients had *Actinomycetes* within the tonsils or adenoids; 75% of these were in the group undergoing adenotonsillectomy for obstructive indications.[159] The authors suggest a role for core tissue colonization with *Actinomycetes* in producing lymphoid tissue hypertrophy in these patients. These data must be viewed with caution, however, since the tonsillitis group may have received more antibiotic treatment prior to surgery. Two other studies, which did not look for *Actinomycetes*, have found no differences in the adenotonsillar microbial flora between the two groups.[160, 161] Isolated IgA deficiency and OSAS have been reported in one child,[162] but this may have been a chance occurrence and there is no evidence that immune abnormalities play a role in the pathogenesis of OSAS in normal children. Heiner states that adenotonsillar hypertrophy with upper airway obstruction "may be caused, or aggravated by, food allergies,"[163] but there are no data to support or refute this contention.

The relationship between allergy and OSAS needs further investigation. Adenoid histamine content has been found to correlate with serous otitis media, mouth breathing, and nasal obstruction in children.[164] Conceivably, inflammatory mediators are released locally into the airway in some children and cause airway dysfunction. Preliminary data, using a multiallergen radioallergosorbent testing (RAST) (Phadiotop Paediatric, Pharmacia Diagnostics), show that 41% of children presenting for evaluation of snoring and OSAS have evidence of allergy.[165] However, PSG evaluation revealed that the presence of allergy was associated with both primary snoring and OSAS and was not specific.[165]

Complications

Complication, as used in this chapter, refers to *another disease or condition that develops during the course of OSAS as a consequence of OSAS* (Table 18–3). Frequently occurring complications, such as suboptimal growth, were discussed under *Associated Features* (see p 171). Major complications of childhood OSAS include failure-to-thrive, developmental delay, cor pulmonale, and death. Because earlier recognition of OSAS in children has reduced the incidence of cor pulmonale to the point that it is an uncommon presenting feature, it is discussed as a *complication* rather than an *associated feature*. As knowledge and diagnostic ability improves, certain *complications* may become *associated* or even *essential features* of childhood OSAS. For example, better recognition of daytime cognitive dysfunction may reveal that it is a common feature. Ventricular dysfunction during OSA in children is not routinely found but it is also not routinely measured. If it were, compromised right ventricular (RV) function might become an essential feature.

Table 18–3. COMPLICATIONS OF CHILDHOOD OSAS

Death:	(? incidence)
Growth:	Failure-to-thrive
	Short stature
	Impaired growth hormone release
Cardiovascular:	Cor pulmonale/pulmonary hypertension
	Polycythemia
	Chronic respiratory acidosis
	Hypertension?
Gastrointestinal:	Feeding difficulties
	Gastroesophageal reflux
Pulmonary:	Chronic aspiration
	Pulmonary edema (postoperative)
	Pectus excavatum
Behavioral:	Developmental delay
	Behavioral problems
	School problems
Neurologic:	Enuresis (? etiology)
	Increased intracranial pressure
	Lethargy/dull affect
	"Hypoxia headache"
Surgical:	Death (intraoperative, RVH/RVD*)
	Death (postoperative)
	Postoperative respiratory compromise

*Right ventricular hypertrophy/right ventricular dilatation.

Cardiovascular

Cor Pulmonale

Early literature on OSAS in children contained numerous reports of OSAS presenting with cor pulmonale.[4, 5, 53–62, 64–66, 68–71, 80, 166, 167] Table 18–4 summarizes the cardiac catheterization data from case reports. It is clear that OSAS will progress in some children to cause severe cor pulmonale, which is reversible after intervention. In many cases pulmonary artery (PA) pressure increased during oxygen breathing. Noonan believed that this was caused by the large increase in $PaCO_2$ that occurred when the inspired oxygen was increased.[4] By approximately 1980, OSAS was beginning to be recognized as a disorder that could present in a milder form before the development of severe complications. In 1982, 55% of cases in the series reported by Brouillette and associates still showed signs of cor pulmonale.[8] Although progress has been made, children still develop cor pulmonale and overt congestive heart failure (CHF) secondary to OSAS. Childhood OSAS should be in the differential diagnosis of any child with unexplained cor pulmonale or CHF. The importance of recognizing OSA as a cause of cor pulmonale becomes even more clear when one considers that improvement occurs in nearly all patients after relief of upper airway obstruction.[168–170]

Down Syndrome, OSAS, and Pulmonary Hypertension

Loughlin and associates pointed out in 1981 that children with congenital heart disease (CHD) and Down syndrome frequently have pulmonary hypertension out of proportion to the severity of the cardiac defects.[84] They proposed that unrecognized OSAS with nighttime hypoxemia in Down syndrome patients might be responsible for the excessively severe pulmonary hypertension and reported on five children with CHD and pulmonary hypertension. All five children had right ventricular hypertrophy; four had CHD and the degree of pulmonary hypertension could not be explained by their cardiac lesion. All five were documented to have OSA. In a 10-year-old patient undergoing cardiac catheterization, awake pulmonary arterial pressure was 30/15 mmHg but rose to 65/35 mmHg during sleep (Table 18–5). Similar findings were reported by Rowland and associates, Levine and Simpser, Kasian and associates and Bloch and asso-

Table 18–4. CARDIAC CATHETERIZATION DATA FROM CASE REPORTS OF CHILDREN WITH OSAS

Author	Age (years)	Preoperative PA Pressure Air Systolic/diastolic (mmHg)	Preoperative PA Pressure Oxygen Systolic/diastolic (mmHg)	Postoperative PA Pressure Air Systolic/diastolic (mmHg)
Noonan[4]	2	55/28	93/65*	—
	4	50/30	—	—
Menashe[54]	9	45–95/5–50**	—	21/7
Cox[53]	1.5	104/67	—	45/16
Luke[55]	4.5	47/14	—	29/9
	3	33/15	—	—
Levy[80]	3	99/66	46/23	38/16
Setliff[58]	3	90/45	85/42	—
Massumi[62]	3	50/30	—	—
Gerald[57]	?	70/20	—	22/12
	?	45/18	—	—
	?	40/15	—	—
Cayler[59]	2.5	45/15	—	—
Macartney[61]	3	76/28	—	30/5
	2	33/4	—	—
Freeman[65]	2.5	30/12	—	—
Thanopoulos[70]	3	65/30	60/28	—
Goodman[5]	1.5	44/8	—	—
	2	44/5	—	19/14
	3	43/5	—	—
Galal[198]	?	85/56	61/28	—
	2	86/47	52/20	—

*$PaCO_2$ increased during O_2 breathing.
**PA pressure varied owing to obstructed breathing.

Table 18–5. CARDIAC CATHETERIZATION DATA FROM CASE REPORTS OF CHILDREN WITH OSAS, DOWN SYNDROME, AND CRANIOFACIAL ABNORMALITIES

| Author | Syndrome | Age (years) | Preoperative | | Postoperative |
			Pa Pressure Air Systolic/diastolic (mmHg)	PA Pressure Oxygen Systolic/diastolic (mmHg)	PA Pressure Air Systolic/diastolic (mmHg)
Loughlin[84]	Down syndrome	3	85/45	55/25	—
	Down syndrome	1.5	65/15	—	—
	Down syndrome	10	65/35	—	25/11*
	Down syndrome	2	40/20	—	—
Rowland[85]	Down syndrome	5	55/25	†	25–10/4
Kasian[171]	Down syndrome	2	86/49	—	45/15
	Down syndrome	1.5	58/25	—	37/21*
Nussbaum[174]	Down syndrome	1	75/40	50/10	—
	Down syndrome	2.5	90/40	—	—
Levine[172]	Down syndrome	2	40/17	—	—
	Down syndrome	2	45/15	—	—
Nussbaum[174]	Pierre Robin	2	100/50	40/10	—

*Postintubation
† states "unresponsive to administration of 100% oxygen" in text

ciates (Table 18–5).[85, 171–173] The response of the pulmonary circulation was variable; oxygen either caused a drop in PA pressure or no change (Table 18–5). Thus, pulmonary hypertension in Down syndrome may be sleep-related, secondary to OSA, and due to airway obstruction and hypoxemia. Only 2 of the 5 patients reported by Loughlin and associates had adenotonsillar hypertrophy, suggesting that OSAS in Down syndrome children is often due to a combination of midfacial hypoplasia, micrognathia, and muscular hypotonia.[84]

Right Ventricular Hemodynamics

Compromised RV function appears to be common in children with OSA, even though overt signs of cardiac dysfunction are absent.[170] Hemodynamics during sleep in children with OSAS can be strikingly abnormal.[5, 55, 59, 62, 71, 174] Besides hypoxemia and hypercapnia, both of which affect peripheral vascular resistance, blood pressure, and cerebral blood flow, children have large swings in intrathoracic pressure during obstructed breathing (intrapleural pressures lower than -90 cmH$_2$O). Numerous investigators performing cardiac catheterization in children with OSA have recorded near zero or subatmospheric right-sided cardiac pressures.[5, 55, 59, 62, 71, 174] RV pressures during the inspiratory phase of breathing can drop below atmospheric pressure, to values as low as -50 cmH$_2$O (Fig. 18–1).[5, 55, 59, 62, 71] Echocardiographic studies in children with OSAS reveal that right systolic ejection is impaired.[174]

In four children studied by Nussbaum and associates, right pre-ejection period/RV ejection times were 0.5, 0.5, 0.66, and 0.37 (normal = 0.24 ± 0.06) preoperatively and 0.25, 0.3, 0.25, and 0.31 after surgical intervention.[174] RV ejection time was found to be markedly prolonged during the inspiratory phase of breathing, consistent with a large RV afterload imposed by subatmospheric intrathoracic pressures.[174] Using radionuclide ventriculography, Tal and associates showed that 10 of 27 children with OSAS (37%) had reduced RV ejection fractions and 18 of 27 (60%) showed RV hypokinesia.[170] Only 2 of the 27 children, aged 9 months to 7.5 years, had cardiac involvement detected by clinical assessment.[170]

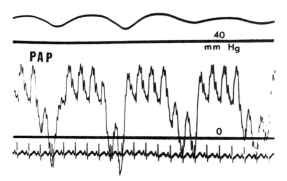

Figure 18–1. Pulmonary artery pressure in a 2-year-old child with adenotonsillar hypertrophy and partial upper airway obstruction while breathing room air. Note that pulmonary artery pressure becomes subatmospheric during obstructed inspiratory efforts. (From Levin DL, Muster AJ, Pachman LM, et al: Cor pulmonale secondary to upper airway obstruction. Chest 68:166, 1975.)

Left Ventricular Hemodynamics

Large swings of intrathoracic pressure must also increase left ventricular (LV) afterload in children with OSAS. Mean LV ejection fraction for the group of patients reported by Tal and associates did not change after surgery; however, in 5 of 11 patients postoperative LV ejection fraction increased markedly.[170] Ross and associates reported on brothers with OSA, systemic hypertension, and prolonged LV systolic time interval ratios.[175] One child died before surgery was performed; after tracheostomy, the other child's RV and LV systolic time intervals[175] returned to normal within 7 months. In the child who died, marked LV hypertrophy was noted on postmortem examination.[175] Serratto and associates described three additional children 2 to 4.5 years of age with upper airway obstruction and systemic blood pressures ranging from 150/100 to 200/100 mmHg.[176]

Cerebral perfusion pressure is determined in part by systemic arterial pressure. Wide swings in intrathoracic pressure, leading to large increases in LV afterload during inspiration, could affect LV ejection fraction, stroke volume, and systemic blood pressure on a breath-by-breath basis. Adverse effects of such fluctuations in perfusion pressure on blood flow distribution, especially to the brain, may be important.

Electrocardiogram and Echocardiogram Abnormalities

The incidence of cardiac complications in children with OSAS is not known. Wilkinson and associates reviewed electrocardiograms (EKG) from 92 children undergoing adenotonsillectomy for all indications.[177] Three (3.3%) were found to have signs of right heart strain and showed snoring and daytime sleepiness. Talaat and Nahhas also searched for cardiopulmonary changes in 30 children with chronic adenotonsillitis and found that two showed signs of right heart strain.[178] Unfortunately, the proportion of children in these studies that actually had OSAS was not reported. Laurikainen and associates, in Finland, studied 19 children "for whom adenotomy and/or tonsillectomy was indicated" using EKG, echocardiogram, and vectorcardiogram.[179] Sleep-related disordered breathing was confirmed using the static charge sensitive bed method.[179] They found that 21% (4/19) had evidence of RV hypertrophy, which corre-

lated with apnea index severity but not with measured adenotonsillar size.[179] Discrepancies in the prevalence of EKG and echocardiographic abnormalities among studies may be explained by patient referral patterns in different countries.

Systemic Hypertension

Except for isolated case reports of systemic hypertension in children with severe OSAS, little is known about OSAS and blood pressure in children, especially blood pressure during sleep.[175, 176]

Blunted Respiratory Drive

Children with OSAS sometimes have low or absent ventilatory responses to hypoxia or hypercarbia. Since it has been demonstrated that children with moderate-severe OSAS have normal awake ventilatory responses to hypercapnia and hypoxia,[180] it is likely that blunting of respiratory drive in these children is secondary to chronic respiratory failure. Several young children (<3 years old) were seen at our institution with severe OSAS and central alveolar hypoventilation with persistent hypoxemia following relief of upper airway obstruction by adenotonsillectomy. These patients were managed with supplemental oxygen at home and were gradually weaned to room air over a period of months. However, Ingram and Bishop reported on four patients 5 to 12 years of age who were found to have blunted ventilatory responses to CO_2 2 or more years after surgical intervention.[181] They suggested that a pre-existing abnormality of CO_2 respiratory drive predisposed them to develop CO_2 retention with upper airway obstruction. However, the children reported by Ingram and Bishop were older, had suffered longstanding severe OSAS, and all had right heart failure.[181] It is possible that these children had developed irreversible blunting of their ventilatory response to CO_2; whereas the patients at Johns Hopkins were younger, diagnosed earlier, and still at a reversible stage of the process. Current data suggest that abnormal chemoreceptor-mediated ventilatory drive is not a primary causative factor in childhood OSAS, although it remains possible that arousal responses to hypoxia and hypercapnia, or drives to upper airway muscles, are abnormal.

Unusual Complications

About 6% of children may develop pulmonary edema following relief of severe acute upper airway obstruction such as laryngotracheobronchitis or epiglottitis[182] and chronic upper airway obstruction including childhood OSAS.[182-184] The mechanism is assumed to be related to large swings of intrathoracic pressure during obstructed breathing but is not really known. Pasterkamp and associates reported on a 16-year-old girl with type II Arnold-Chiari malformation who developed increased intracranial pressure due to OSA.[185] Intracranial pressure monitoring during PSG revealed that rises in pressure followed onset of OSA by 8 to 10 seconds and were associated with severe hypoxemia.[185] Increased cerebral blood flow due to hypoxemia and hypercarbia were presumed to be the mechanism. Early reports of OSAS sometimes mentioned pectus excavatum in association with OSAS. In one child with pectus excavatum and OSAS, surgical repair of pectus excavatum was performed before the OSAS was recognized and corrected.[6] Fan and Murphy reported two toddlers with severe OSAS and pectus excavatum in whom the chest deformity markedly improved following adenotonsillectomy.[186] The mechanism of OSA leading to pectus excavatum is assumed to be related to large negative intrathoracic pressures during obstructed breathing.

Death

The mortality rate in childhood OSAS is not known. Case reports have documented children with OSAS who died[62] but such children must be under-reported in the literature. Often physicians will verbally describe perioperative and postoperative death in children undergoing adenotonsillectomy for OSAS, but these cases are rarely reported in the medical literature (personal observation). In the last 5 years one child at Johns Hopkins was diagnosed with OSAS who died before surgical intervention could be accomplished. Mortality rate in children with undiagnosed OSAS is, of course, unknown. Perioperative complications such as intraoperative death owing to cardiac decompensation and postoperative respiratory arrest may occur in children with OSAS. Some authors believe that OSA is a potential cause of some apparent life-threatening events or even unexpected death in infants.[23, 187-191]

Sickle Cell Disease

Painful Crisis

Because patients with sickle cell (SC) disease are vulnerable to the effects of hypoxemia, even mild OSAS could lead to severe complications. In addition, narcotics and other sedatives prescribed during painful sickle crises (vaso-occlusive crisis) can worsen OSA and hypoxemia by decreasing respiratory drive.[192] Adults with SC disease and frequent sickle crises develop mild hypoxemia during sleep, owing to a decrease in tidal volume, even without sleep-associated upper airway obstruction.[192] Ijaduola and Akinyanju reported on 15 patients with SC disease, ages 6 to 35 years, who underwent tonsillectomy for chronic tonsillitis. The average number of pain crises dropped from 4.7 per year preoperatively to 1.5 per year after tonsillectomy.[193] However, since patients were seen frequently during the 1 year follow-up period and the study did not include a control group, improvement may be attributable to better medical care and not to tonsillectomy. A 12-year-old girl with frequent painful crises and PSG-proven OSAS had no further crises in the 2 years following adenotonsillectomy.[194] Although circumstantial evidence suggests a link between OSAS and frequent crises in SC patients, this relationship remains to be proven. Until more evidence is available it would seem reasonable to perform PSG on any SC patient with snoring or frequent painful crises. Careful attention to preoperative preparation, including exchange transfusion, and intraoperative management makes adenotonsillectomy a relatively safe procedure for these patients.[195, 196]

Stroke

Robertson and associates reported on a 6.5-year-old girl with SC disease who experienced a series of cerebral infarctions and was found to have severe OSAS.[197] Since the peak incidence of stroke in children with SC disease occurs at 6 to 7 years of age, they speculated that OSAS may be a causative or exacerbating factor. Although this is an attractive hypothesis, there is no evidence to support it at the present time.

References

1. Guilleminault C, Eldrige F, Simmons FB, et al: Sleep apnea in eight children. Pediatrics 58:23, 1976.

2. Osler W: Chronic tonsillitis. *In* The Principles and Practice of Medicine. New York, Appleton and Co, 1892, pp 335–339.

3. Spector S, Bautista AG: Respiratory obstruction caused by acute tonsillitis and acute adenoiditis. NY State J Med 56:2118, 1956.

4. Noonan JA: Reversible cor pulmonale due to hypertrophied tonsils and adenoids: studies in two cases. Circulation 32:164, 1965.

5. Goodman RS, Goodman M, Gootman N, et al: Cardiac and pulmonary failure secondary to adenotonsillar hypertrophy. Laryngoscope 86:1367, 1976.

6. Jaffee IS: Adenotonsillectomy as the treatment of serious medical conditions: five case reports. Laryngoscope 84:1135, 1974.

7. Frank Y, Kravath RE, Pollak CP, et al: Obstructive sleep apnea and its therapy: clinical and polysomnographic manifestations. Pediatrics 71:737, 1983.

8. Brouillette RT, Fernbach SK, Hunt CE: Obstructive sleep apnea in infants and children. J Pediatr 100:31, 1982.

9. Brouillette R, Hanson D, David R, et al: A diagnostic approach to suspected obstructive sleep apnea in children. J Pediatr 105:10, 1984.

10. Weninger M, Saletu B, Popow C, et al: Obstructive sleep apnea: a polysomnographic study of sleep apnea before and after tonsillectomy and adenoidectomy. Helv Paediatr Acta 43:203, 1988.

11. Leiberman A, Cohen A, Tal A: Digital signal processing of stridor and snoring in children. Int J Pediatr Otorinolaryingol 12:173–185, 1986.

12. Schafer J, Pirsig W: Digital signal analysis of snoring sounds in children. Int J Pediatr Otorhinolaryngol 20:193, 1990.

13. Carroll JL, McColley SA, Marcus CL, et al: Reported symptoms of childhood obstructive sleep apnea syndrome (OSA) vs. primary snoring. Am Rev Respir Dis 145(Part 2):A177, 1992.

14. Konno A, Togawa K, Hoshino T: The effect of nasal obstruction in infancy and early childhood upon ventilation. Laryngoscope 90:699, 1980.

15. Guilleminault C, Korobkin R, Winkle R: A review of 50 children with obstructive sleep apnea syndrome. Lung 159:275, 1981.

16. Potsic WP, Pasquariello PS, Baranak CC, et al: Relief of upper airway obstruction by adenotonsillectomy. Otolaryngol Head Neck Surg 94:476, 1986.

17. Guilleminault C, Winkle R, Korobkin R, et al: Children and nocturnal snoring: evaluation of the effects of sleep related respiratory resistive load and daytime functioning. Eur J Pediatr 139:165, 1982.

18. Miyazaki S, Itasaka Y, Yamakawa K, et al: Respiratory disturbance during sleep due to adenoid-tonsillar hypertrophy. Am J Otolaryngol 10:143, 1989.

19. Croft CB, Brockbank MJ, Wright A, et al: Obstructive sleep apnoea in children undergoing routine tonsillectomy and adenoidectomy. Clin Otolaryngol 15:307, 1990.

20. Ahlqvist-Rastad J, Hultcrantz E, Svanholm H: Children with tonsillar obstruction: indications for and efficacy of tonsillectomy. Acta Paediatr Scand 77:831, 1988.

21. Mallory GB, Jr, Fiser DH, Jackson R: Sleep-associated breathing disorders in morbidly obese children and adolescents. J Pediatr 115:892, 1989.

22. Weider DJ, Sateia MJ, West RP: Nocturnal enuresis in children with upper airway obstruction. Otolaryngol Head Neck Surg 105:427, 1991.

23. McGrath SA, Carroll JL, McColley SA, Marcus C, et al: Normal sleep structure found in children with obstructive sleep apnea. Am Rev Resp Dis 145:A176, 1992.

24. Leach J, Olson J, Hermann J, et al: Polysomnographic and clinical findings in children with obstructive sleep apnea. Arch Otolaryngol Head Neck Surg 118:741, 1992.

25. McGrath-Morrow SA, Carroll JL, McColley SA, et al: Termination of obstructive apnea in children is not associated with arousal. Am Rev Respir Dis 141:A195, 1990.

26. Zucconi M, Strambi LF, Pestalozza G, et al: Habitual snoring and obstructive sleep apnea syndrome in children: effects of early tonsil surgery. Int J Pediatr Otorhinolaryngol 26:235, 1993.

27. Guilleminault C: Obstructive sleep apnea syndrome in children. *In* Guilleminault C: Sleep and Its Disorders in Children. New York, Raven Press, 1987, pp 213–224.

28. Mauer KW, Staats BA, Olsen KD: Upper airway obstruction and disordered nocturnal breathing in children. Mayo Clin Proc 58:349, 1983.

29. Stradling JR, Thomas G, Warley AR, et al: Effect of adenotonsillectomy on nocturnal hypoxaemia, sleep disturbance, and symptoms in snoring children. Lancet 335:249, 1990.

30. Diagnostic Classification Steering Committee, Thorpy MJC (Chairman): International Classification of Sleep Disorders: Diagnostic and Coding Manual. Rochester, MN, American Association of Sleep Disorders Associations, 1990.

31. Swift AC: Upper airway obstruction, sleep disturbance and adenotonsillectomy in children. J Laryngol Otol 102:419, 1988.

32. Olsen KD, Kern EB, Westbrook PR: Sleep and breathing disturbance secondary to nasal obstruction. Otolaryngol Head Neck Surg 89:804, 1981.

33. Lavie P, Gertner R, Zomer J, et al: Breathing disorders in sleep associated with "microarousals" in patients with allergic rhinitis. Acta Otolaryngol 92:529, 1981.

34. Stool SE, Eavey RD, Stein NL, et al: The "chubby puffer" syndrome. Upper airway obstruction and obesity, with intermittent somnolence and cardiorespiratory embarrassment. Clin Pediatr (Phila) 16:43, 1977.

35. Phillips DE, Rogers JH: Down syndrome with lingual tonsil hypertrophy producing sleep apnoea. J Laryngol Otol 102:1054, 1988.

36. Kahn A, Groswasser J, Sottiaux M, et al: Clinical symptoms associated with brief obstructive sleep apnea in normal infants. Sleep 16:409, 1993.

37. Kahn A, Van de Merckt C, Dramaix M, et al: Transepidermal water loss during sleep in infants at risk for sudden death. Pediatrics 80:245, 1987.

38. Guilleminault C, Stoohs R: Obstructive sleep apnea syndrome in children. Pediatrician 17:46, 1990.

39. Weider DJ, Hauri PJ: Nocturnal enuresis in children with upper airway obstruction. Int J Pediatr Otorhinolaryngol 9:173, 1985.

40. Norgaard JP, Rittig S, Djurhuus JC: Nocturnal enuresis: an approach to treatment based on pathogenesis. J Pediatr 114:705, 1989.

41. Butt W, Robertson C, Phelan P: Snoring in children: is it pathological? Med J Aust 143:335, 1985.

42. Aldrich MS, Chauncey JB: Are morning headaches part of obstructive sleep apnea syndrome? Arch Intern Med 150:1265–1267, 1990.

43. Richardson MA, Seid AB, Cotton RT, et al: Evalua-

tion of tonsils and adenoids in sleep apnea syndrome. Laryngoscope 90:1106, 1980.

44. Weissbluth M, Davis AT, Poncher J, et al: Signs of airway obstruction during sleep and behavioral, developmental, and academic problems. J Dev Behav Pediatr 4:119, 1983.

45. Greenberg GD, Watson RK, Depula D: Neuropsychological dysfunction in sleep apnea. Sleep 10:254, 1987.

46. Findley LJ, Barth JT, Powers C, et al: Cognitive impairment in patients with obstructive sleep apnea and associated hypoxemia. Chest 90:686, 1986.

47. Lind MG, Lundell BP: Tonsillar hyperplasia in children. A cause of obstructive sleep apneas, CO_2 retention, and retarded growth. Arch Otolaryngol 108:650, 1982.

48. Hibbert J: The occurrence of adenoidal signs and symptoms in normal children. Clin Otolaryngol 6:97, 1981.

49. Klein JC: Nasal respiratory function and craniofacial growth. Arch Otolaryngol Head Neck Surg 112:843, 1986.

50. Leighton BC: Aetiology of malocclusion of the teeth. Arch Dis Child 66:1011, 1991.

51. Hultcrantz E, Svanholm H, Ahlqvist-Rastad J: Sleep apnea in children without hypertrophy of the tonsils. Clin Pediatr (Phila) 27:350, 1988.

52. Monoson PK, Fox AW: Preliminary observation of speech disorder in obstructive and mixed sleep apnea. Chest 92:670, 1987.

53. Cox MA, Schiebler GL, Taylor WJ, et al: Reversible pulmonary hypertension in a child with respiratory obstruction and cor pulmonale. J Pediatr 67:192, 1965.

54. Menashe VD, Farrehi C, Miller M: Hypoventilation and cor pulmonale due to chronic upper airway obstruction. J Pediatr 67:198, 1965.

55. Luke MJ, Mehrizi A, Folger GM, et al: Chronic nasopharyngeal obstruction as a cause of cardiomegaly, cor pulmonale, and pulmonary edema. Pediatrics 37:762, 1966.

56. Ainger LE: Large tonsils and adenoids in small children with cor pulmonale. Br Heart J 30:356, 1968.

57. Gerald B, Dungan WT: Cor pulmonale and pulmonary edema in children secondary to chronic upper airway obstruction. Radiology 90:679, 1968.

58. Setliff RC, Puyau FA, Ward PH: Pulmonary hypertension secondary to chronic upper airway obstruction. Laryngoscope 78:845, 1968.

59. Cayler GG, Johnson EE, Lewis BE, et al: Heart failure due to enlarged tonsils and adenoids. Am J Dis Child 118:708, 1969.

60. Formica U, Fiocchi A: Pulmonary heart disease caused by chronic obstruction of the upper respiratory tract due to hypertrophy of adenoids and tonsils. Review of the literature and report of a personal case. Minerva Pediatr 21:908, 1969.

61. Macartney FJ, Panday J, Scott O: Cor pulmonale as a result of chronic nasopharyngeal obstruction due to hypertrophied tonsils and adenoids. Arch Dis Child 44:585, 1969.

62. Massumi RA, Sarin RK, Pooya M, et al: Tonsillar hypertrophy, airway obstruction, alveolar hypoventilation, and cor pulmonale in twin brothers. Dis Chest 55:110, 1969.

63. Reekie RA, Miller CG: Cor pulmonale secondary to chronic nasopharyngeal obstruction in a child. West Indian Med J 20:41, 1971.

64. Edison BD, Kerth JD: Tonsilloadenoid hypertrophy

resulting in cor pulmonale. Arch Otolaryngol 98:205, 1973.

65. Freeman WJ: Adenoid hypertrophy, cyanosis, and cor pulmonale in children with congenital heart disease. Laryngoscope 83:238, 1973.

66. Talbot AR, Robertson LW: Cardiac failure with tonsil and adenoid hypertrophy. Arch Otolaryngol 98:277, 1973.

67. Jaffe IS: Adenotonsillectomy as the treatment of serious medical conditions: five case reports. Laryngoscope 84:1135, 1974.

68. Simmons FB, Hill MW: Hypersomnia caused by upper airway obstructions: a new syndrome in otolaryngology. Ann Otol 83:670, 1974.

69. Djalilian M, Kern EB, Brown HA, et al: Hypoventilation secondary to chronic upper airway obstruction in childhood. Mayo Clin Proc 50:11, 1975.

70. Thanopoulos B, Ikkos DD, Milingos M, et al: Cardiorespiratory syndrome due to enlarged tonsils and adenoids. A case report with discussion regarding medical treatment and pathogenesis. Acta Paediatr Scand 64:659, 1975.

71. Levin DL, Muster AJ, Pachman LM, et al: Cor pulmonale secondary to upper airway obstruction: cardiac catheterization, immunologic, and psychometric evaluation in nine patients. Chest 68:166, 1975.

72. Everett AD, Koch WC, Saulsbury FT: Failure to thrive due to obstructive sleep apnea. Clin Pediatr (Phila) 26:90, 1987.

73. Schiffmann R, Faber J, Eidelman AI: Obstructive hypertrophic adenoids and tonsils as a cause of infantile failure to thrive: reversed by tonsillectomy and adenoidectomy. Int J Pediatr Otorhinolaryngol 9:183, 1985.

74. Bate TW, Price DA, Holme CA, et al: Short stature caused by obstructive apnoea during sleep. Arch Dis Child 59:78, 1984.

75. Williams EF, Woo P, Miller R, et al: The effects of adenotonsillectomy on growth in young children. Otolaryngol Head Neck Surg 104:509, 1991.

76. Goldstein SJ, Wu RH, Thorpy MJ, et al: Reversibility of deficient sleep entrained growth hormone secretion in a boy with achondroplasia and obstructive sleep apnea. Acta Endocrinol (Copenh) 116:95, 1987.

77. Tardif C, Denis P, Verdure-Poussin A, et al: Reflux gastro-oesophagien pendant le sommeil chez l'obese. Neurophysiol Clin 18:323, 1988.

78. Buts JP, Barudi C, Moulin D, et al: Prevalence and treatment of silent gastro-oesophageal reflux in children with recurrent respiratory disorders. Eur J Pediatr 145:396, 1986.

79. Konno A, Hoshino T, Togawa K: Influence of upper airway obstruction by enlarged tonsils and adenoids upon recurrent infection of the lower airway in childhood. Laryngoscope 90:1709, 1980.

80. Levy AM, Tabakin BS, Hanson JS, et al: Hypertrophied adenoids causing pulmonary hypertension and severe congestive heart failure. N Engl J Med 277:507, 1967.

81. Silvestri JM, Weese-Meyer DE, Bass MT, et al: Polysomnography in obese children with a history of sleep-associated breathing disorders. Pediatr Pulmonol 16:124, 1993.

82. Leiberman A, Tal A, Brama I, et al: Obstructive sleep apnea in young infants. Int J Pediatr Otorhinolaryngol 16:39, 1988.

83. Marcus CL, Keens TL, Bautista DB, et al: Obstructive sleep apnea in children with Down syndrome. Pediatrics 88:132, 1991.

84. Loughlin GM, Wynne JW, Victorica BE: Sleep apnea as a possible cause of pulmonary hypertension in Down syndrome. J Pediatr 98:435, 1981.

85. Rowland TW, Nordstrom LG, Bean MS, et al: Chronic upper airway obstruction and pulmonary hypertension in Down syndrome. Am J Dis Child 135:1050, 1981.

86. Jamieson A, Guilleminault C, Partinen M, et al: Obstructive sleep apnea patients have craniomandibular abnormalities. Sleep 9:469, 1986.

87. Cozzi F, Pierro A: Glossoptosis-apnea syndrome in infancy. Pediatrics 75:836, 1985.

88. Spier S, Rivlin J, Rowe RD, et al: Sleep in Pierre Robin syndrome. Chest 90:711, 1986.

89. Bull MJ, Givan DC, Sadove AM, et al: Improved outcome in Pierre Robin sequence: effect of multidisciplinary evaluation and management. Pediatrics 86:294, 1990.

90. Puckett CL, Pickens J, Reinisch JF: Sleep apnea in mandibular hypoplasia. Plast Reconstr Surg 70:213, 1982.

91. Rosen CL, Novotny EJ, D'Andrea L, et al: Klippel-Feil sequence and sleep disordered breathing in two children. Am Rev Resp Dis 147:202, 1993.

92. Friede H, Lopata M, Fisher E, et al: Cardiorespiratory disease associated with Hallermann-Streiff syndrome: analysis of craniofacial morphology by cephalometric roentgenograms. J Craniofac Genet Dev Biol (Suppl) 1:189, 1985.

93. Ryan CF, Lowe AA, Fleetham JA: Nasal continuous positive airway pressure (CPAP) therapy for obstructive sleep apnea in Hallermann-Streiff syndrome. Clin Pediatr (Phila) 29:122, 1990.

94. Johnston C, Taussig LM, Koopmann C, et al: Obstructive sleep apnea in Treacher Collins syndrome. Cleft Palate J 18:39, 1981.

95. Sher AE, Shprintzen RJ, Thorpy MJ: Endoscopic observations of obstructive sleep apnea in children with anomalous upper airways: predictive and therapeutic value. Int J Pediatr Otorhinolaryngol 11:135, 1986.

96. Mixter RC, David DJ, Perloff WH, et al: Obstructive sleep apnea in Apert's and Pfeiffer's syndromes: more than a craniofacial abnormality. Plast Reconstr Surg 86:457, 1990.

97. Cistulli PA, Sullivan CE: Sleep-disordered breathing in Marfan's syndrome. Am Rev Resp Dis 147:645, 1993.

98. Carter M, Stokes D, Wang W: Severe obstructive sleep apnea in a child with osteopetrosis. Clin Pediatr (Phila) 27:108, 1988.

99. Zucconi M, Ferini-Strambi L, Erminio C, et al: Obstructive sleep apnea in the Rubinstein-Taybi syndrome. Respiration 60:127, 1993.

100. Tirosh E, Borochowitz Z: Sleep apnea in fragile X syndrome. Am J Med Genetics 43:124, 1992.

101. Goldberg R, Fish B, Ship A, et al: Deletion of a portion of the long arm of chromosome 6. Am J Med Genet 5:73, 1980.

102. Devine P, Bhan I, Feingold M, et al: Completely cartilaginous trachea in a child with Crouzon syndrome. Am J Dis Child 138:40, 1984.

103. Solomon LM, Medenica M, Pruzanski S, et al: Apert syndrome and palatal mucopolysaccharides. Teratology 8:287, 1973.

104. Smith DF, Mihm FG, Flynn M: Chronic alveolar hypoventilation secondary to macroglossia in the Beckwith-Weidemann syndrome. Pediatrics 70:695, 1982.

105. Smith TH, Baska ER, Francisco CB, et al: Sleep apnea syndrome: diagnosis of upper airway obstruction by fluoroscopy. J Pediatr 93:891, 1978.

106. Stokes DC, Phillips JA, Leonard CO, et al: Respiratory complications of achondroplasia. J Pediatr 102:534, 1983.

107. Reid CS, Pyeritz RE, Kopits SE, et al: Cervicomedullary compression in young patients with achondroplasia. J Pediatr 110:522, 1987.

108. Nelson WF, Hecht JT, Horton WA, et al: Neurological basis of respiratory complications in achondroplasia. Ann Neurol 24:89, 1988.

109. Semenza GL, Pyeritz RE: Respiratory complications of mucopolysaccharide storage disorders. Medicine (Baltimore) 67:209, 1988.

110. Shapiro J, Strome M, Crocker AC: Airway obstruction and sleep apnea in Hurler and Hunter syndromes. Ann Otol Rhinol Laryngol 94:458, 1985.

111. Malone BN, Whitley CB, Duvall AJ, et al: Resolution of obstructive sleep apnea in Hurler syndrome after bone marrow transplantation. Int J Pediatr Otorhinolaryngol 15:23, 1988.

112. Perks WH, Cooper RA, Bradbury S, et al: Sleep apnoea in Scheie's syndrome. Thorax 35:85, 1980.

113. Myer CM: Airway obstruction in Hurler's syndrome: radiographic features. Int J Pediatr Otorhinolaryngol 22:91, 1991.

114. Haponik EF, Givens D, Angelo J: Syringobulbia-myelia with obstructive sleep apnea. Neurology 33:1046, 1983.

115. Chaudhary BA, Elguindi AS, and King DW: Obstructive sleep apnea after lateral medullary syndrome. South Med J 75:65, 1982.

116. Adelman S, Dinner DS, Goren H, et al: Obstructive sleep apnea in association with posterior fossa neurologic disease. Arch Neurol 41:509, 1984.

117. Alcala H, Dodson WE: Syringobulbia as a cause of laryngeal stridor in childhood. Neurology 25:875, 1975.

118. Holinger PC, Holinger LD, Reichert TJ, et al: Respiratory obstruction and apnea in infants with bilateral abductor vocal cord paralysis, meningomyelocele, hydrocephalus, and Arnold-Chiari malformation. J Pediatr 92:368, 1978.

119. Ruff ME, Oakes WJ, Fisher SR, et al: Sleep apnea and vocal cord paralysis secondary to type I Chiari malformation. Pediatrics 80:231, 1987.

120. Kelly DH, Krishnamoorthy KS, Shannon DC: Astrocytoma in an infant with prolonged apnea. Pediatrics 66:429, 1980.

121. Guilleminault C, Simmons FB, Motta J, et al: Obstructive sleep apnea syndrome and tracheostomy: long-term follow-up experience. Arch Intern Med 141:985, 1981.

122. MacNaughton DM, Tewfik TL, Bernstein ML: Hodgkin's disease in the nasopharynx. J Otolaryngol 19:282, 1990.

123. Erwin SA: Unsuspected sarcoidosis of the tonsil. Otolaryngol Head Neck Surg 100:245, 1989.

124. Rodgers GK, Chan KH, Dahl RE: Antral choanal polyp presenting as obstructive sleep apnea syndrome. Arch Otolaryngol 117:914, 1991.

125. Kahn A, Blum D, Hoffman A, et al: Obstructive sleep apnea induced by a parapharyngeal cystic hygroma in an infant. Sleep 8:363, 1985.

126. Brodsky L, Siddiqui SY, Stanievich JF: Massive oropharyngeal papillomatosis causing obstructive sleep apnea in a child. Arch Otolaryngol Head Neck Surg 113:882, 1987.

127. Leiberman A, Yagupsky P, Lavie P: Obstructive sleep apnoea probably related to a foreign body. Eur J Pediatr 144:205, 1985.

128. Fairley JW, Hunt BJ, Glover GW, et al: Unusual lymphoproliferative oropharyngeal lesions in heart and heart-lung transplant recipients. J Laryngol Otol 104:720, 1990.

129. Myer CM, 3d, Reilly JS: Airway obstruction in an immunosuppressed child. Arch Otolaryngol 111:409, 1985.

130. Ali NJ, Pitson D, Stradling JR: The prevalence of snoring, sleep disturbance and sleep related breathing disorders and their relation to daytime sleepiness in 4–5 year old children. Am Rev Respir Dis 143:A381, 1991.

131. Corbo GM, Fuciarelli F, Foresi A, et al: Snoring in children: association with respiratory symptoms and passive smoking. Br Med J 299:1491, 1989 (published erratum appears in Br Med J 300:226, 1990).

132. U.S. Bureau of the Census: Statistical Abstract of the United States: 1991. Washington, DC, U.S. Government Printing Office, 1991.

133. Guilleminault C, Stoohs R: From apnea of infancy to obstructive sleep apnea syndrome in the young child. Chest 102:1065, 1992.

134. el-Bayadi S, Millman RP, Tishler PV, et al: A family study of sleep apnea. Anatomic and physiologic interactions. Chest 98:554, 1990.

135. Strohl KP, Saunders NA, Feldman NT, et al: Obstructive sleep apnea in family members. N Engl J Med 299:969, 1978.

136. Redline S, Tosteson T, Tishler PV, et al: Studies in the genetics of obstructive sleep apnea. Am Rev Respir Dis 145:440, 1992.

137. Carroll JL, McColley SA, Marcus CL, et al: Can childhood obstructive sleep apnea syndrome (OSA) be diagnosed by a clinical symptom score? Am Rev Respir Dis 145(Part 2):A179, 1992.

138. Wilson SL, Thach BT, Brouillette RT, et al: Upper airway patency in the human infant: influence of airway pressure and posture. J Appl Physiol 48:500, 1980.

139. Reed WR, Roberts JL, Thach BT: Factors influencing regional patency and configuration of the human infant upper airway. J Appl Physiol 58:635, 1985.

140. Felman AH, Loughlin GM, Leftridge CA, Jr, et al: Upper airway obstruction during sleep in children. Am J Roentgenol 133:213, 1979.

141. Fernbach SK, Brouillette RT, Riggs TW, et al: Radiologic evaluation of adenoids and tonsils in children with obstructive sleep apnea: plain films and fluoroscopy. Pediatr Radiol 13:258, 1983.

142. Fan LL: Transnasal fiberoptic endoscopy in children with obstructive apnea. Crit Care Med 12:590, 1984.

143. Croft CB, Thomson HG, Samuels MP, et al: Endoscopic evaluation and treatment of sleep-associated upper airway obstruction in infants and young children. Clin Otolaryngol 15:209, 1990.

144. Hagen R, Schrod L: Functional nasopharyngeal fiberoptic endoscopy for pre-therapeutic diagnosis of sleep apnea syndrome in infants. A case report. HNO 39:195, 1991.

145. Suratt PM, Dee P, Atkinson RL, et al: Fluoroscopic and computed tomographic features of the pharyngeal airway in obstructive sleep apnea. Am Rev Respir Dis 127:487, 1983.

146. Brodsky L, Moore L, Stanievich JF: A comparison of tonsillar size and oropharyngeal dimensions in children with obstructive adenotonsillar hypertrophy. Int J Pediatr Otorhinolaryngol 13:149, 1987.

147. Praud JP, D'Allest AM, Delaperche MF, et al: Diaphragmatic and genioglossus electromyographic ac-

148. tivity at the onset and at the end of obstructive apnea in children with obstructive sleep apnea syndrome. Pediatr Res 23:1, 1988.

148. Jeffries B, Brouillette RT, Hunt CE: Electromyographic study of some accessory muscles of respiration in children with obstructive sleep apnea. Am Rev Respir Dis 129:696, 1984.

149. Fukuda K, Matsune S, Ushikai M, et al: A study on the relationship between adenoid vegetation and rhinosinusitis. Am J Otolaryngol 10:214, 1989.

150. Brodsky L, Adler E, Stanievich JF: Naso- and oropharyngeal dimensions in children with obstructive sleep apnea. Int J Pediatr Otorhinolaryngol 17:1, 1989.

151. Maw AR, Jeans WD, Cable HR: Adenoidectomy. A prospective study to show clinical and radiological changes two years after operation. J Laryngol Otol 97:511, 1983.

152. Olson LG, Strohl KP: Airway secretions influence upper airway patency in the rabbit. Am Rev Respir Dis 137:1379, 1988.

153. Hudgel DW: Mechanisms of obstructive sleep apnea. Chest 101:541, 1992.

154. Kuna ST, Sant'Ambrogio G: Pathophysiology of upper airway closure during sleep. JAMA 266:1384–1389, 1991.

155. Sullivan CE, Issa FG: Pathophysiological mechanisms in obstruction sleep apnea. Sleep 3:235–246, 1980.

156. Praud JP, D'Allest AM, Nedelcoux H, et al: Sleep-related abdominal muscle behavior during partial or complete obstructed breathing in prepubertal children. Pediatr Res 26:347–350, 1989.

157. Baker SB, Fewell JE: Heart rate response to arousal and lung inflation following upper airway obstruction in lambs. Sleep 11:233, 1988.

158. Canet E, Gaultier C, D'Allest AM, et al: Effects of sleep deprivation on respiratory events during sleep in healthy infants. J Appl Physiol 66:1158, 1989.

159. Pransky SM, Feldman JI, Kearns DB, et al: Actinomycosis in obstructive tonsillar hypertrophy and recurrent tonsillitis. Arch Otolaryngol Head Neck Surg 117:883, 1991.

160. DeDio RM, Tom LW, McGowan KL, et al: Microbiology of the tonsils and adenoids in a pediatric population. Arch Otolaryngol Head Neck Surg 114:763, 1988.

161. Kielmovitch IH, Keleti G, Bluestone CD, et al: Microbiology of obstructive tonsillar hypertrophy and recurrent tonsillitis. Arch Otolaryngol Head Neck Surg 115:721, 1989.

162. Lim DT, Freel BJ, Ghani M: Isolated IgA deficiency associated with upper airway obstruction, sleep dysrhythmia and failure to thrive: a case report. Ann Allergy 41:299, 1978.

163. Heiner DC: Respiratory disease and food allergy. Ann Allergy 53:657, 1984.

164. Collins MP, Church MK, Bakhshi KN, et al: Adenoid histamine and its possible relationship to secretory otitis media. J Laryngol Otol 99:685, 1985.

165. McColley SA, Carroll JL, Curtis S, et al: High prevalence of allergy in pediatric sleep disordered breathing. Am J Respir Crit Care Med 149(Part 2):A884, 1994.

166. Kravath RE, Pollak CP, Borowiecki B: Hypoventilation during sleep in children who have lymphoid airway obstruction treated by nasopharyngeal tube and T and A. Pediatrics 59:865, 1977.

167. Harrington R: Tonsillar hypertrophy and chronic hypoxia. Med J Aust 2:175, 1978.

168. Hunt CE, Brouillette RT: Abnormalities of breathing

control and airway maintenance in infants and children as a cause of cor pulmonale. Pediatr Cardiol 3:249, 1982.

169. Yates DW: Adenotonsillar hypertrophy and cor pulmonale. Br J Anaesth 61:355, 1988.

170. Tal A, Leiberman A, Margulis G, et al: Ventricular dysfunction in children with obstructive sleep apnea: radionuclide assessment. Pediatr Pulmonol 4:139, 1988.

171. Kasian GF, Duncan WJ, Tyrrell MJ, et al: Elective oro-tracheal intubation to diagnose sleep apnea in children with Down syndrome and ventricular septal defect. Can J Cardiol 2:2, 1987.

172. Levine OR, Simpser M: Alveolar hypoventilation and cor pulmonale associated with chronic airway obstruction in infants with Down syndrome. Clin Pediatr (Phila) 21:25, 1982.

173. Bloch K, Witztum A, Wieser HG, et al: Obstructive sleep apnea syndrome in a child with trisomy 21. Monatsschr Kinderheilkd 138:817, 1990.

174. Nussbaum E, Hirschfeld SS, Wood RE, et al: Echocardiographic changes in children with pulmonary hypertension secondary to upper airway obstruction. J Pediatr 93:931, 1978.

175. Ross RD, Daniels SR, Loggie JM, et al: Sleep apnea-associated hypertension and reversible left ventricular hypertrophy. J Pediatr 111:253, 1987.

176. Serratto M, Harris VJ, Carr I: Upper airways obstruction: presentation with systemic hypertension. Arch Dis Child 56:153, 1981.

177. Wilkinson AR, McCormick MS, Freeland AP, et al: Electrocardiographic signs of pulmonary hypertension in children who snore. Br Med J 282:579, 1981.

178. Talaat AM, Nahhas MM: Cardiopulmonary changes secondary to chronic adenotonsillitis. Arch Otolaryngol 109:30, 1983.

179. Laurikainen E, Aitasalo K, Erkinjuntti M, et al: Sleep apnea syndrome in children—secondary to adenotonsillar hypertrophy? Acta Otolaryngol Suppl 492:38, 1992.

180. Marcus CL, Gozal D, Arens R, et al: Ventilatory responses during wakefulness in children with the obstructive sleep apnea syndrome. Am J Respir Crit Care Med 149:715, 1994.

181. Ingram RH, Bishop JB: Ventilatory response to carbon dioxide after removal of chronic upper airway obstruction. Am Rev Respir Dis 102:645, 1970.

182. Galvis AG: Pulmonary edema complicating relief of upper airway obstruction. Am J Emerg Med 5:294, 1987.

183. Kanter RK, Watchko JF: Pulmonary edema associated with upper airway obstruction. Am J Dis Child 138:356, 1984.

184. Sofer S, Weinhouse E, Tal A, et al: Cor pulmonale due to adenoidal or tonsillar hypertrophy or both in children. Noninvasive diagnosis and follow-up. Chest 93:119, 1988.

185. Pasterkamp H, Cardoso ER, Booth FA: Obstructive sleep apnea leading to increased intracranial pressure in a patient with hydrocephalus and syringomyelia. Chest 95:1064, 1989.

186. Fan L, Murphy S: Pectus excavatum from chronic upper airway obstruction. Am J Dis Child 135:550, 1981.

187. Kelly DH, Shannon DC: Episodic complete airway obstruction in infants. Pediatrics 67:823, 1981.

188. Dunne K, Matthews T: Near-miss sudden infant death syndrome: clinical findings and management. Pediatrics 79:889, 1987.

189. Guilleminault C, Souquet M, Ariagno RL, et al: Five cases of near-miss sudden infant death syndrome and development of obstructive sleep apnea syndrome. Pediatrics 73:71, 1984.

190. Guilleminault C, Heldt G, Powell N, et al: Small upper airway in near-miss sudden infant death syndrome infants and their families. Lancet 1:402, 1986.

191. Kurz R, Kenner T, Reiterer F, et al: Factors involved in the pathogenesis of unexpected near miss events of infants (ALTE). Acta Paediatr Hung 30;435, 1990.

192. Castele RJ, Strohl KP, Chester S, et al: Oxygen saturation with sleep in patients with sickle cell disease. Arch Intern Med 146:722, 1986.

193. Ijaduola CA, Akinyanju OO: Chronic tonsillitis, tonsillectomy and sickle cell crises. J Laryngol Otol 101:467, 1987.

194. Sidman JD, Fry TL: Exacerbation of sickle cell disease by obstructive sleep apnea. Arch Otolaryngol Head Neck Surg 114:916, 1988.

195. Maddern BR, Reed HT, Ohene-Frempong K, et al: Obstructive sleep apnea syndrome in sickle cell disease. Ann Otol Rhinol Laryngol 98:174, 1989.

196. Derkay CS, Bray G, Milmoe GJ, et al: Adenotonsillectomy in children with sickle cell disease. South Med J 84:205, 1991.

197. Robertson PL, Aldrich MS, Hanash SM, et al: Stroke associated with obstructive sleep apnea in a child with sickle cell anemia. Ann Neurol 23:614, 1988.

198. Galal O, Galal I: Cor pulmonale as a sequela of tonsillar hypertrophy. [Cor pulmonale als Folge von Tonsillenhypertrophie]. Monatsschr Kinderheilkd (German) 137:326, 1989.

Obstructive Sleep Apnea Syndrome in Infants and Children: Diagnosis and Management

JOHN L. CARROLL and GERALD M. LOUGHLIN

This chapter deals with the diagnosis and management of childhood obstructive sleep apnea syndrome (OSAS). Primary snoring (PS) is discussed in Chapter 17 and the clinical features and pathophysiology of childhood OSAS are reviewed in Chapter 18.

Diagnosis of Childhood Obstructive Sleep Apnea Syndrome

Physicians likely to see a child with OSAS include family practitioners, pediatricians, sleep medicine specialists, otolaryngologists, pediatric pulmonologists, psychologists, psychiatrists, and neurobehavioral specialists. The primary care physician basically decides which children need referral for evaluation. Keeping in mind that it is a rare child who will have OSAS with *no history of snoring*; it can generally be said that if there is no snoring and no other symptoms then the child probably does not have OSAS. Beyond that, if a child exhibits snoring or difficulty breathing during sleep that prompts a complaint, OSAS cannot be ruled in or out on the basis of history alone and referral for evaluation is indicated. At the specialist level, the sleep medicine specialist and the otolaryngologist should function as a team.

Diagnostic Criteria

The 1990 International Classification of Sleep Disorders[1] (ICSD) diagnostic criteria for OSAS do not apply to children and should not be used for the evaluation of children.[1] ICSD criteria for OSAS *require* a complaint of excessive daytime sleepiness (EDS) and more than five obstructive events per hour lasting longer than 10 seconds.[2] As discussed in Chapter 18, most children with OSAS do not exhibit EDS; EDS is rarely the presenting symptom; children with less than five obstructive episodes per hour can have significant symptoms; children with severe OSAS may not have any obstructive apnea ("event counts" do not work); and a 10 second minimum time limit on obstructive events will result in failure to detect significant events.[3] Suggested diagnostic criteria for childhood OSAS are presented in Table 19–1.

Aims of Evaluation

The aims of evaluation are to establish a provisional diagnosis; determine if complications or associated conditions are present; confirm the diagnosis and the presence of complications by objective testing; determine the severity of symptoms, physiologic abnormalities, and complications; and determine the best treatment and plan for follow-up. Each of these topics is controversial.

OSAS is a clinical diagnosis based on information obtained by clinical history, physical examination, and laboratory studies (of which polysomnography [PSG] is only one). Recommendations for treatment must be based on

Table 19–1. DIAGNOSTIC CRITERIA FOR OSAS IN CHILDREN

A. Caregivers complain of child having noisy or disturbed breathing during sleep and/or inappropriate daytime sleepiness or behavioral problems
B. Episodes of complete or partial airway obstruction during sleep
C. Associated features include
   1. Snoring
   2. Paradoxical chest/abdomen motion and/or retractions
   3. Apnea or difficulty breathing observed by caregivers
   4. Excessive daytime sleepiness
   5. Behavior problems
   6. Adenotonsillar hypertrophy
   7. Daytime mouth breathing
   8. Other features of adenoidal hypertrophy
   9. Failure-to-thrive or obesity
D. Polysomnographic monitoring demonstrates:
   1. Obstructive hypoventilation (see Table 19–4), and/or
   2. One or more obstructive apnea/hour, usually with one or more of the following
      a. Arterial oxygen desaturation below 90–92%
      b. Arousals from sleep associated with upper airway obstruction
      c. An MSLT demonstrating an abnormal sleep latency for age
E. Usually associated with other medical disorders, e.g., adenotonsillar enlargement
F. Other sleep disorders can be present, e.g., narcolepsy

Format for above diagnostic criteria were modeled after the International Classification of Sleep Disorders: Diagnostic and Coding Manual criteria for adult OSAS.[2]

the assessment, duration, and severity of symptoms and the anatomic, structural, and physiologic abnormalities and their associated severity. This can only be accomplished by a comprehensive evaluation of the patient. Recommendations for therapy, including surgery, are based on the *entire clinical picture*, not just results of PSG, and often require the expertise of a specialist in this area.

History

Diagnosis begins with a thorough clinical history. Sleep history should include information pertaining to sleep environment, bedtime, sleep onset, sleep quality, sleeping positions, head positions, movements, arousals or awakenings, parasomnias, morning awakening, and any evidence of daytime sleepiness inappropriate for age. Breathing history should include inquiries about the quality, pattern, and intensity of snoring; gasping, snorting and other noises; observed apnea; cyanosis; difficulty breathing; retractions; sudden awaken-

ings; and other signs of difficulty breathing during sleep. A history of abnormal growth velocity, daytime symptoms, developmental problems, psychosocial interactions, behavior problems, school problems, or personality changes must also be carefully sought. Table 19–2 lists guidelines for establishing the severity of the disorder.

Physical Examination

Physical examination should not only be an evaluation of the airway but should be a general assessment, looking for signs of complications or associated abnormalities. Height, weight, growth velocity, and blood pressure should be determined. The child should be observed for signs of excessive sleepiness, mouth breathing, difficulty breathing while awake, speech abnormalities, or behavior problems. Cranial and facial structure should be evaluated, particularly with respect to midfacial hypoplasia, retrognathia, or micrognathia. Signs of respiratory allergies should be sought. The respiratory examination should determine nasal patency and the presence of structural abnormalities of the nasal airway. Oropharyngeal examination should include evaluation of tongue size and control, oromotor control, the hard and soft palate, dentition, tonsil size and location, adenoid hypertrophy (as much as possible), the gag reflex, and the presence of structural abnormalities. The neck should be examined for abnormal lymphadenopathy or neck masses. Chest examination should provide identification of asthma or other lung disease. Cardiac examination should include an evaluation of the second heart sound for signs of pulmonary hypertension. Finally, neurologic function and development should be assessed.

OSA in children cannot be reliably distinguished from PS by history alone or any combination of history plus testing while awake (see Chapter 17). The history is necessary for making a provisional diagnosis and for planning further evaluation, and not every child needs an echocardiogram, multiple sleep latency test (MSLT), or full developmental evaluation. History and physical examination combined with PSG results in some cases are used to tailor additional workup to each child.

Laboratory Tests to Detect OSAS in Children

Laboratory tests can be roughly divided into two categories: tests to detect and quantify the

Table 19–2. SEVERITY CRITERIA FOR OSAS IN CHILDREN*

	Mild	Moderate	Severe
Daytime symptoms	None or minimal	May be present but not disabling	Functional impairment
Difficulty breathing during sleep	Most of sleep period free of obstruction	Obstruction during 33–66% of sleep period	Obstruction during most of sleep period
Oxygen desaturation and $P_{ET}CO_2$ elevation	Minimal	Present but not life-threatening	Potentially life-threatening
Cor pulmonale, failure-to-thrive, developmental delay	Absent	Absent	May be present

*May vary with underlying condition.

severity of sleep-associated airway obstruction, and tests to detect and quantify the severity of associated features and complications (Table 19–3). Although objective testing is necessary and important, there is a tendency to place excessive emphasis on laboratory tests. It should be remembered that PSG can detect and quantify sleep-associated upper airway ob-

Table 19–3. SUGGESTED GUIDELINES FOR EVALUATION OF CHILD WITH SNORING AND DIFFICULTY BREATHING DURING SLEEP

Evaluation/Test/Action	Comments
Provisional diagnosis History Physical examination	History of snoring, difficulty breathing during sleep, daytime symptoms, and nighttime symptoms allows only a provisional diagnosis of PS or OSAS.
Screening tests Brief observation in clinic Home audiotaping Home videotaping Overnight oximetry Sleep sonography	Screening tests useful to clarify a history of noisy breathing during sleep. Brief observation may fail to detect OSAS. Oximetry during sleep, without continuous observation of the child, does not establish cause of hypoxemia or detect hypercarbia. Sonography cannot distinguish central from obstructive apnea.
Tests to diagnose OSAS PSG Direct patient observation Oximetry, observation	PSG establishes the diagnosis and severity of OSAS. Based on PSG findings, further work-up is planned on a case-by-case basis. Patient observation may fail to detect OSA and obstructive hypoventilation and may underestimate severity.
Tests to locate site of obstruction and identify structural airway abnormalities Upper airway fluoroscopy Upper airway endoscopy Cephalometric x-rays	Not used routinely for otherwise normal children. Most useful for children with craniofacial abnormalities.
Tests to detect daytime symptoms Developmental evaluation Daytime cognitive function	MSLT probably indicated for any child with EDS. Developmental evaluation and cognitive function testing recommended for children with severe OSAS or a specific history of developmental delay or daytime behavior problems (e.g., school failure).
Tests to detect complications and determine severity Bicarbonate level Hematocrit Echocardiogram Electrocardiogram	EKG and echocardiogram are recommended for children with moderate-severe OSAS. Bicarbonate level and hematocrit may help establish severity.
Clinical diagnosis of sleep-associated upper airway obstruction	Physician makes final diagnosis, based on entire clinical picture derived from history, physical examination, and laboratory data.
Recommendations for follow-up	Patients with moderate-severe PS should be advised that OSAS may develop. Postoperative follow-up for OSAS is recommended since adenotonsillectomy may not fully correct problem. Repeat PSG is recommended if difficulty breathing during sleep, nighttime symptoms, or daytime symptoms persist.

struction, but the diagnosis of OSAS can only be made by the clinician, based on the total clinical picture.

Polysomnography

The "gold standard" for the diagnosis of abnormal breathing during sleep is nocturnal, full-night PSG. At present, the cardiorespiratory variables monitored during pediatric PSG are the same as for adults. As knowledge about childhood OSAS increases, it is anticipated that PSG for children will be modified. In pediatrics, arterial oxygen saturation is always recorded continuously and many pediatric laboratories record end-tidal CO_2. Some laboratories also make audiovisual tapes of the patient during the entire PSG. Although not recommended, PSG may be performed during morning or afternoon naps and during drug-induced sleep. PSG definitions for children are presented in Table 19–4.

Special Features of the Pediatric Sleep Laboratory. PSG in children is often attempted, with limited success, in adult-oriented laboratories that are not prepared to cope with the special needs of children. This has lead to the erroneous concept that PSG is too difficult to perform in children. As recently as 1990 investigators stated that the "complex equipment" such as EEG electrodes and airflow sensors "is not well tolerated by the pre-

school child."[4] On the contrary, in a *pediatric* sleep laboratory with *pediatric-oriented* technicians, full PSG can be performed easily and safely in children of any age. When approached correctly, nearly all infants, toddlers, preschoolers, and older children tolerate full 14–22 channel PSG without problems. A child's age should *never* be a reason to forgo PSG testing if it is clinically indicated.

Child-Oriented Polysomnography. Two additional factors are crucial to obtaining successful PSG in children: child-oriented technicians and parental participation in the study. A pediatric sleep laboratory should be a place where children are comfortable, with toys, appropriate room decorations, and a videocassette player. There should not be a cold and frightening laboratory atmosphere. One parent should accompany the child, participate in the preparations for study, and remain with the child all night (in a separate bed). The technician should show the child around the laboratory, reassure him or her appropriately, and answer questions. During the preparation when electrodes and other measuring devices are to be attached, *everything* should be explained in advance to the child's satisfaction. With the technician's reassurance, a gentle approach, and a parent in attendance at all times, PSG is easily performed in children.

Indications for Polysomnography. Any discussion of the clinical diagnosis of childhood

---

Table 19–4. POLYSOMNOGRAPHIC DEFINITIONS FOR CHILDREN

Obstructive apnea. Absence of oronasal airflow in the presence of continued respiratory effort, lasting longer than two respiratory cycle times. Usually, but not always, associated with hypoxemia.

Central apnea. Cessation of respiratory effort lasting at least two respiratory cycle times.

Obstructive hypoventilation.* Partial upper airway obstruction leading to a peak $PETCO_2 \geq 55$ mmHg, or $PETCO_2 > 45$ mmHg for more than 60% of total sleep time (TST), or $PETCO_2 > 50$ mmHg for more than 10% of TST (in the absence of lung disease).

Obstructive hypopnea. Decreased breathing associated with a 50% or greater reduction in airflow at the nose and mouth in the presence of continued respiratory efforts; usually associated with paradoxical chest wall motion (in children) and oxyhemoglobin desaturation. The term hypopnea has been retained for use when "airflow" is detected qualitatively by a nasal-oral thermistor and CO_2 is not measured. If SaO_2 and $PETCO_2$ are measured, the more physiologically descriptive term, obstructive hypoventilation, is preferable.

Nonobstructive hypoventilation. *Subtype: Central.* Decreased breathing due to reduction in CNS respiratory drive, leading to hypercarbia and usually associated with hypoxemia. Respiratory abnormalities are usually worse during sleep than wakefulness and during NREM than REM sleep. *Subtype: neuromuscular.* Decreased breathing caused by peripheral neural abnormalities or muscle weakness (e.g., muscular dystrophy). *Subtype: restrictive.* Decreased breathing caused by chest wall restriction (e.g., severe scoliosis).

Nonobstructive hypopnea. Classically defined as a 50% or greater reduction in airflow at the nose and mouth associated with a 50% or greater reduction in respiratory effort, sometimes associated with oxyhemoglobin desaturation. In children, obstructive hypopnea or hypoventilation is sometimes associated with markedly decreased chest wall *motion*, giving a false impression of decreased respiratory *effort*. Therefore, although transient nonobstructive hypoventilation may occur in children, it cannot be reliably detected using only a nasal thermistor and measurement of chest and abdomen motion. Detection of transient nonobstructive hypopnea in children requires measurement of respiratory effort (such as esophageal pressure). If $PETCO_2$ or minute ventilation is measured, the more physiologically descriptive term, nonobstructive hypoventilation, is applicable.

---

*Based on data of Marcus CL, et al: Normal polysomnographic values for children and adolescents. Am Rev Respir Dis 146:1235, 1992.

OSAS eventually comes around to one question: "Is PSG indicated for the diagnosis of OSAS in all snoring children?" Proponents of PSG emphasize that the final diagnosis and determination of severity are only possible by objective testing, and PSG is the best test available. At the present time no other test has been shown to be superior to or as good as PSG and no screening test has been able to distinguish PS from OSAS. Some opponents suggest that PSG is stressful to children, cumbersome, difficult to perform, and expensive; others believe it is not necessary in all cases to diagnose childhood OSAS.

The ICSD Diagnostic and Coding Manual, states:

In the young child, the signs and symptoms of obstructive sleep apnea are more subtle than in the adult; therefore, the diagnosis is more difficult and should be confirmed by polysomnography.[2]

International standard practice in adults suspected of having OSAS is to establish the diagnosis of OSAS by objective testing prior to institution of relatively benign therapy such as nasal continuous positive airway pressure (CPAP). It would appear to be incongruous not to insist that the diagnosis be confirmed in children by objective testing before exposing them to the risks of general anesthesia, surgery, and postoperative complications. If an adult needs PSG before starting CPAP therapy or undergoing surgery, why not provide the same standard of evaluation for a child?

A common objection from otolaryngologists is that, because of parental complaints of loud snoring, they were "going to remove the tonsils and adenoids anyway. Why perform a sleep study?" Presently, parental annoyance, parental concern, and PS are no longer considered indications for general anesthesia and surgery in a child. If the indication for surgical intervention is sleep-associated upper airway obstruction, then the diagnosis must be established and OSAS must be differentiated from PS.

A significant benefit of PSG is determination of severity. Patients with severe OSA on PSG are at higher risk of postoperative respiratory complications.[5] Finally some patients, especially certain of those with craniofacial abnormalities, do not improve significantly after surgical intervention. In these children it is useful to know how severe their obstructive sleep apnea was before surgery.

The financial aspects of PSG is an important consideration, and no one argues that a less expensive and less cumbersome but equally accurate diagnostic test would be desirable. Consider that about 7 to 9% of children appear to be habitual snorers but only about 1 to 2% of children are believed to have significant OSAS (see Chapter 18). PSG on all habitually snoring children would cost approximately 3 billion dollars per year in the United States alone! A simple test that could identify primary snorers and other children who do not require intervention would be desirable.

Polysomnographic Features of OSAS in Children

Obstructive Apnea. In children with OSAS, respiratory measurements indicate partial or complete upper airway obstruction during continuation of respiratory efforts. Unlike standards for adults with OSAS, "significant" obstructive apnea in children should not be limited only to those greater than 10 seconds duration. Normal respiratory rate varies with age. Infants or young children may show oxyhemoglobin desaturations significant for age but which would be considered insignificant by adult standards (Fig. 19–1). An upper airway obstruction lasting 8 seconds may represent 5 to 6 missed breaths in a 6-month-old infant but only 2 missed breaths in a 16 year old. Therefore, "significant" obstructive apnea in a child can be defined as one lasting more than two times the respiratory cycle time (T_{TOT}). Although published data are not yet available, experience suggests that apnea duration varies with age (infants tend to have shorter obstructive apnea than older children), and desaturation is greater for a given event duration in young children. Infants and young children may have numerous upper airway obstructions lasting less than 10 seconds associated with hypoxemia.

Patterns of Obstruction. Children more often exhibit obstructive hypoventilation (hypopnea) than complete upper airway obstruction (see Chapter 18).[6–9] Obstructive hypoventilation of any duration may be significant. Patterns of obstruction are variable between children and within a night in an individual child. Some children will exhibit a predominant pattern of repetitive obstructive apnea, while others may have continuous obstructive hypoventilation lasting hours. Many children exhibit both obstructive hypoventilation and apnea during a single night.

Patients with neurologic and neuromuscular disease may exhibit hypoventilation due to ab-

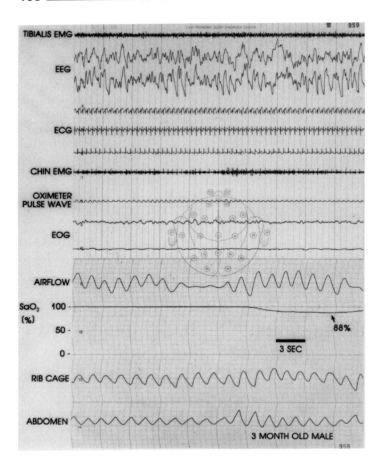

Figure 19–1. Polysomnography tracing from a 3-month-old male infant showing a 4-second obstructive apnea associated with arterial oxygen desaturation to 88%. Paradoxical rib cage motion is continuously present, as expected for a 3-month-old infant.

normalities of the peripheral nervous system, neuromuscular junction, or muscle function. PSG measurement of hypoventilation in these patients does not easily fit into either the central or obstructive category. It may be preferable to classify hypoventilation as *obstructive* versus *nonobstructive*, with subcategories under *nonobstructive* for hypoventilation due to abnormal central breathing regulation, abnormal peripheral motor control, and muscle dysfunction.

Paradoxical Rib Cage Motion. The rib cage is more compliant in infancy and early childhood than at any other time in life. Therefore, infants normally exhibit paradoxical chest wall motion or "paradoxical inward rib cage motion on inspiration" (PIRCM).[10] Infants can have PIRCM in all stages of sleep, but it is most pronounced during REM sleep. The proportion of REM sleep time spent with PIRCM decreases exponentially during the first 3 years of life, so that by about 3 to 4 years of age large amounts of PIRCM are no longer a normal finding. PIRCM occurs during upper airway obstruction due to the large subat-

mospheric intrathoracic pressures. PIRCM occurring in NREM sleep, and in REM sleep in children over about 3 years of age, usually indicates upper airway obstruction.

Hypoxemia. Hypoxemia is usually a feature of OSAS in children, although it has not been well described. Most studies state if hypoxemia occurred, report the lowest SaO_2, or describe the hypoxemia in relative terms (none, mild, moderate, severe). Others arbitrarily define a minimum drop in SaO_2, e.g., >4%, and count the number of drops or "dips" (SaO_2 dipping rate).[11] The prevalence of hypoxemia during sleep in children with OSAS is not known since definitions vary from study to study. Mauer and associates defined obstructive hypopnea and apnea in terms of air flow through the nose or mouth and did not include desaturation in the definition.[7] In their study, all 14 patients showed obstructive hypopnea, obstructive apnea, or both but only four patients exhibited a greater than 4% reduction in SaO_2.[7] Brouillette and associates, using nap PSG studies and recording end-tidal CO_2 ($PETCO_2$) and transcutaneous PO_2 ($PtcO_2$), described 22 infants and children with moderate-severe OSAS.[8] Although 73% of their patients showed evidence of severe sequelae (cor pulmonale, failure-to-thrive, neurologic damage), only 5 of 22 (23%) had hypoxemia during sleep.[8] This study probably underestimates the prevalence and degree of hypoxemia in childhood OSAS since they used $PtcO_2$ measurements, which would not detect brief drops in PaO_2. Nevertheless, it documents that children with severe complications, daytime symptoms, and even hypercarbia during continuous partial airway obstruction may show little or no hypoxemia.[8]

Most hypoxemic episodes experienced by children with OSAS are *not* associated with obstructive apnea according to recent work by Rosen and associates.[3] They reported PSG data from 20 children with symptoms of OSAS and arterial oxygen desaturation during sleep. In spite of thousands of significant desaturation events occurring during sleep in these children (average ~25/hour), only three had apnea indices of 5 or more per hour. Only 9% of severe hypoxemic episodes ($\downarrow$ SaO_2 ≥ 15%

for ≥30 sec) were found to be associated with obstructive apnea scored by adult criteria (i.e., ≥10 sec).[3] These important findings underscore the points that children may have severe sleep-related upper airway obstruction without obstructive apnea, and adult PSG scoring criteria for OSAS do not apply to children.[1, 3]

At the Johns Hopkins Pediatric Sleep Center and elsewhere, children have been documented to have repetitive OSA without hypoxemia (with hypoxemia defined as SaO_2 <92% by oximetry). In addition, children may have significant obstructive hypoventilation without hypoxemia. Figure 19–2 shows respiratory recordings during delta sleep from a 10-year-old child with snoring but no lung disease and a normal $PaCO_2$ while awake. Breathing during sleep was regular, end-tidal CO_2 was ~50 mmHg (higher at other times), and esophageal pressure ranged from −50 to −60 cmH_2O, yet the SaO_2 was 97 to 100% (Figure 19–2). On the other hand, children may also desaturate quite rapidly during brief obstructive apnea or obstructive hypoventilation. Figure 19–3 shows an approximately 6-second

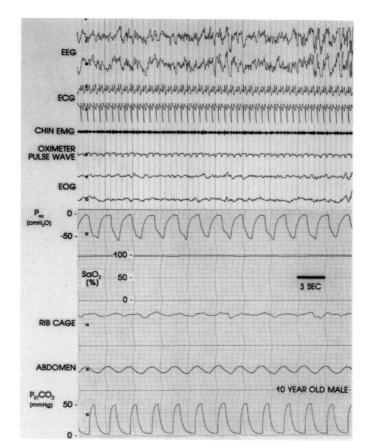

Figure 19–2. Continuous obstructive hypoventilation without hypoxemia in a 10-year-old obese male.

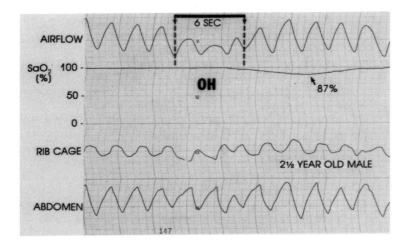

Figure 19–3. Arterial oxygen desaturation to 87% following 6 seconds of obstructive hypoventilation (hypopnea) in a 2 1/2-year-old child.

obstructive hypopnea episode in a 2-year-old child, with SaO₂ falling from 96 to 87% in seconds. Figure 19–4 shows repetitive brief events leading to hypoxemia in a 3-month-old child (arterial desaturation to 79% occurs after a 3–4-sec obstructive apnea). Thus, brief obstructions (that would not be scored as "significant" by adult criteria) can lead to hypoxemia in children.

It is widely believed that hypoxemia is worse during REM sleep than NREM sleep. However, because older studies predated widespread availability of pulse oximetry, and many did not stage sleep, there has been little study of this specific question. Observations in our sleep laboratory indicate that children experience hypoxemia in all sleep stages but that the worst hypoxemia tends to occur during REM

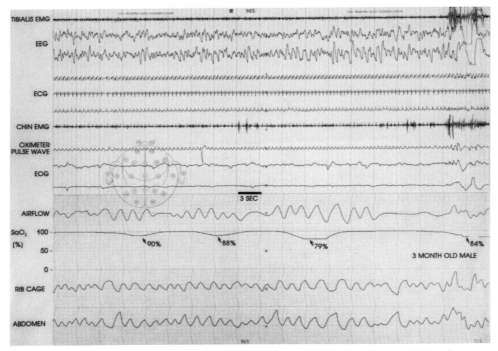

Figure 19–4. Repetitive obstructive episodes in a 3-month-old infant with childhood OSAS. Infants especially can exhibit rapidly developing hypoxemia following very brief obstructive events. Note continuous paradoxical inward rib cage motion typical of infants this age. Also note lack of arousal from sleep until the end of the 10-second obstructive apnea at the far right.

sleep. This is not surprising in view of the effects of REM sleep on functional residual capacity (FRC) and body oxygen stores in children. However, studies of OSAS in children of different ages are needed.

Hypercarbia. Much less is known about hypercarbia than hypoxemia in children with OSAS. Case reports of OSAS with hypercarbia abound in the older literature but these tend to reflect an advanced stage of OSAS with severe complications. Brouillette and associates found that 11 of 22 children with OSAS exhibited hypercarbia ($PaCO_2$ >45 mmHg) during PSG. Hypercarbia due to OSAS was severe in some children, with $PaCO_2$ values as high as 85 mmHg.[8] Rowe and associates measured transcutaneous PCO_2 ($PtcCO_2$) in five children with OSAS due to a variety of causes; only two were due to adenotonsillar hypertrophy.[12] They found that highest $PtcCO_2$ values ranged from normal to 45 to 55 mmHg.[12] Miyazaki and associates also reported that $PtcCO_2$ in children with OSAS may be elevated above 60 or 70 mmHg for hours but unfortunately only reported results for a few cases.[9] Recently Rosen and associates found that peak $PETCO_2$ values in children with OSAS ranged from 50 to 68 mmHg, even though their awake values were 35 to 45 mmHg.[3] These data, combined with the finding by Marcus and associates that peak $PETCO_2$ values in normals should not exceed 53 mmHg,[13] show that a peak $PETCO_2$ greater than 53 mmHg during pediatric PSG may indicate sleep-related upper airway obstruction (see discussion of normal values under Interpretation of Polysomnography). This is valid only for children without nonobstructive hypoventilation or hypercarbia due to lung disease.

Disturbed Sleep. Very little has been published on the quantification of disturbed sleep by PSG in children. Although some normal values exist for arousal, awakenings, sleep efficiency and other sleep variables in children, most of these reports are based on small numbers of patients whose PSG did not include cardiorespiratory monitoring. The effects of anxiety, the "first night effect," thermistors, $PETCO_2$ catheters, and other respiratory recording devices on sleep quality in the laboratory are not yet known. Until better information is available, it seems reasonable to consider a sleep efficiency of 85% or less abnormal. Awakenings, arousal, movements, and other sleep behavior is assessed on a case-by-case basis.

Instrumentation and Scoring

Before a PSG can be used to diagnose OSAS it must first be scored. This requires tremendous data reduction since a PSG consists of nearly 1000 pages of continuous recording of 14 to 22 channels. This record must be reviewed, pertinent information identified, and data extracted in a usable form. In pediatrics there are no standards for cardiorespiratory sleep studies and no consensus about how to score, interpret, or report PSG findings.

Detection of Airflow. By definition, airflow at the nose and mouth must be monitored in order to detect obstructive apnea. In adult laboratories usually a nasal-oral thermistor or thermocouple is used for semiquantitative detection of airflow. This is acceptable in the adult setting since adults show predominantly obstructive apnea. However, when obstructive hypoventilation predominates, such detection of airflow is inadequate. Children may be encountered with significant partial obstruction and hypercarbia that would not have met the criteria for "obstructive hypopnea" as defined by the ICSD.[2] Therefore, most pediatric laboratories monitor $PETCO_2$ in order to detect obstructive hypoventilation. When $PETCO_2$ is measured at the nose, it is advisable to use a thermistor or thermocouple to detect mouth breathing. Since not all sleep laboratories have end-tidal gas monitoring capabilities, a definition of obstructive hypopnea (using a nasal-oral thermistor for flow detection) is included (see Table 19–4).

Detection of Hypercarbia. Carbon dioxide tension can be detected during sleep by an indwelling arterial catheter, transcutaneous measurement, or $PETCO_2$ monitoring. The indwelling arterial catheter is only safe to use in an intensive care setting and not practical for routine PSG. $PtcCO_2$ monitoring detects trends well but fails to detect transient changes in $PaCO_2$. Expired CO_2 monitoring is capable of detecting breath-to-breath changes in $PETCO_2$, although it may seriously underestimate arterial PCO_2 in the child with lung disease (i.e., bronchopulmonary dysplasia). $PETCO_2$ monitoring is prone to artifact and great care must be taken to ensure a consistently high-quality signal.

Expired CO_2 can be used to evaluate obstructive apnea in several ways. During obstructive apnea there is no airflow, and no CO_2 is expired for the duration of complete upper airway obstruction. Therefore, for apnea detection the expired CO_2 signal is used only to detect the absence of airflow, which can be done just as well with a nasal-oral thermistor. Some laboratories measure the $P_{ET}CO_2$ from the first postobstruction breath, which some believe can yield a measure of the severity of gas exchange derangements. However, this can be misleading. Experience indicates that children often have obstructive apnea with normal $P_{ET}CO_2$ measured from the first 1 or 2 postapnea breaths. The explanation for this is not clear. The postapnea breaths may also be partially obstructed and/or the expired air may not reflect true alveolar PCO_2.

Expired CO_2 monitoring is much more useful for detecting obstructive hypoventilation. Due to the sigmoidal shape of the oxyhemoglobin saturation curve, it is possible for a child to show an elevation in expired CO_2 with a minimal change in SaO_2. Therefore, expired CO_2 monitoring may slow obstructive hypoventilation undetectable by nasal thermistor plus oximetry. One way to quantify hypoventilation is to take the highest or peak $P_{ET}CO_2$ (2 consecutive breaths) associated with an obstructive event.[13] This method has the advantage of simplicity. Another way is to measure the proportion of sleep time spent with $P_{ET}CO_2$ above 45 or 50 mmHg.[13] This method was used by Marcus and associates in recent studies of normal children[13] and children with Down syndrome.[14] This method has the advantages of addressing the problem of variability and of having normal values for comparison. Unfortunately, measurement of percent of time spent with $PaCO_2$ greater than 45 or 50 mmHg is time consuming. Finally, one can compare $PaCO_2$ in patients while awake with peak $PaCO_2$ while asleep. However, the usefulness of this measurement has not been confirmed and normal values do not yet exist.

Consistently good quality expired CO_2 monitoring is only possible with meticulous attention to technique by a conscientious technician. Artifact is common and, at least at present, artifacts must be visually identified and rejected during scoring. Some expired CO_2 monitors will save and output a "trend" recording, but the information may be erroneous since artifact rejection is primitive on most instruments. Some laboratories use $PtcCO_2$ monitoring. It is technically easier, provides a trend that may be less prone to artifact, and allows easy quantification of "duration of hypoventilation." However, because of its slow response time, it does not detect transient elevations (although it is not known if brief or transient hypercarbia is harmful to children).

In addition, $PtcCO_2$ does not correlate well with arterial PCO_2 (and skin perfusion changes may change this relationship further); sleep may be disturbed when the electrode site is changed; the electrode may cause skin burns; and $PtcCO_2$ measurement is particularly ill-suited for use in obese children. Nevertheless, several laboratories have used skin surface CO_2 monitoring with success (despite the current lack of normal values for children).[9]

In spite of the potential for artifacts, because both $PtcCO_2$ and $P_{ET}CO_2$ measurements may be helpful, it has been suggested that both be recorded during pediatric PSG.

Detection of Hypoxemia. Nearly all laboratories use pulse oximetry to detect hypoxemia during sleep. Technology has advanced so that probes are small, lightweight, can be taped to fingers or toes, and are well-tolerated by children. Artifact rejection has also improved but is far from perfect. In addition to the SaO_2, the oximetry "pulse wave" may be recorded so that false readings can be easily detected (often critical in infants and young children). Oximetry has several advantages over $PtcO_2$ monitoring: oximetry detects transient or brief desaturations, is easier to use, does not require calibration, and is free of most complications. Pulse oximeters will now store data in microchip memory and output "trend" information. Some laboratories have also used computers to record SaO_2 overnight and produce a "saturogram" showing percentage of time spent in the hypoxemic range. Although this is attractive, there are no studies on the significance of such data in children. Age-specific normal values will be necessary (since infants, for example, normally desaturate to less than 92% for brief periods).

Detection of Respiratory Effort. Methods used to detect chest wall motion are essentially the same for adults and children. Respiratory inductance plethysmography and strain gauges work well in children but still detect only respiratory movements, not actual respiratory effort. The problem with only detecting chest and abdomen movement is that in children the chest may expand very little during obstructed breathing. As a result, PSG may show decreased oronasal airflow and markedly *decreased* chest and abdomen movement. By adult PSG definitions this would erroneously be classified as "central hypopnea." In order to better detect true respiratory "effort," some laboratories measure intercostal EMG using surface electrodes. Essentially this provides another respiratory effort channel that may be helpful in distinguishing obstructive hypoventilation from transient central hypoventilation (central hypopnea).

Monitoring of esophageal pressure is not part of standard PSG in the United States but is used routinely by some investigators in other countries.[9] It should be considered when conventional PSG fails to adequately detect suspected obstructive hypoventilation. Esophageal pressure monitoring may be especially useful in obese children who exhibit pseudocentral apnea or hypoventilation.

Quantification of Upper Airway Obstruction. Scoring the PSG of an adult with OSAS is relatively straightforward. Compared with children, adults tend to exhibit obstructive apnea that is longer and more frequent, and obstructive "hypopnea" is easier to identify using a thermistor (personal observations). However, the utility of obstructive event counts or indices in children is not clear. Although in children the number and duration of obstructive apneas is easily determined and expressed as the obstructive apnea index (number of apneas per hour of sleep time), obstructive hypoventilation is much more difficult to evaluate. Some children exhibit numerous discrete obstructive hypoventilation episodes that can be counted and measured as with apnea. However, children often exhibit continuous obstructive hypoventilation, sometimes for hours, with no clear-cut transition between obstructive hypoventilation and nonobstructed breathing. Often at the end of an episode, obstructive hypoventilation simply gradually fades into less obstructed breathing (i.e., into severe PS). Even when it is possible to define the onset and end of obstructive hypoventilation episodes, in such children counting such episodes as "events" is of little value and the "obstructive event index" does not accurately reflect the severity of the obstructed breathing. Some children exhibit obstructive apnea events embedded in continuous obstructive hypoventilation. Others exhibit continuous mixed apnea or obstructive periodic breathing (central apnea alternating with obstructive hypoventilation) for prolonged periods. A key feature of childhood OSAS is the heterogeneity of obstructed breathing patterns during sleep.

At present, there are no standards for scoring of cardiorespiratory sleep studies in children. At Johns Hopkins pediatric laboratory, obstructive apnea is quantitated by calculation of an obstructive apnea index as follows:

$$\text{Obstructive apnea index} = \frac{\text{Number of obstructive apneas}}{\text{Total sleep time (minutes)}} \times 60$$

Obstructive hypoventilation is quantitated by recording expired CO_2 and measuring PETCO_2 for each epoch. This is then used to determine percentage of (nonapnea) total sleep time (TST) spent with PETCO_2 greater than 50 mmHg (Tables 19–1, 19–4, and 19–5). This can be calculated as:

$$\text{Duration of hypoventilation (\%)} = \frac{\text{Time with } \text{PETCO}_2 > 50 \text{ mmHg}}{\text{TST}} \times 100$$

"Duration of hypoventilation" refers to the percentage of breathing that was associated with an PETCO_2 greater than 50 mmHg (hypoventilation). Ideally, time spent in apnea should be subtracted from TST. However, this form of the equation is practical for routine use because the total apnea duration for children is usually negligible compared with TST. Thus, the "duration of hypoventilation" yielded by the above equation is sufficiently accurate for clinical purposes. However, if a child exhibits numerous and/or prolonged obstructive apneas, then the following equation would yield a more accurate index of hypoventilation:

$$\text{Duration of hypoventilation (\%)} = \frac{\text{Time with } \text{PETCO} > 50 \text{ mmHg}}{\text{TST} - \text{Total apnea time}} \times 100$$

Although measuring the duration of hypoventilation is labor intensive, so is sleep staging. A more practical approach may be to determine average PETCO_2 for each epoch (30 sec) and calculate the proportion of epochs (expressed as %) with PETCO_2 greater than 50 mmHg. The advantages of determining "duration of hypoventilation" (time spent with hypercarbia) are that is physiologically meaningful, it allows quantification of obstructive hypoventilation in studies showing continuous prolonged partial obstruction, and it avoids the problem of misleading event "indices." A practical advantage of determining duration of hypoventilation using the equations above is that normal values have been reported for children.[13] Finally, maximum or peak PETCO_2, defined as the highest PETCO_2 for two consecutive breaths associated with upper airway obstruction, can easily be measured. None of these methods have been validated in large clinical trials.

Table 19–5. SUGGESTED NORMAL VALUES FOR PSG IN CHILDREN

	Normal Values	Comments
Obstructive apnea index	≤ 1 apnea/hour 0 apneas > 10 sec duration 0 apneas > 15 sec duration	Probably valid for children > 3 months of age (> 3 months of age) (< 3 months of age)
Maximum $PaCO_2$	≤ 55 mmHg during study	Only useful in children without underlying lung disease
% TST spent with $P_{ET}CO_2 > 50$ mmHg	≤ 10% of TST	Only useful in children without underlying lung disease
% TST spent with $P_{ET}CO_2 > 45$ mmHg	≤ 60% of TST	Only useful in children without underlying lung disease
Minimum SaO_2	≥ 92%	Evaluate on case-by-case basis in children with lung disease
Maximum ΔSaO_2	≤ 8%	Does not apply to children with cyanotic heart disease

Based on data from Gaultier C: Respiratory adaptation during sleep from the neonatal period to adolescence. _In_ Guilleminault C (ed): Sleep and Its Disorders in Children. New York, Raven Press, 1987, pp 67–98, and Marcus CL, et al: Normal polysomnographic values for children and adolescents. Am Rev Respir Dis 146:1235, 1992.

Determining Validity of Results. PSG may be uninterpretable without knowing if the child's sleep and breathing on the night of the study were representative of his or her _usual_ sleep and breathing. Children referred for snoring may not snore during a single night of PSG. In pediatrics a prestudy and "morning-after" questionnaire is important. The prestudy questionnaire builds a profile of the parent's perception of how the child sleeps and breathes at home. The morning-after questionnaire determines if the parent thought the night's sleep and breathing to be representative of what is _usual_ for the child. This information becomes part of the PSG data and is essential for interpretation.

Interpretation of Polysomnography

The ICSD states in the diagnostic criteria for OSA that PSG monitoring must demonstrate "more than five obstructive apneas, greater than 10 seconds' duration, per hour of sleep. . . ."[2] Children may exhibit severe sleep-associated upper airway obstruction without _any_ obstructive apnea (Fig. 19–5). Children with obstructive hypoventilation may show markedly abnormal intrathoracic pressures and hypercapnia without discrete obstructive "events" or even hypoxemia (see Fig. 19–2). Finally, obstructive events less than 10 seconds' duration are often associated with hypoxemia in children (see Fig. 19–4). Therefore, the adult diagnostic criteria for OSAS do not apply to children and should not be used for that purpose.

Role of Polysomnography. Although many consider the role of PSG to be confirmation of the provisional diagnosis, it does not stop there. PSG also identifies specific problems so that further evaluation and treatment can be appropriately focused and provides a measure of severity that is also useful in planning additional evaluation, treatment, and appropriate follow-up. A patient with mild OSAS needs little additional evaluation, treatment is straightforward, and follow-up can be managed by the general pediatrician. A child with severe OSAS requires cardiac, hematologic, and developmental evaluation; pediatric anesthesia consultation; an optimal surgical approach; intensive postoperative monitoring; and long-term follow-up focused on problem areas (including neurodevelopmental). PSG is an invaluable aid to making these judgments.

Limitations of the Traditional Laboratory Approach. Once data from PSG have been "scored" and extracted, it must be interpreted. This requires knowledge of what is normal or at least the ability to identify _some_ features that are clearly abnormal. It is also important to understand the limitations of the testing techniques. There are fundamental difficulties with the conventional approach to evaluating sleep-disordered breathing in children. Interpretation of PSG has focused on three major features: hypoxemia, the amount of upper airway obstruction, and sleep disruption. Traditionally, based on some method of quantifying these features, a sleep study would be classified as "normal" or "abnormal." The premise underlying this approach is that hypoxemia, airway obstruction, and sleep disruption are "bad" for a child; few would argue the point. However, we know very little about how frequently and for how long each of these must

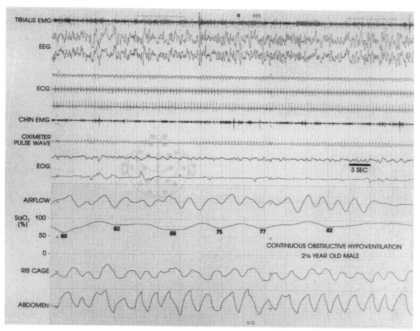

Figure 19–5. Obstructive hypoventilation in a 2 1/2-year-old child. Except for obstructive apnea embedded in obstructive hypoventilation (far right), discrete obstructive "events" are not easily discernible. Event "counts" or indices are difficult if not impossible to determine accurately in children with this pattern of obstructed breathing during sleep.

occur to produce a particular adverse outcome.

It is also assumed that PSG measures the correct parameters. Conventional (adult) PSG does not quantitate hypercarbia or impaired cardiac function, which may be important determinants of adverse outcome. Another assumption is that it is appropriate to force a dichotomous conclusion (normal or abnormal, positive or negative) onto PSG in children. The utility of interpreting PSG as either normal or abnormal would appear to be questionable, since manifestations are variable and little is known about which PSG values are normal and which values predict positive or negative outcomes. At least in pediatrics, clinical judgment is still required.

General Approach to the Polysomnogram. The interpretation of PSG in children requires considerable judgment. First, determine if the child's sleep and breathing were "representative." Various data are reviewed to determine that sleep disruption is present; to determine whether awake breathing, SaO_2, and $PaCO_2$ are normal; and to determine the amount of upper airway obstruction and duration and degree of hypoxemia and hypercarbia during sleep. The EKG is reviewed for evidence of arrhythmia. Snoring is rated according to intensity, duration, and quality. Parasomnias or other events noted by technicians can be reviewed on videotape. Sleep and breathing are judged to be normal, probably normal, probably abnormal, or abnormal. All of this information is then integrated with the parent's impressions of how "representative" the data are, and the final interpretation is summarized.

Sleep Disruption. There are relatively few guidelines available for assessing sleep disturbance. The ICSD defines restlessness during sleep as "persistent or recurrent body movements, arousals, and brief awakenings in the course of sleep."[2] However, many normal children are "restless" during sleep and normal values for numbers of arousals, body movements, movement time, and other measures of disturbed sleep are not available. Similarly, the ICSD defines sleep fragmentation as "the interruption of any stage of sleep due to the appearance of another stage or to wakefulness, leading to disrupted NREM-REM sleep cycles."[2] Again, age-specific normal values are lacking. Sleep efficiency is an easy number to determine but, currently, not a determination of abnormality. Markers of sleep disturbance vary between different laboratories and even between technicians within the same laboratory. Until better normal values for children are available, determination of sleep disruption remains largely a matter of experience and judgment.

Breathing During Sleep. Breathing during sleep is slightly easier to assess than sleep disruption but also is made difficult by a lack of data on normal children. There is a large amount of normal data for newborns and infants, some for older children and adolescents, and little on children between 1 year of age and adolescence.[15–18] Canet and associates studied infants 1 to 6 months of age (mean age = 3.6 ± 1 month) and found an obstructive apnea index of 0.04 ± 0.13 apneas per hour, an obstructive hypoventilation index of 0.4 ± 0.64 events per hour, and total obstructive respiratory event index of 0.4 ± 0.8 events per hour (mean ± 1 SD).[16] From these and data of others[15, 19, 20] it can be said that after the first several months of life, mixed and obstructive apnea index in children should be less than one event per hour, desaturations over 4% are rare, SaO_2 should remain above 95%, and the maximal change in SaO_2 should not exceed about 6%. Mallory and associates considered $PETCO_2$ greater than 50 mmHg for more than 5% of TST to be abnormal in children based on their "estimate of clinical significance."[21] Marcus and associates studied 50 normal children, ages 1 to 17 years of age, using polysomnography.[13] They found that only 18% of the children had any obstructive apnea and none showed mixed apnea. PSG in these children showed no obstructive apnea longer than 10 seconds' duration and the average obstructive apnea index was 0.1 ± 0.5 events per hour.[13] They agreed with Gaultier's findings and recommended a normal value of less than one obstructive apnea per hour for children.[13] With respect to gas exchange, they found minimum SaO_2 to be $96 \pm 2\%$ and the average maximal change in SaO_2 during the study to be $4 \pm 2\%$. Mean peak $PETCO_2$ (defined as the highest of two consecutive values associated with upper airway obstruction) was 46 ± 4 mmHg and $PETCO_2$ was greater than 50 mmHg for $0.5 \pm 4\%$ of total sleep time.[13] Based on these and other data, suggested normal values for scoring obstructed breathing during sleep are listed in Table 19–5.

Based on their study of PSG in normal children, Marcus and associates recommended that obstructive hypoventilation could be diagnosed if a child spent 60% or more of TST with a $PETCO_2$ equal to or greater than 45 mmHg and/or 8 to 10% or more of TST with a $PETCO_2$ equal to or greater than 50 mmHg.[13] That study was published in 1992. Since then we now have a 2-year experience using the diagnostic criteria recommended by the authors; measuring percent of TST spent with a $PETCO_2$ equal to or greater than 45 mmHg and $PETCO_2$ equal to or greater than 50 mmHg. Our impression, after using these criteria for more than 500 PSGs in children, is that the most useful measurement is percent of TST spent with $PETCO_2$ equal to or greater than 50 mmHg. In our experience, measuring the percent of TST spent with $PETCO_2$ equal to or greater than 45 mmHg is exceedingly time consuming for technicians scoring PSGs, and many children without OSA or sleep-related airway obstruction spend more than 60% of TST with $PETCO_2$ values between 45 and 49 mmHg. In contrast, the criterion of 8 to 10% or more of TST with a $PETCO_2$ equal to or greater than 50 mmHg has proven useful and appears to reliably distinguish snoring from obstructive hypoventilation (personal observations). At the present time, only the higher $PETCO_2$ criterion (% TST spent ≥ 50 mmHg) for scoring of obstructive hypoventilation in children is recommended.[13a]

Polysomnography Report. PSG results are usually summarized in a 1 or 2 page report. At present there are no standards for reporting pediatric PSG results. At Johns Hopkins the practice is to include patient data, a very brief summary of pertinent history and indications for study, a summary of techniques used, awake breathing data, sleep architecture, arousal and movement counts, some measure of actual snoring, central and obstructive apnea indices, SaO_2 and $PETCO_2$ data, and a summary of technician's comments. From this information and from reviewing the PSG tracing, videotapes, and other available information, the results are interpreted. Conclusions are made regarding whether the child's sleep and breathing were perceived by parent(s) to be representative, evidence of sleep disturbance and upper airway obstruction during sleep, and amount and degree of hypoxemia and hypoventilation. Then, with respect to sleep and breathing, the study is classified as normal or consistent with PS or OSAS. The interpretation usually includes specific comments on the pattern(s) of obstruction, hypoxemia, hypercarbia, central apnea, sleep disruption, parasomnias or any other notable findings. Occasionally a study performed for suspected OSAS yields unexpected results that should be described and interpreted in context.

Severity. There are no guidelines for rating the severity of PSG findings. For sleep disruption, severity is entirely a matter of experience and clinical judgment. For breathing during sleep, "flexible" severity criteria may be used (see Table 19–2). These criteria are intended only as a rough clinical guide for the clinician. More precise severity criteria must await studies associating specific PSG findings with outcome.

Nap Studies, Sleep Deprivation, and Sedation

A number of laboratories perform PSG during daytime naps instead of overnight. This approach would have obvious advantages if it could be validated. Because children often do not sleep easily during the day, some workers have employed prior sleep deprivation or sedatives such as chloral hydrate. There are potential problems with all of these approaches. With respect to naps, daytime sleep may not be the same as nighttime sleep. Furthermore, many children are worse during the latter half of the night. Nap studies would thus tend to underdetect obstructed breathing and underestimate severity. One could argue that nap studies could be used as preliminary tests if they clearly show sleep-associated airway obstruction, then no further PSG would be needed. Data from Marcus and associates suggests that nap PSG (using chloral hydrate) has a positive predictive value of 100% but a negative predictive value of only 17%.[22] They suggested that nap studies are useful when clearly abnormal, but overnight PSG should be performed if the nap study is "negative" or inconclusive.[22] Given the 4 to 5:1 ratio of PS to OSAS children, one would expect many nap studies to be negative or inconclusive. Sleep deprivation prior to PSG has been shown to cause or worsen OSAS[16] and should not be used. Sedation may preferentially suppress upper airway dilator muscle function and is probably best avoided. Biban and associates recently described two children (~2 years of age) with OSAS who developed life-threatening respiratory compromise when sedated with chloral hydrate (80 mg/kg).[23] Although it seems clear that sedation can worsen upper airway obstruction in children with OSAS, it is less clear whether sedation (using appropriate doses) induces OSA in children without OSAS or other predisposing factors.

Other Tests to Detect OSAS in Children

Several investigators have searched for simple methods to diagnose childhood OSAS that would by-pass the need for PSG. Most have focused on one aspect, such as snoring[24] or hypoxemia.[4, 25] However, the determinants of adverse outcome due to OSAS are only crudely known and the risk in all limited diagnostic techniques is that at worst the wrong parameter is measured or at best the measurement is incomplete. Even PSG, the gold standard, does not provide measurements for some variables that may be important (such as the effect of obstructed breathing on cardiac function).

Home Audiotaping. Although used by some practitioners, the value of home audiotaping as a diagnostic tool has never been evaluated. Occasionally, it may be used if the history of snoring is doubtful and daytime symptoms are absent. Parents are instructed to tape the child's worst snoring for approximately 10 to 15 minutes and then send it to the practitioner. If breathing sounds during sleep are not clearly normal, the child undergoes further evaluation (the final diagnosis of OSAS should never be based on home audiotaping).

Home Videotaping. Families can videotape the child's breathing during sleep for evaluation by Sleep Center physicians. Home videotaping is useful in several situations. Sometimes parents describe bizarre movements, arousals, or other events that are best evaluated by observation. Occasionally, a physician is not sure a referral is really needed, and viewing a videotape of what the parents perceive as the child's worst breathing during sleep can be useful for advising the referring physician. Videotaping may be useful but has not been evaluated as a screening or diagnostic tool.

Observation, Physical Examination, and Oximetry. Some authors have suggested that examination of the sleeping child in the physician's office is sufficient to make the diagnosis of OSAS.[8] This is clearly true of the patient with severe OSAS who may fall asleep on the examination table and demonstrate severe apnea and cyanosis. However, the usefulness of direct observation in clinic has not been demonstrated for children with mild to moderate OSAS. Some children will sleep for several hours before onset of obstructed breathing. Other clinicians have advocated hospital admission for observation of the child's breathing during sleep by nurses and other personnel.[26–28] However, both untrained and trained observers (including physicians) frequently fail to detect OSA in children and nearly always underestimate its severity. Direct observation of the sleeping child, perhaps combined with pulse oximetry, can be an alternative for patients and physicians in remote areas without access to a pediatric sleep center.

van Someren and associates recently suggested that hypoxemia during sleep in children undergoing adenotonsillectomy could reliably be predicted by a combination of noisy mouth breathing and SaO_2 less than 94 to 96% while awake.[25] However, many patients will have normal SaO_2 values while awake and marked hypoxemia and OSAS during sleep. They presumed desaturation was caused by upper airway obstruction and did not perform polysomnography, and only patients already scheduled for adenotonsillectomy were evaluated.[25] It remains to be shown that any combination of daytime SaO_2, historic features, or physical examination is useful for screening or diagnosing OSAS.

Stradling and associates have reported using history, physical examination, overnight oximetry, and overnight videotaping with movement analysis to diagnose OSAS in children awaiting adenotonsillectomy.[11] They found that hypoxemia and movement during sleep were much more common before surgery than after.[11] However, this was a selected group of patients, PSG was not performed, videotaping was performed before and after surgery in less than half of the study group, and the positive or negative predictive value of the screening tests were not established.

A recent report describes automated analysis of nasal capnography (without PSG) for diagnosing upper airway obstruction during sleep.[29] However, to date the number of patients reported is insufficient to allow evaluation of this technique.

Fluoroscopic Evaluation. A number of investigators have described the use of upper airway fluoroscopy in children with OSAS.[6, 30–32] Although fluoroscopy of the sleeping child can determine the site of obstruction, it is not indicated for otherwise normal children with OSAS, because, at the present time, knowing the precise site of obstruction does not change the treatment approach for normal children with OSAS. Radiologic evaluation is most useful in children with craniofacial abnormalities in which adenotonsillar hypertrophy are not believed to play a major role and treatment is not straightforward.

Endoscopic Evaluation. Transnasal endos-copy of the child during sleep has been advocated as a tool to diagnose OSAS in children. Fan has reported that endoscopic examination "influenced therapeutic interventions,"[33] and Croft and associates reported that it "allowed a rational and successful management plan."[34] However, both studies included many patients with airway abnormalities other than adenotonsillar hypertrophy, and neither study systematically compared endoscopic evaluation with other methods. Endoscopic evaluation appears to be most useful for children with craniofacial abnormalities or structural airway problems other than large tonsils and adenoids.

Cephalometric X-rays. Although cephalometric x-rays have been used in children with OSAS, they have not been shown to add substantially to the evaluation of an otherwise normal child with symptoms of OSAS.[6] The otolaryngologist should examine the airway endoscopically, since subtle findings on cephalometry will not change the treatment approach in normal children with adenotonsillar hypertrophy. At the present time, cephalometric x-rays are most useful in evaluating children with craniofacial abnormalities and other structural abnormalities of the upper airway.

Sleep Sonography. Sleep sonography has been proposed by Potsic[24] and Marsh and associates[35] as a "reliable method for evaluating patients (children) with upper airway obstruction." This technique, which consists of recording the child's breathing sounds during sleep and analyzing the sounds for "regularity" of respiration and pauses, has been shown to agree with PSG findings in children with OSAS.[24] Advantages include ease of use, lower cost, and the ability to study the child at home. The disadvantages are the inability to distinguish central from obstructive apnea and unknown predictive value.

Multiple Sleep Latency Testing. The MSLT is currently the most popular and widely used test for EDS. Although there are no firm guidelines on the use of MSLT in children, at Johns Hopkins an MSLT is obtained for all children with a history of EDS. Several children (mostly adolescents) have been identified with EDS, OSAS, and narcolepsy. Persistence of EDS after successful treatment for OSAS should always suggest the possibility of narcolepsy, even in children. Major drawbacks, at present, are the lack of normative data on large numbers of children of all ages, and the fact that MSLT cannot detect effects of sleep disruption or nighttime hypoxemia on daytime cognitive function.

Tests to Detect Complications or Associated Features of OSAS

Tests to detect complications of OSAS are listed in Table 19–3. Although there have been studies of EKG and echocardiographic abnormalities in children awaiting adenotonsillectomy[36] and in OSAS patients with cor pulmonale, the use of these tests is still largely a matter of local practice and clinical experience. At our institution children undergoing adenotonsillectomy for OSAS have been studied to determine risk factors for postoperative respiratory complications.[5] Results indicated that young age (<3 years of age), high obstructive event index (>10 obstructive events/hour), failure-to-thrive, craniofacial abnormalities, or an abnormal EKG or echocardiogram were significant risk factors for developing postoperative respiratory compromise.[5] The utility of awake arterial blood gases or an elevated bicarbonate level or hematocrit is not precisely defined; abnormal findings mainly signify that evaluation for severe hypoxemia and respiratory failure is indicated.

Role of the Pediatric Sleep Specialist—the Clinical Diagnosis of OSAS

Suggested diagnostic criteria for OSAS are listed in Table 19–1. OSAS remains a clinical, not a PSG, diagnosis. The role of the clinician, after the history, physical examination, and evaluation of laboratory data, is to assess the entire clinical picture, characterize the child's manifestations of the syndrome, determine the severity of OSAS and the presence and severity of complications, and make recommendations for treatment and follow-up. Each child manifests OSAS in a slightly different manner.

Treatment

Treatment for OSAS has included: nothing (follow-up only), medical/pharmacologic (theophylline), surgical (tracheostomy, adenotonsillectomy), mechanical therapy (positive airway pressure, tongue retainers), and a few unusual approaches that are now of historic interest only (radiation therapy to the nasopharynx).[37] Early reported cases were treated by surgical relief of upper airway obstruction,

and the surgical approach has remained the most popular. Adenotonsillectomy is easily performed in most hospitals, is straightforward, and is effective in most pediatric cases of OSAS (at least short-term).

There is little scientific information and no consensus on treatment for childhood OSAS. Current practice is based largely on what seems reasonable to practitioners rather than on scientific data. Whether some children with mild OSAS should be followed carefully without surgical intervention is not known. At present there are no published guidelines suggesting appropriate indications for nasal sprays and decongestants; tonsillectomy, adenoidectomy, adenotonsillectomy or other surgical procedures; special perioperative management; or postoperative follow-up.

Surgical Treatment of Childhood OSAS

Adenotonsillectomy. "If the tonsils are large and the general state is evidently influenced by them," stated William Osler speaking of childhood OSAS in 1892, "they should be at once removed. The treatment of the adenoid growths in the pharynx is of greatest importance."[38] Osler not only understood the value of tonsillectomy, but realized the importance of adenoid hypertrophy in these patients. However, it would be 73 years before case reports would document that relief of sleep-associated upper airway obstruction alleviates symptoms of severe OSAS in children.[37, 39–58] Later studies involving larger series of patients established the efficacy of adenotonsillectomy for childhood OSAS in patients with a wider range of severity.[7, 8, 11, 26, 27, 59–62] Since the 1970s, the percentage of tonsillectomies and adenoidectomies for childhood OSAS has risen dramatically.[63]

Although there are no firm guidelines, current general practice is to recommend adenotonsillectomy for any child with OSAS thought to be associated with adenotonsillar hypertrophy. The combined procedure (tonsillectomy and adenoidectomy) is recommended by most since, as Potsic states, "If only the most obvious culprit, either tonsils or adenoids, is removed, obstruction often recurs, requiring a second procedure."[24] At some institutions when OSAS is the indication for adenotonsillectomy, postoperative management is routinely carried out in a pediatric intensive care unit. Such practices, although likely valid, were established largely on the basis of experience, not scientific study.

Complications of adenotonsillectomy include postoperative death, hemorrhage, pain, airway compromise, and respiratory distress.[5, 64–66] Many centers assume that children undergoing adenotonsillectomy for OSAS are at higher risk for postoperative complications and, therefore, perform all such procedures on an inpatient basis. Williams and associates recently reported a postoperative complication rate of 27% for children undergoing adenotonsillectomy for OSAS.[65] Children under 3 years of age have been shown to have a higher incidence of airway complications after adenotonsillectomy for OSAS.[66] McColley and associates have shown that an increased likelihood of postadenotonsillectomy respiratory compromise is associated with young age, OSA frequency of more than 10 per hour documented on PSG, suboptimal growth, EKG or echocardiogram abnormalities, or craniofacial deformities.[5] Price and associates recently reported a respiratory complication rate of approximately 19% in children undergoing tonsil and adenoid surgery for upper airway obstruction.[67] They described several preoperative "danger signals" of postoperative complications including severity of OSA, EDS, cardiomegaly, and "urgent admission for T and A."[67] The presence of a neuromuscular disorder also increases the likelihood of postoperative respiratory compromise.[68] Patients with pulmonary hypertension are at high risk for intraoperative complications including death,[36] and postoperative complications including full respiratory arrest.[69]

Although current literature supports the contention that adenotonsillectomy for childhood OSAS should be performed on an inpatient basis,[5, 36, 65, 66, 69] there is still debate about the merits of outpatient versus inpatient surgery for these children.[70, 71] Reiner and associates recently reported that if patients are carefully selected most adenotonsillectomies (even for OSAS) can be performed on an outpatient basis.[70] In addition, they found no association between complication rates and indication for surgery, age, gender, and type of procedure, stating that ". . . there is no increased risk associated for outpatient surgery in those patients with the diagnosis of obstructive sleep apnea."[70] Because the implications of this statement are far-reaching, it is worth asking whether such a conclusion can be reached at the present time. Abundant anecdotal reports of death and other serious complications following adenotonsillectomy for childhood OSAS suggest that caution is warranted. First, the diagnosis of OSAS in the study of Reiner and associates was not established by PSG but by a history of snoring and observed apnea or labored breathing.[70] Therefore, the OSA group in this study most likely was a mixed sample consisting of some children with benign (primary) snoring and others with OSAS. Second, this study only looked at traditional complications, with no specific focus on respiratory complications. Airway compromise, hypoxemia, and hypercarbia in children not being continuously monitored for these complications will be underestimated. Third, according to study design, 60% of the patients spent their first postoperative night outside of the hospital, unobserved by medical personnel. Sleep-related airway compromise and hypoxemia would not be detected by many if not most parents. Finally the study group, although composed of 1000 patients, was not large enough to evaluate the rate of death as a complication of adenotonsillectomy for OSAS.

It seems reasonable to anticipate that the risk of postoperative respiratory compromise would be high in a group of patients whose indication for undergoing airway surgery is upper airway obstruction; several studies support this contention.[5, 65, 66, 69] Price and associates recommended evaluating each child for preoperative "danger signals" in order to determine which children may be candidates for outpatient surgery.[67] Until better information is available and firm guidelines are developed, it seems reasonable to recommend that adenotonsillectomy be performed on an inpatient basis when the indication for surgery is OSAS. Patients should be monitored postoperatively in a manner and setting in which hypoxemia and airway compromise can be rapidly detected and managed. At Johns Hopkins, children considered to be at very high risk, such as those with severe OSAS, cor pulmonale, failure-to-thrive, young age, neuromuscular disorders, or craniofacial abnormalities, undergo a thorough preoperative evaluation and are monitored postoperatively in the pediatric intensive care unit.[5]

Based on the analysis of 37 patients, Rosen and associates[71a] suggest that postoperative respiratory compromise is more likely in the following groups: children less than 2 years of age and those with craniofacial anomalies; failure-to-thrive; hypotonia; cor pulmonale; morbid obesity; previous trauma to the upper airway; severe apnea confirmed by PSG (respiratory distress index >40 or nadir SaO_2 <70%); or if uvulopalatopharyngoplasty (UPPP) is done in addition to the adenotonsillectomy. Nasal CPAP or bilevel positive airway pressure (BiPAP) were used successfully to manage upper airway obstruction in both the immediate preoperative and postoperative periods in some of the patients.

Follow-up after adenotonsillectomy is important in all children and essential in high-risk groups. At our institution, OSAS patients are scheduled for a return visit approximately 4 to 6 weeks after surgery. If there is any evidence from history or physical examination that sleep-associated airway obstruction persists, then PSG is performed. It should also be kept in mind that the long-term outcome of these children is not yet known. Parents should be counseled that symptoms may recur during respiratory tract infections, with age, or with drugs (sedation) that affect upper airway motor function.

Uvulopalatopharyngoplasty. UPPP may be effective in adults with OSAS.[72] Except for a report of a single patient,[73] there are no studies evaluating the indications for, or efficacy of, this procedure in children with OSAS. Furthermore, the long-term complications of palatal resection (e.g., velopharyngeal insufficiency) in a growing child are not known.

Tracheostomy. Tracheostomy is indicated for children with severe and/or complicated OSAS in whom other treatment approaches are either not possible or not successful. Securing a stable airway by tracheostomy may also be necessary as part of certain plastic surgery procedures in complicated patients (such as those with craniofacial abnormalities). In most children, other therapeutic approaches are successful or can at least be attempted before resorting to tracheostomy. Occasionally, tracheostomy may be performed urgently in children with severe OSAS, severe complications, and no other treatment options. Sleep-associated airway obstruction may persist even after tracheostomy. Fedok and associates reported on an 8-year-old obese child whose submental and neck panniculus was large enough to occlude a tracheostomy that had been performed earlier due to OSAS.[74] Suction-assisted lipectomy was successfully employed to reduce the bulk of neck tissues and produce a widely patent stomal area.[74]

Other Surgical Approaches. Other approaches to OSAS have been described, including inferior sagittal osteotomy of the mandible with hyoid myotomy and suspension;

maxillary, mandibular, and hyoid advancement[75]; modified UPPP; tongue "debulking" (midline partial glossectomy); partial epiglottectomy; hyoid expansion plasty[76]; and lingual tonsillectomy.[76–78] Some of these procedures have been used in selected children but have not been systematically studied. The treatment of patients with craniofacial abnormalities is complex and requires a coordinated multidisciplinary approach involving oral and plastic surgery, otolaryngology, a pediatric sleep specialist and sleep laboratory, genetics, pediatric anesthesia, and critical care.[79–84]

Mechanical Therapy

Continuous Positive Airway Pressure. CPAP has been successfully used to treat children with OSAS.[85–87] Because adenotonsillectomy is an effective treatment for OSAS in most children, CPAP has usually been reserved for children in whom surgical therapy has either failed or was not indicated or in whom it has been used in the perioperative period.[71a] Thus, for the treatment of childhood OSAS in otherwise normal children without tonsillar and adenoid hypertrophy, CPAP is currently viewed as one alternative to tracheostomy.[85, 86] Since a nasal mask or nasopharyngeal tube is used in CPAP, it is not well tolerated by some children, requires highly motivated parents, and can be easily disconnected during sleep by an active child. In spite of these disadvantages, CPAP by nasal mask has been successfully used in children as young as 3 years of age.[85] The experience at our institution is that CPAP is more likely to be successful if the child undergoes "training," which involves getting accustomed to the mask over several weeks before starting therapy. Involvement of behavioral specialists is sometimes necessary and may be a key factor for success with CPAP in some children.

A recent survey of 8 major pediatric sleep laboratories revealed that CPAP or BiPAP is more commonly used now than previously.[87a] Common indications for treating childhood OSAS with CPAP were obesity (26% of 78 OSAS patients being treated with CPAP), craniofacial anomalies (19%), OSAS persisting after adenotonsillectomy (15%), and Down syndrome (15%).[87a] CPAP therapy for OSAS was deemed successful in 78% of the children and was said to be "safe, effective, and well-tolerated" by children and adolescents.[87a] Although this was not an actual study of the safety or efficacy of CPAP use in children for

OSAS, it clearly shows that CPAP is being used in the United States and Canada to treat children with OSAS. We routinely use BiPAP for treatment of complicated OSAS in children because of increased patient compliance with its use. Patients report that BiPAP is much more comfortable to use than CPAP, and children tolerated BiPAP better than CPAP in our experience. In addition, we and others[71a] now use CPAP and BiPAP in children with severe OSAS awaiting surgery and to treat persistent sleep-related upper airway obstruction in the postoperative period.

Intraoral Appliances. Although a variety of mechanical devices aimed at reducing airway obstruction during sleep are marketed for adults with OSAS, none have been shown to be effective in children with OSAS. Since craniofacial abnormalities are more common in adults with OSA,[87a] it is intriguing to speculate whether orthodontic treatment of high-risk children might prevent the development of adult OSA. What would constitute such a high risk is presently unknown.

Medical Therapy

Weight Loss. To date there have been no studies of weight loss and OSAS in children. Obese children with OSAS do not necessarily improve after adenotonsillectomy. Attempts to obtain improvement of sleep-associated airway obstruction by dietary restriction and weight loss have been unrewarding. Very obese children, especially those with complications (e.g., cor pulmonale), may require tracheostomy. Intensive dietary counseling and follow-up may be effective in some cases; treatment often will be unsuccessful unless the entire family is involved. Extremely obese children may require inpatient dietary restriction, long-term dietary counseling, and long-term psychotherapy.

Supplemental Oxygen. At present, there is no evidence supporting the use of supplemental oxygen as a *primary* treatment for childhood OSAS. Oxygen may worsen obstructive hypoventilation. Levin and associates reported on three children with OSAS in which supplemental oxygen was given preoperatively, worsening obstructive hypoventilation and necessitating emergency assisted ventilation.[56] Supplemental oxygen used preoperatively in children with severe OSAS should be given carefully in a controlled setting with continuous monitoring, at least initially. Supplemental

oxygen has a clearer role in the immediate postoperative period. At our institution, experience shows that, when it is looked for, at least 10% of children undergoing adenotonsillectomy for OSAS have postoperative respiratory compromise defined as arterial oxyhemoglobin desaturation to 70% or less, hypercapnia, or bradycardia due to partial upper airway obstruction or nonobstructive hypoventilation.[5] A recent study of postoperative respiratory compromise in children with OSA by Rosen and associates reported similar results and risk factors.[71a] Price and associates reported an approximately 19% respiratory complication rate after adenotonsillectomy for childhood OSAS.[67] Finally, several children have shown persistent nonobstructive (central) hypoventilation for several months after surgical correction of OSAS. These children can be sent home on supplemental oxygen and followed with serial measurements of pulse oximetry during sleep until it is no longer necessary.

Pharmacologic Approaches. Numerous drugs have been evaluated for the treatment of OSAS in adults, including nasal vasoconstrictive sprays, nasal decongestants, medroxyprogesterone, acetazolamide, nicotine, almitrine, perchlorazine, tricyclic antidepressants, naloxone, theophylline, and L-tryptophan.[88] None of these agents has been shown to be effective in treating childhood OSAS. When OSA occurs in a child with chronic nasal obstruction, a trial of nasal decongestants and topical steroids seems reasonable. Experience suggests this is rarely a long-term solution. Premature infants with obstructive apnea may benefit from treatment with theophylline.[89] However, it is now known that intermittent obstructive apnea is normal in premature infants,[90] and firm guidelines for treatment in this age group have not yet been established.

Special Subgroups

Children with Severe OSAS. Patients with severe OSAS comprise a high-risk group. Many will show signs of cor pulmonale and some will exhibit overt heart failure, placing them at high risk for general anesthesia.[69] Because intraoperative death has been reported in children with severe cor pulmonale and OSAS,[36] at our institution children with severe cor pulmonale due to OSAS receive supplemental oxygen and aggressive treatment of heart failure prior to general anesthesia. Children with severe OSAS are often extremely sensitive to the effects of sedation or anesthesia on upper airway patency and must be managed carefully during induction of general anesthesia. Postoperatively these children may continue to have upper airway obstruction and hypoxemia during sleep for days, sometimes requiring up to a 2-week stay in hospital. Experience suggests that children with severe OSAS are less likely to be cured by simple adenotonsillectomy and may be more prone to a recurrence over time. Although these clinical impressions remain to be validated, it would seem prudent to anticipate and attempt to avoid complications. Brown and associates have published guidelines for the perioperative management of children with cor pulmonale due to OSAS.[69]

Pharyngeal Flap Surgery. Patients undergoing pharyngeal flap surgery are at high risk of developing severe OSA or obstructive hypoventilation postoperatively. Kravath and associates described elective surgical correction of velopharyngeal insufficiency in a 4-year-old girl who developed severe OSAS during the immediate postoperative period and died 4 weeks after surgery during an acute respiratory illness (for which she received a phenothiazine and cough medicine containing codeine).[91] Orr and associates described five children undergoing pharyngeal flap surgery, all of whom showed no upper airway obstruction during sleep before surgery and severe OSAS after surgery.[92] Management of these children is complex, ideally utilizing a team approach involving the pediatric sleep laboratory and plastic and reconstructive surgery.[93] Specific guidelines for the management of these patients have been published.[92, 94]

Craniofacial Abnormalities. Children with craniofacial abnormalities such as Pfeiffer's, Apert's, Crouzon, or Treacher Collins syndrome are at increased risk of developing OSAS. Treatment of OSAS in such children is complex, sometimes involving reconstructive facial surgery[79–83, 95, 96] with tracheostomy often as a first stage in a series of reconstructive procedures. CPAP may be effective in selected cases. Some of these children are likely to have lower respiratory problems as well. Ideally, a team approach should be taken. These children should be referred to centers with expertise in the management of craniofacial abnormalities.

Achondroplastic Dwarfism. OSAS is often seen in children with achondroplastic dwarfism. The anatomic configuration of the head, neck, and airway in combination with a small thorax and possible brainstem compression, places these children at high risk for developing OSAS and makes intubation, anesthesia, and surgery risky. Simple adenotonsillectomy is not effective in most of these children. Craniocervical decompression, which theoretically could decrease obstructed breathing during sleep, remains experimental at present.

Down Syndrome. Many children with Down syndrome and OSAS may not be effectively treated by simple adenotonsillectomy.[14, 97, 98] For any surgical procedure in these children, tongue volume (macroglossia), muscular hypotonia, and midface abnormalities must be considered. In these children, various published surgical approaches stress that the anatomic structure of each child must be assessed individually and surgery planned accordingly.[97, 98]

Neuromuscular Disorders and Mental Insufficiency. Children with mental retardation and cerebral palsy may exhibit OSAS owing to muscular hypotonia, macroglossia, and soft palate abnormalities in the absence of adenotonsillar hypertrophy.[99] Seid and associates recently outlined a surgical approach to such children.[99] On the other hand, these children do develop adenotonsillar hypertrophy but are at increased risk of complications following adenotonsillectomy.[68] Grundfast and associates recently published guidelines for the management of these patients.[68]

References

1. Carroll JL, Loughlin GM: Diagnostic criteria for obstructive sleep apnea syndrome in children. Pediatr Pulmonol 14:71, 1992.
2. Diagnostic Classification Steering Committee, Thorpy MJ (Chairman): International Classification of Sleep Disorders: Diagnostic and Coding Manual. Rochester, MI, American Association of Sleep Disorders, 1990.
3. Rosen CL, D'Andrea L, Haddad GG: Adult criteria for obstructive sleep apnea do not identify children with serious airway obstruction. Am Rev Respir Dis 146:1231, 1992.
4. van Someren VH, Hibbert J, Stothers JK, et al: Identification of hypoxaemia in children having tonsillectomy and adenoidectomy. Clin Otolaryngol 15:263, 1990.
5. McColley SA, April M, Carroll JL, et al: Predictors of respiratory compromise (RC) after adenotonsillectomy (T&A) in children with obstructive sleep apnea. Arch Otolaryngol Head Neck Surg 118:940, 1992.
6. Fernbach SK, Brouillette RT, Riggs TW, et al: Radiologic evaluation of adenoids and tonsils in children with obstructive sleep apnea: plain films and fluoroscopy. Pediatr Radiol 13:258, 1983.
7. Mauer KW, Staats BA, Olsen KD: Upper airway ob-

struction and disordered nocturnal breathing in children. Mayo Clin Proc 58:349, 1983.

8. Brouillette RT, Fernbach SK, Hunt CE: Obstructive sleep apnea in infants and children. J Pediatr 100:31, 1982.

9. Miyazaki S, Itasaka Y, Yamakawa K, et al: Respiratory disturbance during sleep due to adenoid-tonsillar hypertrophy. Am J Otolaryngol 10:143, 1989.

10. Gaultier C: Respiratory adaptation during sleep in infants. Lung 168:905, 1990.

11. Stradling JR, Thomas G, Warley AR, et al: Effect of adenotonsillectomy on nocturnal hypoxaemia, sleep disturbance, and symptoms in snoring children. Lancet 335:249, 1990.

12. Rowe LD, Hansen TN, Nielson D, et al: Continuous measurements of skin surface oxygen and carbon dioxide tensions in obstructive sleep apnea. Laryngoscope 90:1797, 1980.

13. Marcus CL, Omlin KJ, Basinski DJ, et al: Normal polysomnographic values for children and adolescents. Am Rev Respir Dis 146:1235, 1992.

13a. Marcus CL: Personal communication, 1994.

14. Marcus CL, Keens TL, Bautista DB, et al: Obstructive sleep apnea in children with Down syndrome. Pediatrics 88:132, 1991.

14a. Morielli A, Desjardins D, Brouillette RT: Transcutaneous and end-tidal carbon dioxide pressures should be measured during pediatric polysomnography. Am Rev Resp Dis 148:1599, 1993.

15. Guilleminault C, Eldrige F, Simmons FB, et al: Sleep apnea in eight children. Pediatrics 58:23, 1976.

16. Canet E, Gaultier C, D'Allest AM, et al: Effects of sleep deprivation on respiratory events during sleep in healthy infants. J Appl Physiol 66:1158, 1989.

17. Gaultier C: Respiratory disorders during sleep in children. [Troubles respiratoires au cours du sommeil de l'enfant] Rev Prat 39:21, 1989.

18. Gaultier C: Respiratory adaptation during sleep from the neonatal period to adolescence. *In* Guilleminault C (ed): Sleep and Its Disorders in Children. New York, Raven Press, 1987, pp 67–98.

19. Chipps GA, Mak H, Schuberth KC, et al: Nocturnal oxygen saturation in normal and asthmatic children. Pediatrics 65:1157, 1980.

20. Smith TF, Hudgel DW: Arterial oxygen desaturation during sleep in children with asthma and its relation to airway obstruction and ventilatory drive. Pediatrics 66:746, 1980.

21. Mallory GB Jr, Fiser DH, Jackson R: Sleep-associated breathing disorders in morbidly obese children and adolescents. J Pediatr 115:892, 1989.

22. Marcus CL, Keens TG, Davidson Ward SL: Comparison of nap and overnight polysomnography in children. Pediatr Pulmonol 13:16, 1992.

23. Biban P, Baraldi E, Pettenazzo A, et al: Adverse effect of chloral hydrate in two young children with obstructive sleep apnea. Pediatrics 92:461, 1993.

24. Potsic WP: Comparison of polysomnography and sonography for assessing regularity of respiration during sleep in adenotonsillar hypertrophy. Laryngoscope 97:1430, 1987.

25. van Someren VH, Hibbert J, Stothers JK, et al: Identifying hypoxaemia in children admitted for adenotonsillectomy. Br Med J 298:1076, 1989.

26. Swift AC: Upper airway obstruction, sleep disturbance and adenotonsillectomy in children. J Laryngol Otol 102:419, 1988.

27. Butt W, Robertson C, Phelan P: Snoring in children: is it pathological? Med J Aust 143:335, 1985.

28. Weider DJ, Sateia MJ, West RP: Nocturnal enuresis in children with upper airway obstruction. Otolaryngol Head Neck Surg 105:427, 1991.

29. Smith TC, Proops DW, Pearman K, et al: Nasal capnography in children: automated analysis provides a measure of obstruction during sleep. Clin Otolaryngol 18:69, 1993.

30. Smith TH, Baska ER, Francisco CB, et al: Sleep apnea syndrome: diagnosis of upper airway obstruction by fluoroscopy. J Pediatr 93:891, 1978.

31. Felman AH, Loughlin GM, Leftridge CA Jr, et al: Upper airway obstruction during sleep in children. AJR Am J Roentgenol 133:213, 1979.

32. Richardson MA, Seid AB, Cotton RT, et al: Evaluation of tonsils and adenoids in sleep apnea syndrome. Laryngoscope 90:1106, 1980.

33. Fan LL: Transnasal fiberoptic endoscopy in children with obstructive apnea. Crit Care Med 12:590, 1984.

34. Croft CB, Thomson HG, Samuels MP, et al: Endoscopic evaluation and treatment of sleep-associated upper airway obstruction in infants and young children. Clin Otolaryngol 15:209, 1990.

35. Marsh RR, Potsic WP, Pasquariello PS: Reliability of sleep sonography in detecting upper airway obstruction in children. Int J Pediatr Otorhinolaryngol 18:1, 1989.

36. Wilkinson AR, McCormick MS, Freeland AP, et al: Electrocardiographic signs of pulmonary hypertension in children who snore. Br Med J 282:579, 1981.

37. Noonan JA: Reversible cor pulmonale due to hypertrophied tonsils and adenoids: studies in two cases. Circulation 32:164, 1965.

38. Osler W: Chronic Tonsillitis. *In* The Principles and Practice of Medicine. New York, Appleton and Co, 1892, pp 335–339.

39. Menashe VD, Farrehi C, Miller M: Hypoventilation and cor pulmonale due to chronic upper airway obstruction. J Pediatr 67:198, 1965.

40. Cox MA, Schiebler GL, Taylor WJ, et al: Reversible pulmonary hypertension in a child with respiratory obstruction and cor pulmonale. J Pediatr 67:192, 1965.

41. Luke MJ, Mehrizi A, Folger GM, et al: Chronic nasopharyngeal obstruction as a cause of cardiomegaly, cor pulmonale, and pulmonary edema. Pediatrics 37:762, 1966.

42. Levy AM, Tabakin BS, Hanson JS, et al: Hypertrophied adenoids causing pulmonary hypertension and severe congestive heart failure. N Engl J Med 277:507, 1967.

43. Ainger LE: Large tonsils and adenoids in small children with cor pulmonale. Br Heart J 30:356, 1968.

44. Setliff RC, Puyau FA, Ward PH: Pulmonary hypertension secondary to chronic upper airway obstruction. Laryngoscope 78:845, 1968.

45. Gerald B, Dungan WT: Cor pulmonale and pulmonary edema in children secondary to chronic upper airway obstruction. Radiology 90:679, 1968.

46. Cayler GG, Johnson EE, Lewis BE, et al: Heart failure due to enlarged tonsils and adenoids. Am J Dis Child 118:708, 1969.

47. Macartney FJ, Panday J, Scott O: Cor pulmonale as a result of chronic nasopharyngeal obstruction due to hypertrophied tonsils and adenoids. Arch Dis Child 44:585, 1969.

48. Formica U, Fiocchi A: Pulmonary heart disease caused by chronic obstruction of the upper respiratory tract due to hypertrophy of adenoids and tonsils. Review of the literature and report of a personal case. Minerva Pediatr 21:908, 1969.

49. Massumi RA, Sarin RK, Pooya M, et al: Tonsillar hypertrophy, airway obstruction, alveolar hypoventilation, and cor pulmonale in twin brothers. Dis Chest 55:110, 1969.

50. Freeman WJ: Adenoid hypertrophy, cyanosis and cor pulmonale, in children with congenital heart disease. Laryngoscope 83:238, 1973.

51. Talbot AR, Robertson LW: Cardiac failure with tonsil and adenoid hypertrophy. Arch Otolaryngol 98:277, 1973.

52. Edison BD, Kerth JD: Tonsilloadenoid hypertrophy resulting in cor pulmonale. Arch Otolaryngol 98:205, 1973.

53. Simmons FB, Hill MW: Hypersomnia caused by upper airway obstructions: a new syndrome in otolaryngology. Ann Otol 83:670, 1974.

54. Djalilian M, Kern EB, Brown HA, et al: Hypoventilation secondary to chronic upper airway obstruction in childhood. Mayo Clin Proc 50:11, 1975.

55. Thanopoulos B, Ikkos DD, Milingos M, et al: Cardiorespiratory syndrome due to enlarged tonsils and adenoids. A case report with discussion regarding medical treatment and pathogenesis. Acta Paediatr Scand 64:659, 1975.

56. Levin DL, Muster AJ, Pachman LM, et al: Cor pulmonale secondary to upper airway obstruction: cardiac catheterization, immunologic, and psychometric evaluation in nine patients. Chest 68:166, 1975.

57. Goodman RS, Goodman M, Gootman N, et al: Cardiac and pulmonary failure secondary to adenotonsillar hypertrophy. Laryngoscope 86:1367, 1976.

58. Kravath RE, Pollak CP, Borowiecki B: Hypoventilation during sleep in children who have lymphoid airway obstruction treated by nasopharyngeal tube and T and A. Pediatrics 59:865, 1977.

59. Guilleminault C, Korobkin R, Winkle R: A review of 50 children with obstructive sleep apnea syndrome. Lung 159:275, 1981.

60. Guilleminault C, Winkle R, Korobkin R, et al: Children and nocturnal snoring: evaluation of the effects of sleep related respiratory resistive load and daytime functioning. Eur J Pediatr 139:165, 1982.

61. Frank Y, Kravath RE, Pollak CP, et al: Obstructive sleep apnea and its therapy: clinical and polysomnographic manifestations. Pediatrics 71:737, 1983.

62. Potsic WP, Pasquariello PS, Baranak CC, et al: Relief of upper airway obstruction by adenotonsillectomy. Otolaryngol Head Neck Surg 94:476, 1986.

63. Rosenfeld RM, Green RP: Tonsillectomy and adenoidectomy: changing trends. Ann Otol Rhinol Laryngol 99:187, 1990.

64. Rasmussen N: Complications of tonsillectomy and adenoidectomy. Otolaryngol Clin North Am 20:383, 1987.

65. Williams EF, Woo P, Miller R, et al: The effects of adenotonsillectomy on growth in young children. Otolaryngol Head Neck Surg 104:509, 1991.

66. Wiatrak BJ, Myer CM, 3d, Andrews TM: Complications of adenotonsillectomy in children under 3 years of age. Am J Otolaryngol 12:170, 1991.

67. Price SD, Hawkins DB, Kahlstrom EJ: Tonsil and adenoid surgery for airway obstruction: perioperative respiratory mobidity. Ear Nose Throat J 72:526, 1993.

68. Grundfast K, Berkowitz R, Fox L: Outcome and complications following surgery for obstructive adenotonsillar hypertrophy in children with neuromuscular disorders. Ear Nose Throat J 69:756, 1990.

69. Brown OE, Manning SC, Ridenour B: Cor pulmonale secondary to tonsillar and adenoidal hypertrophy:

management considerations. Int J Pediatr Otorhinolaryngol 16:131, 1988.

70. Reiner SA, Sawyer WP, Clark KF, et al: Safety of outpatient tonsillectomy and adenoidectomy. Otolaryngol Head Neck Surg 102:161, 1990.

71. Shott SR, Myer CM, 3rd, Cotton RT: Efficacy of tonsillectomy and adenoidectomy as an outpatient procedure: a preliminary report. Int J Pediatr Otorhinolaryngol 13:157, 1987.

71a. Rosen GM, Muckle RP, Mahowald MW, et al: Postoperative respiratory compromise in children with obstructive sleep apnea syndrome: can it be anticipated? Pediatrics 93:784, 1994.

72. Shepard JW, Olsen KD: Uvulopalatopharyngoplasty for treatment of obstructive sleep apnea. Mayo Clin Proc 65:1260, 1990.

73. Abdu MH, Feghali JG: Uvulopalatopharyngoplasty in a child with obstructive sleep apnea. A case report. J Laryngol Otol 102:546, 1988.

74. Fedok FG, Houck JR, Manders EK: Suction-assisted lipectomy in the management of obstructive sleep apnea. Arch Otolaryngol Head Neck Surg 116:968, 1990.

75. Riley RW, Powell N, Guilleminault C: Current surgical concepts for treating obstructive sleep apnea syndrome. J Oral Maxillofac Surg 45:149, 1987.

76. Fujita S: Pharyngeal surgery for obstructive sleep apnea and snoring. *In* Fairbanks DNF (ed): Snoring and Obstructive Sleep Apnea. New York, Raven Press, 1987, pp 101–128.

77. Phillips DE, Rogers JH: Down's syndrome with lingual tonsil hypertrophy producing sleep apnoea. J Laryngol Otol 102:1054, 1988.

78. Guarisco JL, Littlewood SC, Butcher RB, 3d: Severe upper airway obstruction in children secondary to lingual tonsil hypertrophy. Ann Otol Rhinol Laryngol 99:621, 1990.

79. Kuo PC, West RA, Bloomquist DS, et al: The effect of mandibular osteotomy in three patients with hypersomnia sleep apnea. Oral Surg Oral Med Oral Pathol 48:385, 1979.

80. Mixter RC, David DJ, Perloff WH, et al: Obstructive sleep apnea in Apert's and Pfeiffer's syndromes: more than a craniofacial abnormality. Plast Reconstr Surg 86:457, 1990.

81. Schafer ME: Upper airway obstruction and sleep disorders in children with craniofacial anomalies. Clin Plast Surg 9:555, 1982.

82. Lauritzen C, Lilja J, Jarlstedt J: Airway obstruction and sleep apnea in children with craniofacial anomalies. Plastic Reconstr Surg 77:1, 1986.

83. McGill T: Otolaryngologic aspects of Apert syndrome. Clin Plast Surg 18:309, 1991.

84. Colmenero C, Esteban R, Albarino AR, et al: Sleep apnoea syndrome associated with maxillofacial abnormalities. J Laryngol Otol 105:94, 1991.

85. Guilleminault C, Nino-Murcia G, Heldt G, et al: Alternative treatment to tracheostomy in obstructive sleep apnea syndrome: nasal continuous positive airway pressure in young children. Pediatrics 78:797, 1986.

86. Klein M, Reynolds LG: Relief of sleep-related oropharyngeal airway obstruction by continuous insufflation of the pharynx. Lancet 1:935, 1986.

87. Ryan CF, Lowe AA, Fleetham JA: Nasal continuous positive airway pressure (CPAP) therapy for obstructive sleep apnea in Hallermann-Streiff syndrome. Clin Pediatr (Phila) 29:122, 1990.

87a. Marcus CL, Brooks LJ, Ward SLD, et al: CPAP use for treatment of childhood obstructive sleep apnea syndrome. Am J Respir Crit Care Med 149:A886, 1994.

87b. Pracharktam N, Hans MG, Strohl KP, et al: Upright and supine cephalometric evaluation of obstructive sleep apnea syndrome and snoring subjects. Angle Orthod 64:63, 1994.

88. Strohl KP, Cherniack NS, and Gothe B: Physiologic basis of therapy for sleep apnea. Am Rev Respir Dis 134:791, 1986.

89. Roberts JL, Mathew OP, Thach BT: The efficacy of theophylline in premature infants with mixed and obstructive apnea and apnea associated with pulmonary and neurologic disease. J Pediatr 100:968, 1982.

90. Barrington KJ, Finer NN: Periodic breathing and apnea in preterm infants. Pediatr Res 27:118, 1990.

91. Kravath RE, Pollak CP, Borowiecki B, et al: Obstructive sleep apnea and death associated with surgical correction of velopharyngeal incompetence. J Pediatr 96:645, 1980.

92. Orr WC, Levine NS, Buchanan RT: Effect of cleft palate repair and pharyngeal flap surgery on upper airway obstruction during sleep. Plast Reconstr Surg 80:226;230, 1987.

93. Barot LR, Pearlman M, Freed G, et al: Nasal airway blockage caused by displaced premaxilla mimicking posterior pharyngeal flap obstruction. Ann Plast Surg 21:77, 1988.

94. Randall P: Effect of cleft palate repair and pharyngeal flap surgery on upper airway obstruction during sleep (discussion). Plast Reconstr Surg 80:231, 1987.

95. Shapiro J, Strome M, Crocker AC: Airway obstruction and sleep apnea in Hurler and Hunter syndromes. Ann Otol Rhinol Laryngol 94:458;461, 1985.

96. Ruckenstein MJ, Macdonald RE, Clarke JTR, et al: The management of otolaryngological problems in the mucopolysaccharidoses: a retrospective review. J Otolaryngol 20:177;183, 1991.

97. Donaldson JD, Redmond WM: Surgical management of obstructive sleep apnea in children with Down syndrome. J Otolaryngol 17:398, 1988.

98. Strome M: Obstructive sleep apnea in Down syndrome children: a surgical approach. Laryngoscope 96:1340, 1986.

99. Seid AB, Martin PJ, Pransky SM, et al: Surgical therapy of obstructive sleep apnea in children with severe mental insufficiency. Laryngoscope 100:507, 1990.

Sleep and Respiratory Disease in Children

GERALD M. LOUGHLIN and JOHN L. CARROLL

Alterations in breathing that occur during sleep[1,2] and in response to circadian rhythms,[3] are typically of little consequence in children with normal lungs. However, for children with underlying lung disease and limited pulmonary reserve, the normal effects of sleep on breathing can lead to clinically significant ventilatory and gas exchange abnormalities.[1,4-6] As medical care of premature infants has improved, the number of infants surviving with chronic lung disease has grown. Childhood asthma affects as many as 15 to 20% of children in industrialized countries, and its prevalence and severity may even be increasing.[7] Children with cystic fibrosis (CF), a genetically transmitted disorder of the lungs and pancreatic exocrine function, are surviving longer, but still suffer from life-long chronic lung disease. Pediatricians and sleep medicine specialists evaluating and caring for children should be aware of the effects of sleep on the pathophysiology and clinical course of chronic lung disease. This chapter reviews what is known about the interaction between sleep and breathing in normal infants and children and those with common chronic pulmonary diseases, including bronchopulmonary dysplasia (BPD), and asthma.

Breathing During Sleep in Normal Children

Minute ventilation decreases, breathing patterns change, PaO_2 decreases, and $PaCO_2$ increases during sleep in normal children. Several mechanisms occurring alone or in combination are responsible for these sleep-related changes in breathing. During sleep, lung volume decreases; specifically, functional residual capacity (FRC) (resting end-expiratory lung volume) declines during sleep. Because the lungs are the major reservoir of oxygen for the body, a sleep-related decline in FRC means that total body oxygen stores are lower during sleep. A decline in FRC may also alter ventilation/perfusion relationships, decreasing the overall ability of the lungs to take up oxygen and expel CO_2. Finally, the increased muscular effort associated with paradoxical inward rib cage motion (PIRCM) may contribute to increased oxygen consumption during sleep.[8]

There are also age-dependent mechanical factors that affect breathing and gas exchange during sleep. The rib cage of the infant and toddler is circular shaped and does not achieve a mature ellipsoid configuration until after 4 years of age. This circular shape of the thorax causes the angle of diaphragm insertion to be horizontal in the infant versus oblique in the adult. In children older than 4 years of age, diaphragm contraction lifts the rib cage, pivoting the ribs at their attachments to the vertebral column, and thereby expanding the chest. In infants, because the diaphragm attachment is perpendicular rather than oblique, contraction of the diaphragm is inefficient, partially wasting energy in chest wall distortion instead of expanding the thorax.[9] Lung diseases that cause hyperinflation may aggravate this situation by shifting the diaphragm muscle to an even less efficient position on its length-tension curve.[10] FRC in adults and older children is the result of a balance between the inward elastic recoil forces of the lung and the outward pull of the chest wall. However, in infants, because the chest wall is more compliant, the outward pull of the rib cage is less, and FRC is relatively lower than in older children. The effect of this would be marginally adequate oxygen stores and atelectasis were it not for the fact that infants actively maintain FRC at a higher volume than passive end-expiratory lung volume.[10, 11] For the most part, this is achieved by a combination of active glottic narrowing during expiration and initiation of the next inspiration before passive expiration is complete.[10, 11] Although awake infants can easily compensate for the high chest wall compliance and inefficient mechanical arrangement of the diaphragm, the ability of sleeping infants to compensate may be decreased, especially in REM sleep. The tonic activity of the diaphragm muscles are reduced during REM sleep. In normal infants and young children, the highly compliant rib cage is actively stabilized by contraction of the intercostal muscles during inspiration. Thus, infants expend energy to prevent the rib cage from collapsing during the inspiratory phase of breathing. During REM sleep, when tonic and phasic activity of the intercostal muscles are absent, the rib cage is no longer actively stabilized and therefore moves inward during inspiration.[12] Because the rib cage should normally expand during inspiration, the inward movement of the rib cage during inspiration is called paradoxical inward rib cage movement (PIRCM) (Fig. 20–1). In children with normal lung function, PIRCM occurs predominantly but not exclusively during REM sleep.[12] The frequency of paradoxical breathing decreases over the first year of life (Fig. 20–2) and PIRCM is not found in normal adolescents.[13] Other mechanisms, such as the active maintenance of FRC above passive end-expiratory lung volume, are also affected by sleep. However, little is known about the extent to which sleep and sleep states affect the upper airway component of this active system. The observation that pharyngeal muscle tone decreases during REM sleep suggests that the contribution of the upper airway may also be altered during REM sleep.[14] The effects of sleep and, in particular, sleep states on lung volume and gas exchange in infants and children remain controversial. Hendersen-Smart found decreases in FRC of up to 30% associated with the onset of REM sleep in infants.[15] However, in other studies this finding could not be confirmed in either term[16] or preterm infants,[17]

and the decreases in FRC observed in these studies were considerably smaller than that reported by Hendersen-Smart.[15] Differences between these studies may be reconciled if one looks at the occurrence of asynchronous breathing, since in a subsequent study FRC was shown to decrease significantly during periods of PIRCM in both sleep states.[18] It would appear that in infants PIRCM may be a more important determinant of lung volume than sleep stage per se.

The findings in adolescents and young adults are somewhat more consistent. Muller and associates, although not measuring FRC directly, concluded from shifts in the position of the rib cage and abdomen, recorded by uncalibrated magnetometers, that the decrease in SaO_2 seen in normal controls (mean age 26.2 yr) was due to a lowering of FRC associated with REM sleep.[19] Similarly, Hudgel and coworkers[20] demonstrated small but statistically significant decreases in FRC from the awake baseline during both REM and Stage 3–4 NREM sleep in normal young adults. There was no difference in FRC between REM and stage 3–4 NREM sleep in this study. Changes in FRC were small and not sufficient to cause clinically significant effects on gas exchange. It was not stated if PIRCM was present during REM sleep in this group, but it is unlikely since these subjects were adults.[21] More work is needed in children of all ages to determine, in the same subject, the effects of transition from wakefulness to REM and NREM sleep, correlated with identification of PIRCM in each of these sleep states.

These changes in lung volume cause minimal alterations in gas exchange in normal children. Oxygenation may be more affected than CO_2 exchange because oxygen exchange is more affected by ventilation/perfusion mismatching. In normal neonates, $TcPO_2$ was on the average approximately 7 mmHg less during the asynchronous breathing of active sleep than during the regular breathing of quiet sleep.[8] In contrast, no significant change in $TcPO_2$ occurs during PIRCM in older infants (7–31 mo) without lung disease.[12] In older children and adolescents, small decreases in oxygen saturation during sleep have been reported. Chipps and associates,[22] in a study of children with asthma, identified in the normal control group a mean maximal change in SaO_2 of 2.2% associated with the onset of sleep assessed behaviorally. In a study of normal adolescents (5 males, 4 females, mean age 15 yr), Tabachnik and coworkers reported a mean fall

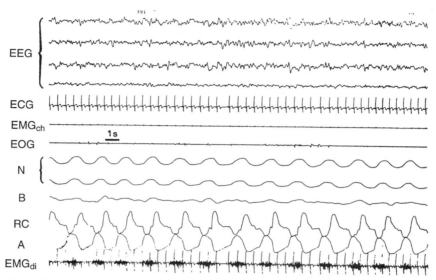

Figure 20–1. Sleep recording of a 10-month-old infant during REM sleep. PIRCM on inspiration was present during the inspiratory phasic diaphragmatic activity. Electroencephalogram (EEG), electro-oculogram (EOG), chin electromyogram (EMGch), nasal (N) and buccal (B) thermistors, rib cage (RC) and abdominal (A) anteroposterior diameters (magnetometers), and diaphragmatic electromyographic activity (EMG$_{di}$) (surface electrodes). (From Gaultier C, et al: Paradoxical inward rib cage motion during rapid eye movement sleep in infants and young children. J Dev Physiol 9:391, 1987.)

in SaO_2 from the awake baseline of 1.5% during NREM sleep and 1.4% during REM sleep.[13] Smith and associates found greater changes in saturation (mean maximal changes from baseline of 5.6%) in the normal control population of children and adolescents with asthma (the large changes they found have been attributed to the effects of altitude).[23]

There are limited data on $PaCO_2$ during

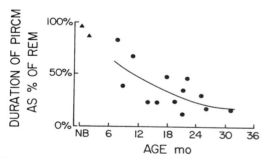

Figure 20–2. Age in months is displayed on the abscissa (NB, newborns). Duration of PIRCM on inspiration expressed as a percentage of REM sleep time is displayed on the ordinate. Full circles are individual values of PIRCM in the tested infants from 7 to 31 months. Duration of PIRCM decreased significantly with age as a power function (r = −.66, P<0.02). Triangles are data from published values in neonates. (From Gaultier C, et al: Paradoxical inward rib cage motion during rapid eye movement sleep in infants and young children. J Dev Physiol 9:391, 1987.)

sleep in children. Marcus and associates reported end-tidal CO_2 in a group of children (mean age 9.7 ± 4.6 years) without underlying lung disease during overnight PSG.[24] End-tidal CO_2 values greater than 50 mmHg were seen in 6% of these normal children. These authors used the standard definition of hypoventilation, PCO_2 greater than 45 mmHg, and found that normal children "hypoventilate" for up to 60% of total sleep time.[24] Although reference values will likely change as more data becomes available, it appears that, if the current standard definition is used, mild hypoventilation occurs in some normal children during sleep, especially during NREM sleep, and appears to occur without clinical consequence. There were no sleep state specific data included in this report.[24] However, a study in normal adolescents demonstrated a state-dependent variation in minute ventilation during sleep; a mean decrease of 8% was observed in minute ventilation at the transition from awake to NREM sleep and a mean increase of 4% with the change to REM from NREM sleep.[12] These changes are of little consequence in children with normal lung function, but, as shown in adults, periods of mild hypoventilation during sleep may contribute to gas exchange abnormalities in patients with obstructive lung disease.[6, 24–26]

How the child responds to respiratory challenges is also affected by sleep. In neonates, the response to hypoxia is biphasic (an initial increase in minute ventilation followed by a decrease) when the infant is awake and in REM sleep.[27] During NREM sleep the ventilatory response to hypoxia has been reported to be better sustained than in REM sleep.[27] Adult males demonstrate a decreased hypoxic response during both REM and NREM sleep,[28] although adult females have a decreased hypoxic response only during REM sleep.[29] How this data applies to prepubertal children is unclear, but one might anticipate that the gender differences might not exist.

In adults and children, the response to CO_2 is decreased compared with the awake state in both NREM and REM sleep.[30, 31] A decreased CO_2 response in REM sleep has been found in some but not all studies of infants.[32, 33]

There are limited data on the response to loaded breathing in infants and children. In neonates, the response to a resistive load is characterized by an increase in ventilation in NREM but not in REM sleep.[34] Work by Issa and Sullivan demonstrated a progressive increase in respiratory effort in response to airway occlusion in NREM sleep and a change in breathing pattern to one characterized by rapid shallow breathing in REM sleep.[35] However, a decrease in the ventilatory response to both acute and sustained resistive loaded breathing was seen in NREM sleep in young adults.[36] How chronic lung disease and the accompanying hypoxemia, hypercapnia, or increased airway resistance during infancy affects the maturation of these normal responses is unknown. Abnormalities of normal ventilatory defense mechanisms during sleep may play a role in complications of chronic lung disease, such as the increased incidence of sudden death during sleep in infants with BPD.

Circadian Factors

Some changes in minute ventilation and lung function that have been attributed to sleep are actually related to normal circadian variability and not sleep per se.[3] The lowest peak expiratory flow rate of the day is seen during the early morning hours. Since circadian variability appears to have its greatest impact on asthma, it will be discussed in more detail in that section. However, it should be kept in mind that circadian rhythms will affect lung function in all patients, especially those with underlying airway hyperreactivity.

Specific Disease Conditions

Bronchopulmonary Dysplasia

BPD is a form of chronic lung disease in infants and young children, arising as a consequence of an acute lung injury in the newborn period and as a complication of the therapy required to treat it. Major criteria for the diagnosis of BPD include persistent respiratory abnormalities (clinical and radiographic) and the need for supplemental oxygen beyond 1 month of age.[37]

BPD may result in persistent gas exchange and pulmonary function abnormalities for years, although supplemental oxygen can be discontinued in most infants by about 1 year of age.[37, 38] Gas exchange abnormalities may be most severe during sleep.[6] Garg and associates, in a study of 14 infants with BPD, demonstrated sleep-related decreases in SaO_2.[6] The mechanisms responsible for desaturation during sleep were not determined except to rule out central apnea as a cause of the hypoxemia.[6] Since this study did not measure nasal airflow or end-tidal CO_2, it is possible that obstructive hypoventilation or apnea contributed to the hypoxemia. However, Rome and associates could not confirm this hypothesis.[39] They found PIRCM during both active and quiet sleep in a group of infants with BPD; controls only exhibited PIRCM during active sleep. The effect of active sleep (REM) on gas exchange was the same in both groups. However, the BPD group had lower SaO_2 and higher CO_2 values than controls in all sleep states. The differences in these studies may be explained by differences in severity of underlying lung disease and by the shorter duration of monitoring (< 2 hr) in the study of Rome and associates.[39]

Hypoxemia during sleep may also be seen in older children with a past history of BPD. Loughlin and associates reported on children with BPD (3–5 yr in age) who were found on repeated measurements to have adequate awake SaO_2 (>93%), but when studied overnight in the PSG laboratory had marked and prolonged desaturation episodes (Fig. 20–3).[40] The pattern of oxygen desaturation was similar to that seen in adults with chronic obstructive lung disease (COPD), with the worst episodes of desaturation in REM sleep. SaO_2 was maintained in all cases for at least 30 minutes after falling asleep, before a decline in saturation was observed. The same finding was also noted by Gaultier and coworkers who also reported

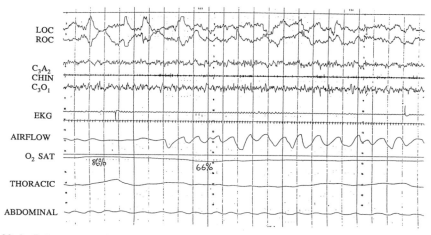

Figure 20–3. Polysomnography during REM sleep from a child with resolving BPD (SaO_2 >94%) Note diminished airflow, thoracic signal, and desaturation associated with REM sleep. LOC and ROC, left and right electro-oculograms; Chin, electromyogram; C_3A_2 and C_3O_1, electroencephalogram.

REM sleep-related increases in $PtcCO_2$, PIRCM, and episodes of obstructive apnea.[41]

The experience at the Johns Hopkins Pediatric Sleep Center is that sleep-related hypoxemic episodes in infants with lung disease may be clinically significant and affect cardiac function. Several children have been encountered with BPD (age 3–4 yr) who experienced worsening of cor pulmonale after being weaned off of supplemental oxygen (based on saturation values obtained during wakefulness).[40] These children were found to have extended periods of desaturation below 90% during sleep. Values as low as 60% were found during REM sleep. Even mild hypoxemia (SaO_2 between 90 and 95%) may have effects on the variability of heart rate.[41a]

Although undetected hypoxemia is a common cause of cardiac complications in infants with BPD, it is not the only culprit. Work by Praud and associates using radionuclide evaluation of cardiac function in a comparably aged group of children with BPD, demonstrated marked effects on cardiac function of PIRCM during sleep (Fig. 20–4).[42] Both the left and right ventricular ejection fractions (LVEF, RVEF) were significantly reduced during sleep, although effects on the RV were greater. In the two subjects with the most significant PIRCM and desaturation, RVEF was reduced by approximately 56%.[42] These findings provide strong evidence for a relationship between sleep-related breathing changes and the development of cor pulmonale seen in infants with BPD. Other consequences of the LV dysfunction seen in these patients are not as well

described, but reduced cerebral blood flow leading to insufficient brain oxygen delivery is a potentially important possibility.

Several studies have reported an increase in the occurrence of sudden death in infants recovering from BPD.[43–45] Those infants were often those who required long-term supplemental oxygen therapy. Possible mechanisms underlying the higher rate of sudden unexpected death are not known, but it is likely that abnormal ventilatory and/or arousal responses during sleep are a factor. Garg and associates showed that infants with BPD have very abnormal responses to hypoxic challenge.[46] In their study, infants with BPD, previously weaned from supplemental oxygen, were challenged by having them breathe a hypoxic gas mixture while asleep. Although 11 of the 12 infants eventually aroused from sleep, the arousal response was not normal; all of the infants required vigorous stimulation and supplemental oxygen following the challenge.[46] This suggests that normal defense mechanisms, such as the ability to arouse from sleep during hypoxia, may be defective in infants with BPD. Since infants with BPD are known to develop occult episodes of hypoxemia during sleep, defective hypoxic arousal is a plausible mechanism for explaining sudden unexpected death. Arousal responses to hypoxia depend, in large part, on the carotid chemoreceptors. This suggests that infants with BPD may have abnormalities in hypoxia chemoreflex responses during sleep.[47, 48]

A comprehensive discussion of BPD management is beyond the scope of this chapter.

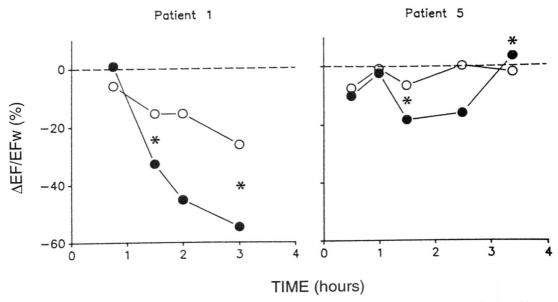

Figure 20–4. Variation of LVEF (open circles) and RVEF (closed circles) during sleep in patient 1 with oxygen desaturation and in patient 5 without oxygen desaturation. On the abscissa, zero time is the time of 99mTc injection. Each LVEF and RVEF value is reported as the relative variation (ΔEF/EFw) from the value measured during wakefulness (EFw). (*) data obtained during REM sleep. Note the large decrease in LVEF and RVEF measurements in patient 1 who had the lower SaO_2 values during sleep compared with patient 5. (From Praud JP, et al: Radionuclide evaluation of cardiac function during sleep in children with bronchopulmonary dysplasia. Chest 100:721, 1991.)

However, it is important to discuss those aspects of management potentially affected by sleep. Currently there is no consensus on how best to determine daytime and nighttime supplemental oxygen needs in these patients. If SaO_2 is abnormal while the infant is awake, then it is very likely to be worse during sleep. Even if SaO_2 is normal while the infant is awake, it still may be abnormal during sleep. Therefore, all infants with BPD, whose awake SaO_2 is in a low-normal range (90–95%), should have SaO_2 recorded by pulse oximetry during an extended period while asleep. Although there is no agreement on the precise definition of how long an "extended period" should last, brief (several minutes) or intermittent (spot checking) of oxygen saturation during sleep is likely to miss episodes of desaturation and lead to underestimation of the severity of hypoxemia.[49, 50] Our recommendation is to monitor SaO_2 during sleep for an entire night if possible, or at least during a nap that includes one or more REM periods. Because monitoring for an entire night is not always practical, it may be acceptable to screen infants by measuring SaO_2 while the infant is awake (approximately 10–15 min) and during a nap (for a similar time period). However,

the minimal amount of testing for adequately assessing day and nighttime oxygenation has not been established by scientific study.

Criteria for when to decrease or discontinue oxygen therapy are also not yet standardized. If the SaO_2 on a particular inspired oxygen concentration (FIO_2) is found to be consistently above 95%, decreasing the FIO_2 can be attempted. Daytime (awake) supplemental oxygen is usually weaned first. However, measuring SaO_2 for several minutes during a clinic visit can be misleading. The authors have discontinued daytime supplemental oxygen in infants who exhibit a normal saturation after 20 minutes off oxygen during a clinic visit only to find on extended oximetry a progressive decline in SaO_2 over the following 48 hours. Follow-up of these infants is extremely important after supplemental oxygen has been discontinued.

What constitutes adequate oxygenation during sleep in children with BPD is unclear.[51] Studies have shown that maintaining SaO_2 above 92% in infants with resolving BPD was successful in facilitating growth and minimizing the risk of cor pulmonale.[38] During the course of weaning from supplemental oxygen, the child's neurodevelopmental progress, growth, cardiorespiratory status, and hematocrit should be checked regularly. Deterioration from the pattern established on the higher oxygen concentration warrants a more thorough evaluation of the child's oxygenation, including measurement during an extended sleep period. This can be done in a sleep laboratory or in the child's home using a portable oximeter coupled to a data storage device. Intermittent abbreviated oxygenation measurements during sleep are inadequate and may give misleading information.[50] Monitoring can be of daytime naps if that is all that can be obtained, but all sleep monitoring (night and day) should be sufficiently long to include periods of REM sleep since these are the most likely times for significant hypoxemia to occur.[40, 41]

Cardiorespiratory monitoring should be considered for all infants with BPD on supplemental oxygen. This recommendation is based on studies suggesting an increased mortality from sudden unexplained death in this population[43-45] and on the data of Garg and associates that demonstrated potentially life-threatening responses to hypoxic episodes in these infants.[46] Monitoring is usually continued for about one month after oxygen therapy is discontinued.

Management of BPD should also include control of gastroesophageal reflux (GER) and nocturnal bronchoconstriction, conditions that may worsen pulmonary function during sleep in these infants.[52] Clinical experience suggests that GER is common in infants with BPD. However, the mere presence of GER on a barium esophogram does not implicate reflux as the cause of the child's pulmonary disease. Whenever possible, the relationship between GER and respiratory worsening should be established by correlating lower esophageal pH (using a pH probe) with SaO_2 and clinical symptoms, such as cough or wheeze. Management includes positioning to minimize GER, thickened feedings, medications, and if medical therapy fails, surgery.[52]

Treatment of bronchoconstriction during sleep should aim to control symptoms at night with minimal disruption of the child's and family's normal nighttime sleep patterns (see section on asthma).

Cystic Fibrosis

CF is the most common lethal genetic disease affecting the Caucasian population.[53] It is inherited in an autosomal recessive fashion and causes a characteristic chronic lung disease that begins in infancy with progressive destruction of functional lung tissue throughout life. It causes premature death with the median survival just into the third decade. The lung disease is manifested by chronic cough and pulmonary infection.

In many instances, obvious chronic lung dysfunction is not apparent until late childhood and adolescence; consequently, most of the information available on the interaction between breathing and sleep in this disease comes from studies of older patients. In 1980, two groups reported arterial oxygen desaturation during sleep in patients (primarily adults) with CF.[54, 55] Stokes and associates[54] found minor changes in SaO_2 (mean change 7.8%) in five patients with moderately severe lung disease (FEV_1 = 31–63% predicted). One patient with severe disease (FEV_1 = 17%) was hypoxemic while awake and experienced a 25% fall in SaO_2 during sleep. Both studies found that the largest dips in saturation occurred during REM sleep. Hypoxemia during sleep in these patients is thought to be due to the decrease in O_2 stores secondary to decreased FRC during REM sleep coupled with $\dot{V}/\dot{Q}$ mismatching. The effects of decreased lung volume are further exacerbated by periodic phasic inhibition of respiratory muscle activity, which causes an additional decrease in SaO_2. Tepper and associates[56] confirmed a sleep-related decline in minute ventilation. They found it was related to a decrease in the contribution of the rib cage to tidal volume breathing, which led to a decrease in lung volume and to episodes of desaturation (Fig. 20–5). Changes in oxygenation during sleep in CF patients are similar to those reported in adults with chronic bronchitis and COPD.[23, 24]

A number of investigators have suggested that nocturnal hypoxemia may play a role in the pathogenesis of cor pulmonale in patients with CF.[57, 58] Although the duration and severity of the desaturation episodes reported in most of the patients would not be considered sufficiently severe to warrant therapy, there is evidence that even brief episodes of desaturation can increase pulmonary artery pressure[57, 58] and that recurrent hypoxemic periods may be a more potent stimulus to the development of pulmonary hypertension than are isolated sustained periods of hypoxemia.[57, 59] Bradley and coworkers concluded that the duration of hypoxemia during both sleeping and waking was critical to the development of cor

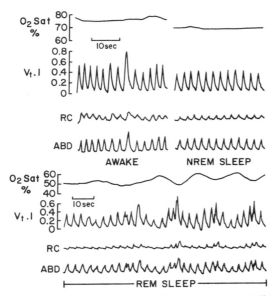

Figure 20–5. Demonstration of the role of hypoventilation and decrease in the rib cage (RC) contribution to tidal volume (V_T) in patients with CF. (Upper panel) Awake and NREM sleep record from a patient with CF illustrating oxygen saturation (O_2 sat%), V_T, RC, and abdominal (ABD) contributions to V_T. (Lower panel) REM sleep (tonic and phasic). Note decrease in RC contribution to V_T during REM sleep in the same patient. (From Tepper RS, et al: Ventilation and oxygenation changes during sleep in cystic fibrosis. Chest 84:388, 1983.)

pulmonale in adults with OSA.[60] More work is needed in patients with CF to define the natural history and role of nocturnal hypoxemia in the pathogenesis of cor pulmonale in CF.

Sleep quality can be affected in patients with CF in ways similar to what has been reported in adults with COPD.[61–63] Spier and coworkers found decreased sleep efficiency, more sleep state changes, and more wakenings (> 5 min) per hour of sleep time in patients with CF.[61] These patients also spent less time in REM sleep than did controls (9.4 vs 16.6%). These results differ from earlier studies that reported nearly normal REM sleep time (approximately 18% of total sleep time).[54, 56]

The cause of the sleep disturbance seen in CF patients is unclear. In the study of Spier and coworkers, CF patients did not have more transient arousals than controls; however, their longer arousals often coincided with coughing paroxysms.[61] Since coughing episodes were a factor in the sleep disruption reported by Stokes and associates,[55] it may be that the sleep disturbance reported by Spier simply reflects the presence of more coughing. Unfortunately, they did not quantify coughing or its

relation to arousals.[61] Future studies of sleep quality in patients with CF should include an assessment of disease severity and the amount of coughing, since these are likely to be important determinants of sleep quality. Although hypoxemia conceivably contributes to sleep disturbance, available data does not support this hypothesis: Boysen and associates found that in young adults with CF, arousals usually did not occur in response to hypoxemia[58]; and in patients with CF and in adults with COPD, supplemental oxygen did not improve sleep quality, although it was effective in alleviating the episodes of desaturation.[61, 63]

The degree of oxygen desaturation during sleep cannot be predicted from awake pulmonary function[64] or exercise testing[65] or from disease severity scores. However, measurement of arterial blood gases during waking may help identify those who should be screened for hypoxemia during sleep. Patients with CF with awake PaO_2 values of less than 60 mmHg were found to spend over 80% of their sleep time with SaO_2 below 90%. Conversely, those patients with PaO_2 values above 70 mmHg spent less than 20% of their sleep time with SaO_2 below 90%.[64] Documentation of hypoxemia during sleep can be provided by continuous monitoring of oxygen saturation in the home or in a sleep laboratory. Although monitoring at home is less disruptive to usual sleep habits, it does not provide any data on the presence of upper airway obstruction. Since oxygen requirements are usually greater in sleep than awake, SaO_2 values should be monitored during sleep at the initiation of therapy, as well as during and following acute pulmonary exacerbations.

Since data are limited, it is difficult to develop guidelines for therapy of hypoxemia during sleep in patients with CF. There have been no studies on the long-term use of supplemental oxygen during sleep in patients with CF comparable to studies in adults with COPD.[66–68] The natural history of hypoxemia during sleep and its role in the pathogenesis of cor pulmonale are unknown. The one study that has attempted to answer these questions did not demonstrate a beneficial effect of nocturnal oxygen therapy in reducing morbidity and mortality in patients with CF (mean age, 23 ± 6 yr).[69] In this study, by Zinman and associates, the mean PaO_2 while awake was approximately 60 mmHg in both patients and matched control groups.[69] Supplemental oxygen was administered at night using oxygen concentrators, but the mean duration of oxygen therapy was only 6.2 hours per day. Results of previous oxygen trials in adults with COPD demonstrated that to have any effect, supplemental oxygen had to be used at least 13 hours a day.[66, 67] Therefore, it is not surprising that Zinman and associates found no effect from supplemental oxygen in their patients with CF. On the other hand, their CF patients who received supplemental oxygen showed better attendance at school and work, compared with the group who did not receive oxygen. Also, compliance with the use of oxygen was considerably better than with the placebo (compressed air).[69] Therefore, it seems that supplemental oxygen even when used for brief intervals during sleep in patients with CF is not without some benefit.

At the present time, the indications for supplemental oxygen during sleep in children and adolescents with CF are unclear except for those patients with severe disease and marked hypoxemia ($PaO_2 < 60$ mmHg). In patients with an adequate PaO_2 awake (i.e., $PaO_2 > 60$ mmHg), decisions regarding supplemental oxygen must be individualized. It is essential that the attending physician know the patient's breathing pattern and oxygen saturation measurements during sleep. At what point should therapy be started? Although waiting for right ventricular (RV) failure to develop is clearly inappropriate, it is not known if patients with evidence of isolated RV hypertrophy and episodic desaturation should be treated with nocturnal oxygen supplementation. Such practice could add considerably to the cost of medical care. Unfortunately, the long-term consequences of brief episodes of oxygen desaturation during sleep are not known. For example, it is not known if short drops in oxygen desaturation to values below 80% are more significant clinically and physiologically than more frequent or longer lasting, yet less severe episodes. The baseline saturation must also be considered in any decision, since a lower baseline SaO_2 places patients with CF on the steep portion of the oxygen-hemoglobin dissociation curve where small changes in PaO_2 may result in more significant effects on hemoglobin saturation. Oxygen therapy is safe and is not associated with excessive CO_2 retention in most patients.[70, 71] Despite the fact that the effects of oxygen on sleep quality are difficult to identify, the importance of assisting patients in maintaining normal daily activities cannot be overstated.[69]

Nasal CPAP has been evaluated in young adult CF patients.[71a] This treatment improved oxygenation in both REM and NREM sleep, although CPAP is not well-tolerated by all patients. Controlled trials are required to establish if this type of treatment has a role in younger CF patients.

Because the already compromised mucociliary transport function in CF patients may worsen during sleep,[72] aggressive pulmonary toilet and control of infection are critical to improving gas exchange and minimizing the disruptive effects of coughing. Airway hyperreactivity is increased in patients with CF and attention must be focused on identifying and controlling nocturnal bronchoconstriction. Theophylline has been shown to decrease desaturation episodes in children with CF, but its adverse effects on sleep patterns may limit its usefulness.[73]

There are essentially no data on breathing during sleep in infants and young children with CF. The natural history of hypoxemia during sleep and the incidence of OSA in this population are unknown. Patients with CF frequently develop nasal polyps that may obstruct nasal airflow and possibly predispose some of these patients to OSA. It is not even known if the progression of cor pulmonale is altered by judicious use of supplemental oxygen during sleep. Additional study is required. With better therapy, survival rates of patients with CF will continue to improve. As CF patients live longer, the effects of sleep on their breathing may become progressively more important.

Asthma (Reactive Airways Disease)

Children often have exacerbations of asthma at night. This is most likely because of normal circadian variation in lung function rather than from the effects of sleep per se.[1, 3] Normal lung function varies throughout the day: it is best around 4:00 PM and worst around 4:00 AM.[74] In normal individuals, this variability is usually small with changes in peak flow averaging between 8 and 10%. In asthmatic children and adults, the decrease in peak flow rate is considerably greater, approaching 50%,[74, 75] and may be associated with drops in SaO_2 of over 10%.[12, 74, 75] Sleep may compound these changes. In a study of adolescents with asthma, the transition from NREM to REM sleep was associated with a reduction in intercostal EMG activity of 43%, a concomitant increase in diaphragmatic activity, a decrease in minute ventilation, and a mean maximal drop in SaO_2 of 3.9%. In addition, these patients developed PIRCM, which is atypical for normal adolescents.[12]

In patients with asthma, changes in pulmonary function parallel changes in circulating hormone and mediator levels that are known to affect lung function. Epinephrine levels are lowest at 4:00 AM, when lung function reaches a circadian nadir, while histamine levels are increased.[76, 77] Cyclic-AMP levels decrease over the night while cyclic-GMP and vagal neural tone increases.[76, 77] Endogenous steroid production also demonstrates diurnal variability, with lowest levels in the early morning hours. However, low steroid levels do not appear to play a role in these changes in lung function.[76] Soutar and associates demonstrated that the intravenous infusion of glucocorticoid in the early morning did not block the decreases in peak flow in adults.[79] Sleep itself does not appear to be a major factor in the variability in pulmonary function in asthma,[80] but it may contribute to the problem in that certain pulmonary defenses, such as the response to hypoxemia and loaded breathing, may be decreased during REM sleep.[27, 35, 37]

A patient with asthma, in whom airway reactivity is already heightened or airflow already severely obstructed, may be highly susceptible to the effects of traditional triggers of asthma such as aeroallergens or environmental irritants.[81] This interaction needs more study in children, since removal of the offending agent does not always result in the resolution of symptoms. Cold air, on the other hand, a potent trigger of asthma symptoms while awake, does not appear to contribute to worsening asthma symptoms during sleep.[82] Another potential trigger is the onset of a late phase reaction from an exposure earlier in the day. This has been reported in adults exposed to Western Red Cedar, but there are no comparable exposure studies in children.[83] The role of GER is not clear.[53, 84] One study of adults with asthma demonstrated a dramatic reduction in nocturnal symptoms following successful treatment of GER.[85] However, Hughes and associates could not confirm an association between GER and chronic asthma symptoms in a group of adolescents with asthma.[86]

Children with asthma have also been shown to have abnormal sleep patterns. Kales and associates studied a group of 10 asthmatic children on two successive nights and demonstrated a significant reduction in stage 4 sleep and increased awakenings and arousals compared with nonasthmatic children.[87] Episodes of asthma, defined clinically as dyspnea severe enough to wake the child, did not occur during the first third of the sleep period. This corresponds to a time when stage 3 and 4 predominates. In fact, no episodes were recorded during stage 4 sleep. It is not clear from this study whether stage 4 sleep imparts protection from asthma exacerbations or, since episodes were defined by their ability to wake the patient, whether there is simply a blunted arousal response to increases in airflow obstruction. A similar pattern has been reported in adults.[88] Unfortunately, there are several key limitations to the study in children. The age range of the patients studied was wide (5–15 yr); there were no measurements of baseline lung function; no respiratory variables were measured during sleep; and the effects of therapy were not clarified. These patients were managed with chronic theophylline and ephedrine containing compounds. However, these medications were stopped 6 hours before the start of the study in most patients, which may have contributed to the increased occurrence of asthma episodes in the early morning hours. In contrast, a recent report by Avital and coworkers on a group of adolescents with controlled, moderately severe asthma demonstrated a normal sleep architecture that was apparently unaffected by the use of theophylline.[89] Theophylline therapy also appeared to protect these patients from oxygen desaturation episodes secondary to central apnea. Similarly, the work of Smith and Hudgel[22] suggested that the episodes of desaturation that they encountered in their adolescent patients during sleep could be abolished with better asthma control. However, data from adults with asthma suggests that even when their asthma is well-controlled, patients have less efficient sleep, more wake time at night, and less stage 4 sleep than do normal individuals.[88] More data is needed to define the sleep patterns of children with asthma both on and off therapy.

Respiratory abnormalities during sleep may contribute to some complications of asthma. Fitzpatrick and associates demonstrated that adults with stable asthma not only exhibit poor sleep quality but also have impaired daytime cognitive function.[90] Data is limited, but the experience from children with OSA suggests that (at least in that condition) altered daytime performance is a consequence of disturbed sleep.[91] Of greater concern is the possible relationship between death and sleep-associated asthma.[92, 93] In a case controlled study of deaths associated with asthma attacks, onset of the attack during sleep was one of the few factors that was significantly associated with a fatal outcome.[94] Unfortunately, since the time of night that these attacks began was not reported, it is impossible to speculate if these episodes represent an abnormal response to circadian variability or a blunted response to airway challenge that allowed an asthma attack to reach a critical level before waking the patient.

Comprehensive management of the pediatric patient with asthma must take into account the potential for significant variability in the severity of asthma during sleep.[6, 95] A detailed history of the timing and nature of nocturnal symptoms is essential in order to plan an appropriate therapeutic strategy. Clinical manifestations of asthma exacerbations during sleep include coughing, wheezing, shortness of breath, and chest tightness or pain sufficient to wake the child from sleep. Increased obstruction in large or small airways may be severe enough to produce episodes of desaturation.[8, 22] A diary may be useful for charting the night's events. Objective confirmation of patients' reporting can be obtained by use of home peak flow meter recordings. Measurements should be obtained at night, in the morning on waking up and, if possible, if the patient wakes during the night with symptoms. It is also helpful to obtain another reading after therapy to determine the degree of recovery and the need for additional therapy.

The goals of asthma therapy are multiple, and control of nocturnal symptoms should be given equal weight to other aspects of management. This is easier said than done in pediatric patients who often have long sleep periods. The ideal nocturnal bronchodilator is one with minimal nonspecific CNS stimulatory effects that also reaches peak effect about 6 to 8 hours after ingestion.[95] The β_2 adrenergic formulations currently available for most children are poorly suited to control symptoms occurring early in the morning. Medications administered by aerosol or in oral liquid preparations have a rapid onset of action, but the duration of effectiveness is relatively short and many patients develop symptoms in the early morning hours. Although these medications may be quite effective acutely, most parents are reluctant to awaken sleeping children to administer medications. Long-acting β_2 agonists that have been shown to be effective in adults[96] are not currently available in dosage strength or formulations that would permit their use in young children.

Despite side effects, the long-acting theophylline preparations are best suited for treating nocturnal symptoms in children. Unfortunately, they may produce undesirable changes in temperament and personality and worsen GER. Children may become hyperactive and restless; side effects that parents have a difficult time tolerating especially at night. However, if tolerated, such treatment can be quite effective in controlling nocturnal symptoms.[89, 97]

If the child's symptoms are not controlled with theophylline or if a patient on theophylline exhibits acute symptoms, a serum theophylline level should be measured. However, a theophylline level obtained during the day may not reflect the nocturnal level, since theophylline metabolism and absorption are different during sleep than when awake and nocturnal levels may be considerably lower than those seen in the day.[98]

The interval between doses is also important since the child's medications are often administered at more regular intervals during the day than the night. Generally, all doses are administered during the child's usual waking hours. Thus, the longest interval without medication, the one at night, is also the time when the level is at a nadir and symptoms are more likely to occur.

Other measures to control asthma symptoms at night should be included in the nocturnal plan of care.[95] Environmental controls are essential. Anti-inflammatory agents are usually administered in the morning in order to reduce adrenal suppression. However, the lowest endogenous steroid levels are found in the early morning at a time well before exogenous steroids are typically administered. In adults, administration of steroids at night did not alter the occurrence of nocturnal symptoms.[79] Since there is no comparable data in children, twice daily dosing of steroids may be worthwhile in children with nocturnal asthma symptoms. Similarly, the effect of sodium cromolyn in controlling nocturnal symptoms is not clear. However, since airway hyperreactivity appears to worsen at night, nocturnal administration of cromolyn sodium is suggested. Supplemental oxygen during sleep is rarely needed in children with asthma. Desaturation during sleep in asthmatic children appears to respond readily to institution of more appropriate and effective asthma therapy.[22, 89]

Conclusion

Eugene Robin's caveat over 30 years ago about the potential impact of sleep on the natural history of disease is particularly relevant to pediatrics: "The sleeping patient is still a patient."[1] In the past, there has been a tendency to overlook the affects of sleep on breathing and on the clinical course of lung disease in children. However, data indicate that what happens during sleep in children of all ages cannot be ignored, especially since the sleep period is likely to be considerably longer in the child. Furthermore, it cannot be assumed that observations on adults with lung disease are applicable to children. In fact, the experience in children with OSAS strongly suggests that breathing disorders associated with sleep are significantly different in children.[99] Not only must one account for the interactions among sleep, circadian rhythms, and disease processes, but in children, the clinician must account for the influences of age, growth, development, and the effects of disease on the maturation of breathing control systems.

References

1. Robin ED: Some inter-relations between sleep and disease. Arch Int Med 102:669, 1958.
2. Phillipson EA: Respiratory adaptations in sleep. Ann Rev Physiol 40:133, 1978.
3. McFadden ER: Circadian rhythms. Am J Med 85(Suppl 1B):2, 1988.
4. Petty TL: Circadian variations in chronic asthma and chronic obstructive pulmonary disease. Am J Med 85(Suppl 1B):21, 1988.
5. Martin RJ: Nocturnal asthma. Immunol Allergy Pract 12:15, 1990.
6. Garg M, Kurzner SI, Bautista DB, et al: Clinically unsuspected hypoxia during sleep and feeding in infants with bronchopulmonary dysplasia. Pediatrics 81:635, 1988.
7. Burney PGJ, Chinn S, Rona RJ: Has the prevalence of asthma increased in children? Evidence from a national study of health and growth 1973–86. Br Med J 300:1306, 1990.
8. Martin RJ, Okken A, Rubin D: Arterial oxygen tension during active and quiet sleep in the normal neonate. J Pediatr 94:271, 1979.
9. Gaultier C: Respiration au course du sommeil pendant la croissance: Physiologic et pathologie. Bull Eur Physiopath Respir 21:55, 1985.
10. Wohl ME, Mead J: Age as a factor in respiratory disease. In Chernick V (ed): Kendig's Disorders of the Respiratory Tract in Children. WB Saunders, Philadelphia, 1990, pp 175–182.
11. LeSouef PN, England SJ, Bryan C: Passive respiratory mechanics in newborns and children. Am Rev Resp Dis 129:552, 1984.
12. Gaultier C, Praud JP, Canet E, et al: Paradoxical in-

ward rib cage motion during rapid eye movement sleep in infants and young children. J Dev Physiol 9:391, 1987.
13. Tabachnik E, Muller NL, Bryan AC, et al: Changes in ventilation and chest wall mechanics during sleep in normal adolescents. J Appl Physiol 51:557, 1981.
14. Hudgel DW: Mechanisms of obstructive sleep apnea. Chest 101:541, 1992.
15. Hendersen-Smart DJ, Read DJC: Reduced lung volume during behavioral active sleep in the newborn. J Appl Physiol 46:1081, 1979.
16. Beardsmore CS, MacFadyen UM, Moosavi SS, et al: Measurement of lung volumes during active and quiet sleep in infants. Pediatr Pulmonol 7:71, 1989.
17. Moriette G, Chaussain M, Radvanyi-Bouvet MF, et al: Functional residual capacity and sleep states in the premature newborn. Biol Neonate 43:125, 1983.
18. Walti H, Moriette G, Radvanyi-Bouvet MF, et al: Influence of breathing pattern on functional residual capacity in sleeping newborn infants. J Dev Physiol 8:167, 1986.
19. Muller NL, Francis PW, Gurwitz D, et al: Mechanism of hemoglobin desaturation during rapid eye movement sleep in normal subjects and in patients with cystic fibrosis. Am Rev Resp Dis 121:463, 1980.
20. Hudgel DW, Devadatta P: Decrease in functional residual capacity during sleep in normal humans. J Appl Physiol 57:1319, 1984.
21. Morgan AD, Rhind GB, Connaughton JJ, et al: Breathing and oxygenation during sleep in patients with nocturnal asthma. Thorax 42:600, 1987.
22. Chipps BE, Mak H, Schuberth KC, et al: Nocturnal oxygen saturation in normal and asthmatic children. Pediatrics 65:1157, 1980.
23. Smith TF, Hudgel DW: Arterial oxygen desaturation during sleep in children with asthma and its relation to airway obstruction and ventilatory drive. Pediatrics 66:746, 1980.
24. Marcus CL, Omlin KJ, Basinski DJ, et al: Normal polysomnographic volumes for children and adolescents. Am Rev Resp Dis 146:1235, 1992.
25. Catterall JR, Calverley PMA, MacNee W, et al: Mechanism of transient nocturnal hypoxemia in hypoxic chronic bronchitis and emphysema. J Appl Physiol 59:1698, 1985.
26. Hudgel DW, Martin RJ, Capehart M, et al: Contribution of hypoventilation to sleep oxygen desaturation in chronic obstructive pulmonary disease. J Appl Physiol 55:669, 1983.
27. Rigatto H: Control of ventilation in the newborn. Ann Rev Physiol 46:661, 1984.
28. Douglas NJ, White DP, Weil JV, et al: Hypoxic ventilatory response decreases during sleep in normal men. Am Rev Resp Dis 125:286, 1982.
29. White DP, Douglas NJ, Pickett CK, et al: Hypoxic ventilatory response during sleep in normal women. Am Rev Resp Dis 126:530, 1982.
30. Douglas NJ, White DP, Weil JV, et al: Hypercapnic ventilatory response in sleeping adults. Am Rev Resp Dis 126:758, 1982.
31. Berthon-Jones M, Sullivan CE: Ventilation and arousal responses to hypercapnia in normal sleeping adults. J Appl Physiol 57:59, 1984.
32. Davi M, Sankaran K, MacCallum M, et al: The effect of sleep state on chest distortion and on the ventilatory response to CO_2 in neonates. Pediatr Res 13:982, 1979.
33. Moriette G, van Reempts T, Moore M, et al: The effect of breathing CO_2 on ventilation and diaphragmatic

electromyography in newborn infants. Respir Physiol 62:387, 1985.

34. Knill R, Andrews W, Bryan AC, et al: Respiratory load compensation in infants. J Appl Physiol 40:357, 1976.
35. Issa FG, Sullivan CE: Arousal and breathing responses to airway occlusion. J Appl Physiol 55:1113, 1983.
36. Iber C, Berssenbrugge A, Skatrud JB, et al: Ventilatory adaptations to resistive loading during wakefulness and non-REM sleep. J Appl Physiol 52:607, 1982.
37. O'Brodovitch HM, Mellins RB: Bronchopulmonary dysplasia: unresolved neonatal acute lung injury. Am Rev Resp Dis 132:694, 1985.
38. Hudak BB, Allen MC, Hudak NL, et al: Home oxygen therapy for chronic lung disease in extremely premature infants. Am J Dis Child 143:357, 1989.
39. Rome ES, Miller MJ, Goldthwart, et al: Effect of sleep state on chest wall movement and gas exchange in infants with resolving bronchopulmonary dysplasia. Pediatr Pulmonol 3:259, 1987.
40. Loughlin GM, Allen RP, Pyzik P: Sleep related hypoxemia in children with bronchopulmonary dysplasia (BPD) and adequate oxygen saturation awake. Sleep Res 16:486, 1987.
41. Gaultier C, Praud JP, Clement A, et al: Respiration during sleep in children with COPD. Chest 87:168, 1985.
41a. Filtchev SI, Curzi-Dascalova L, Spassov L, et al: Heart rate variability during sleep in infants with bronchopulmonary dysplasia: effects of mild decrease in oxygen saturation. Chest 106:1711, 1994
42. Praud JP, Cavailloles F, Boulhadour K, et al: Radionuclide evaluation of cardiac function during sleep in children with bronchopulmonary dysplasia. Chest 100:721, 1991.
43. Werthammer J, Brown ER, Neff RK, et al: Sudden infant death syndrome in infants with bronchopulmonary dysplasia. Pediatrics 69:301, 1982.
44. Kuekarn P, Hall RT, Rhodes PG, et al: Post neonatal infant mortality in infants admitted to a neonatal intensive care unit. Pediatrics 62:178, 1978.
45. Southall DP, Richards JM, Rhoden KJ, et al: Prolonged apnea and cardiac arrythmia in infants discharged from neonatal intensive care units: failure to predict an increased risk for sudden infant death syndrome. Pediatrics 70:844, 1982.
46. Garg M, Kurzner SI, Bautista D, et al: Hypoxic arousal responses in infants with bronchopulmonary dysplasia. Pediatrics 81:635, 1988.
47. Fewell JE, Kondo CS, Dascalu V, et al: Influence of carotid denervation on the arousal and cardiopulmonary response to rapidly developing hypoxemia in lambs. Pediatr Res 25:473, 1989.
48. Fewell JE, Taylor BJ, Kondo CS, et al: Influence of carotid body denervation on the arousal and cardiopulmonary response to upper airway obstruction in lambs. Pediatr Res 28:374, 1990.
49. Rome ES, Stork EK, Carlo WA, et al: Limitations of transcutaneous CO_2 and PCO_2 monitoring in infants with bronchopulmonary dysplasia. Pediatrics 74:217, 1984; 82:59, 1988.
50. Poets CF, Stebbins VA, Samuels MP, et al: Oxygen saturation and breathing patterns in children. Pediatrics 92:686, 1993.
51. Dudell G, Cornish JD, Bartlett RH: What constitutes adequate oxygenation. Pediatrics 85:39, 1990.
52. Orenstein SR, Orenstein DM: Gastroesophageal reflux and respiratory disease in children. J Pediatr 112: 847, 1988.
53. MacLusky I, Levison H: Cystic fibrosis. In Chernick V

(ed): Kendig's Disorders of the Respiratory Tract in Children. WB Saunders, Philadelphia, 1990, pp 692–703.
54. Stokes DC, McBride JT, Wall MA, et al: Sleep hypoxemia in young adults with cystic fibrosis. Am J Dis Child 134:741, 1980.
55. Francis PWJ, Muller NL, Gurwitz D, et al: Hemoglobin desaturation: its occurrence during sleep in patients with cystic fibrosis. Am J Dis Child 134:734, 1980.
56. Tepper RS, Skatrud JB, Dempsey JA: Ventilation and oxygenation changes during sleep in cystic fibrosis. Chest 84:388, 1983.
57. Block AJ, Boysen PG, Wynne JW: The origins of cor pulmonale: an hypothesis. Chest 75:109, 1979.
58. Boysen PG, Block AJ, Wynne JW: Nocturnal pulmonary hypertension in patients with chronic obstructive pulmonary disease. Chest 76:536, 1979.
59. Unger M, Atkins M, Briscoe WA, et al: Potentiation of pulmonary vasoconstrictor response with repeated intermittent hypoxia. J Appl Physiol 43:662, 1977.
60. Bradley TD, Rutherford R, Grossman RF, et al: Role of daytime hypoxemia in the pathogenesis of right heart failure in the obstructive sleep apnea syndrome. Am Rev Resp Dis 131:835, 1985.
61. Spier S, Rivlin J, Hughes D, et al: The effect of oxygen on sleep, blood gases and ventilation in cystic fibrosis. Am Rev Resp Dis 129:712, 1984.
62. Cormick W, Olson LG, Hensley MJ, et al: Nocturnal hypoxemia and quality of sleep in patients with chronic obstructive lung disease. Thorax 41:846, 1986.
63. McKeon JL, Murree-Allen K, Saunders NA: Supplemental oxygen and quality of sleep in patients with chronic obstructive lung disease. Thorax 44:184, 1989.
64. Coffey MJ, Fitzgerald MX, McNicholas WT: Comparison of oxygen desaturations during sleep and exercise in patients with cystic fibrosis. Chest 100:659, 1991.
65. Tilkian AG, Guilleminault C, Schroeder J, et al: Hemodynamics in sleep induced apnea studies during wakefulness and sleep. Ann Intern Med 85:714, 1976.
66. Nocturnal Oxygen Therapy Trial Group: Continuous or nocturnal oxygen therapy in hypoxemic chronic obstructive lung disease: a clinical trial. Ann Intern Med 93:391, 1980.
67. Medical Research Council Working Party: Long-term domiciliary oxygen therapy in chronic hypoxic cor pulmonale complicating chronic bronchitis and emphysema. Lancet 1:681, 1981.
68. Stark RD, Finnegan P, Bishop JM: Long-term domiciliary oxygen in chronic bronchitis with pulmonary hypertension. Br Med J 3:467, 1973.
69. Zinman R, Corey M, Coates AL, et al: Nocturnal home oxygen in the treatment of hypoxemic cystic fibrosis patients. J Pediatr 114:368, 1989.
70. Hazinski TA, Hanson TN, Simon JA, et al: Effect of oxygen administration during sleep on skin surface oxygen and carbon dioxide tensions in patients with chronic lung disease. Pediatrics 67:626, 1981.
71. Montgomery M, Wiebicke W, Bibi H, et al: Home measurement of oxygen saturations during sleep in patients with cystic fibrosis. Pediatr Pulmonol 7:29, 1989.
71a. Regnis JA, Piper AJ, Henke KG, et al: Benefits of nocturnal nasal CPAP in patients with cystic fibrosis. Chest 106:1717, 1994
72. Bateman JRM, Pavia N, Clarke SW: The retention of lung secretions during the night in normal subjects. Clin Sci 55:523, 1978.
73. Avital A, Sanchez I, Holbrow J, et al: Effect of theophylline on lung function tests, sleep quality, and night-

time SaO$_2$ in children with cystic fibrosis. Am Rev Resp Dis 144:1245, 1991.

74. Hetzel MR, Clark TJH: Comparison of normal and asthmatic circadian rhythms in peak expiratory flow rate. Thorax 35:732, 1980.

75. Clark TJH, Hetzel MR: Diurnal variation of asthma. Br J Dis Chest 71:87, 1977.

76. Barnes P, Fitzgerald G, Brown M, et al: Nocturnal asthma and changes in circulating epinephrine, histamine and cortisol. N Eng J Med 303:263, 1980.

77. Soutar CA, Carruthers M, Pickering CAC: Nocturnal asthma and urinary adrenaline and noradrenaline excretion. Thorax 32:677, 1977.

78. Reinhardt D, Schuhmacher P, Fox A, et al: Comparison of the effects of theophylline, prednisolone and sleep withdrawal on airway obstruction and urinary cyclic AMP/cyclic GMP excretion of asthmatic children with and without nocturnal asthma. Intl J Clin Pharmacol, Ther Toxicol 18:399, 1980.

79. Soutar CA, Costello J, Ijadualo O, et al: Nocturnal and morning asthma: relationship to plasma corticosteroids and response to cortisol infusion. Thorax 30:436, 1975.

80. Hetzel MR, Clark TJH: Does sleep cause nocturnal asthma. Thorax 34:749, 1979.

81. Martin RJ, Cicutto LC, Ballard RD: Factors related to the nocturnal worsening of asthma. Am Rev Resp Dis 141:33, 1990.

82. Thomson AH, Pratt C, Simpson H: Nocturnal cough in asthma. Arch Dis Child 62:1001, 1987.

83. Busse WW: Pathogenesis and pathophysiology of nocturnal asthma. Am J Med 85(Suppl 1B):24, 1985.

84. Simpson H, Hampton F: Gastroesophageal reflux and the lung. Arch Dis Child 66:277, 1991.

85. Goodall RJR, Earis JE, Cooper DN, et al: Relationship between asthma and gastroesophageal reflux. Thorax 36:116, 1981.

86. Hughes DM, Spier S, Rivlin J, et al: Gastroesophageal reflux during sleep in asthmatic patients. J Pediatr 102:666, 1983.

87. Kales A, Kales JD, Sly RM, et al: Sleep patterns of asthmatic children: all night electroencephalographic studies. J Allergy 46:300, 1970.

88. Montplaisir J, Walsh J, Malo JL: Nocturnal asthma: features of attacks, sleep and breathing patterns. Am Rev Resp Dis 125:18, 1982.

89. Avital A, Steljes DG, Pasterkamp H, et al: Sleep quality in children with asthma treated with theophylline or cromolyn sodium. J Pediatr 119:979, 1991.

90. Fitzpatrick MF, Engleman H, Whyte KF, et al: Morbidity in nocturnal asthma: sleep quality and daytime cognitive performance. Thorax 46:559, 1991.

91. Guilleminault C, Korobkin R, Winkle R: A review of 50 children with obstructive sleep apnea syndrome. Lung 159:275, 1981.

92. Hetzel MR, Clark TJH, Branthwaite MA: Asthma analysis of sudden deaths and ventilatory arrests in hospital. Br Med J 1:808, 1977.

93. Cochrane GM, Clark JA: A survey of asthma mortality in patients between 35 and 64 in the greater London hospitals in 1971. Thorax 30:300, 1975.

94. Miller BD, Strunk RC: Circumstances surrounding the deaths of children due to asthma. Am J Dis Child 143:1294, 1989.

95. Reed CF, Li JTC: Nocturnal asthma: approach to the patient. Am J Med 85:14, 1988.

96. Stewart IC, Rhind GB, Power JT, et al: Effect of sustained released terbutaline on symptoms and sleep quality in patients with nocturnal asthma. Thorax 42:797, 1987.

97. Zwillich CW, Neagley SR, Cicutto L, et al: Nocturnal asthma therapy: inhaled bitolterol vs. sustained release theophylline. Am Rev Resp Dis 139:470, 1989.

98. Martin RJ, Cicutto LC, Ballard RD, et al: Circadian variations in theophylline concentrations and the treatment of nocturnal asthma. Am Rev Resp Dis 139:475, 1989.

99. Carroll JL, Loughlin GM: Diagnostic criteria for obstructive sleep apnea syndrome in children. Pediatr Pulmonol 14:71, 1992.

Sleep and the Sudden Infant Death Syndrome

STEVEN F. GLOTZBACH, RONALD L. ARIAGNO, and RONALD M. HARPER

Sudden Infant Death Syndrome (SIDS) is the leading cause of death in infants between the ages of 1 and 12 months in the United States and has been the focus of many recent reviews and symposia.[1–5] SIDS, which is a diagnosis of exclusion, peaks between 2 and 4 months of age, coinciding with a time of significant changes in sleep organization and central nervous system (CNS) maturation. Although SIDS deaths apparently occur during periods of sleep, or in close temporal relationship to sleep, specific state-related pathology leading to SIDS is unknown. In this chapter, attention will be directed to the question: What specifically can be learned about the etiology of SIDS from studies of sleep? Also, early postnatal changes in sleep organization and homeostatic and arousal responses during sleep will be reviewed in an effort to better understand infant vulnerability to intrinsic factors and external challenges. This knowledge is essential in developing efficacious screening tests, interventions, and home cardiorespiratory monitoring procedures for infants presumed to be at high risk for SIDS.

Historic Perspective

The definition of SIDS has been recently updated by a National Institutes of Health Panel as: "SIDS is defined as the sudden death of an infant under 1 year of age which remains unexplained after a complete postmortem examination, including an investigation of the death scene and a review of the case history. Cases failing to meet the standards of this definition, including those without postmortem examinations, should not be diagnosed as SIDS." This revised definition emphasizes the necessity for autopsy and death scene evaluation. Thus, some of the uncertainty in SIDS diagnoses that was previously due to differences in diagnostic practices of coroners and law enforcement officers at the local level should be reduced.

In the early 1970s, Steinschneider articulated the "apnea hypothesis" for SIDS based on the observation that some SIDS victims had presented with a prior diagnosis of life-threatening apnea and cyanosis.[6] Consistent with the apnea hypothesis, Naeye and coworkers reported that SIDS victims had an increase in the diameter of small pulmonary vessels compared with controls,[7] which suggested that SIDS infants may not be entirely normal but rather have undetected, preexisting clinical problems associated with chronic hypoxemia.[8] An increase in home cardiorespiratory monitoring for prolonged apnea and/or bradycardia detection as a possible prevention for SIDS occurred subsequent to these findings; however, after 20 years of active investigation, the relationship between apnea and SIDS remains unclear. Monitor design is under review,[9] and the usefulness of monitoring intervention for the prevention of SIDS is currently the focus of a multicenter study sponsored by the National Institutes of Health.

The incidence of SIDS is linked to a consistent pattern of maternal and infant epidemiologic risk factors, including low socioeconomic status, young maternal age, high parity, multiple births, short intervals between births, male gender, race, low birth weight, and maternal tobacco use. In fact, recent studies suggest that postnatal exposure to passive smoking increases SIDS risk.[10, 11] Although these epidemiologic data suggest significant elements that are associated with an increased SIDS risk, they are not prevalent findings in the majority of SIDS cases and are not useful in predicting the vulnerability for SIDS in individuals. Consequently, most SIDS victims are not in "at-risk" groups, and in more than 90% of SIDS victims, prolonged apnea or cyanosis had not been noted prior to the SIDS event. Bentele and Albani[12] reviewed published clinical studies and concluded that tests once proposed to be predictive of SIDS, including EKG, pneumocardiography, polysomnography (PSG), and respiratory control system challenges (ventilatory or arousal responses), have not had sufficient *specificity* or *sensitivity* to identify individuals at risk. In most of the reports reviewed, the conclusions were drawn without regard for the variability that may be introduced by sleep states. Apnea detection in practice has not provided sufficient sensitivity to identify risk of SIDS. Nevertheless, monitor technology and compliance in the use of monitors are under intense scrutiny, as apnea or cardiorespiratory failure is still considered the most likely terminal event in SIDS.

Some research programs are currently focused on the interaction of homeostatic regulatory systems that develop with respiration, such as systems controlling arousal states, circadian rhythms, and body temperature.[1, 13–15] In the adult, profound interactions occur between these regulatory systems, but little is known about the interdependence of these integrative functions in the infant. Because of the striking sleep-related changes that occur in all regulatory systems and because of the dynamic changes in infant sleep that appear during the first months of life, the development of sleep and sleep-related homeostasis in normal infants and in infants presumed to be at "high risk" for SIDS will be addressed.

Sleep and Arousal Hypotheses

In addition to the temporal association between the SIDS event and sleep, any theory that suggests a mechanism of death for SIDS must explain why the majority of deaths occur during a relatively narrow developmental window at 2 to 4 months postnatal age. During this period, significant changes occur both in

sleep organization and in the modulation of brainstem centers involved in respiratory and arousal state control by the forebrain.[16]

The temporal association of the SIDS event with sleep suggests that wakefulness (AW) provides protective mechanisms for survival and that arousal from sleep to waking, or a transition from one sleep state to another when confronted with a life-threatening challenge, confers such protection. This hypothesis has been supported by studies suggesting raised arousal thresholds for respiratory, tactile, and visual stimuli during sleep in infants at risk for SIDS.[17–20] Knowledge of state organization may thus elucidate the role of sleep as a factor in SIDS in infants.

The most notable changes in sleep that occur in the early postnatal period include a decrease in the percentage and bout length of active sleep (AS or REM sleep), an increase in the percentage and episode length of quiet sleep (QS or NREM sleep), and an increase in the consolidation of sleep into the nighttime hours.[21–25] For example, in the Los Angeles data set, AS as a percentage of total recording time (AS/TRT) was 57%, 46%, 32%, and 26% at 1 week, 2 months, 3 months, and 6 months, respectively. QS/TST showed the opposite trend, increasing from 25% at 1 week to 36%, 44%, and 49% at 2, 3, and 6 months, respectively.[23] In comparing infant sleep studies, it is important to consider how the recording protocol may influence the results, particularly with respect to: (a) time of day, (b) type of recording, (c) length of the recording, (d) recording environment, and (e) infant factors. Examples of environmental factors include modulators of sleep and arousal such as temperature, noise, photoperiod, and any disturbances due to the presence of the recording equipment or procedures. Infant factors include the health of the infant and the quality and timing of sleep and feeding preceding the recording.

Two additional points regarding the assessment of infant sleep should be mentioned. First, each of the investigations discussed below, which were designed to compare sleep in normal infants with sleep in infants belonging to epidemiologically high-risk groups or SIDS victims, have been done with the infant sleeping in isolation from the mother or caregiver, a practice that is common in modern western cultures. A new perspective on infant sleep as it relates to SIDS, offered by McKenna[26, 27] (see also Chapter 2), posits that infant-parent co-sleeping (the anthropologic "norm") may optimize infant development and reduce SIDS risk through the interchange of a number of stimulus modalities between mother and infant during sleep. Curiously, the infant's sleep in a co-sleeping environment is characterized by more frequent arousals, apparently in contrast to the notion that consolidated sleep is developmentally more mature and "healthy." It should be noted that SIDS also occurs in co-sleeping environments, and the relative incidence of SIDS for co-sleeping vs isolated sleeping is unknown. Second, several techniques have been developed for quantifying infant sleep that are less invasive than PSG, such as video analysis[28] and the utilization of a mattress sensitive to movement and breathing.[29] Although these procedures have unique analytic, artifact, and sensitivity problems, they allow recordings in the home environment and should be considered for direct comparison of the development of state organization in normal infants and in high-risk groups.

In the last decade, a number of investigators have compared sleep in normal infants with infants who later succumbed to SIDS and with two classes of infants presumed to be at higher-risk for SIDS: siblings of SIDS (SIBS) victims and infants "near-miss" (NM) for SIDS. NM refers to cases in which the infant presented with a history of apnea, cyanosis or pallor, was usually limp, and apparently needed resuscitation by vigorous stimulation or mouth-to-mouth ventilation. The supposition that followed was that had the intervention not occurred, the NM infant would have died of SIDS, and, therefore the surviving infant should be considered at higher risk for SIDS. The "near miss for SIDS" terminology has been replaced by the term "apparent life threatening event" (ALTE), defined at the 1987 NIH Consensus Development Conference on Infantile Apnea and Home Monitoring as: "an episode that is frightening to the observer and that is characterized by some combination of apnea (central or occasionally obstructive), color change (usually cyanotic or pallid but occasionally erythematous or plethoric), marked change in muscle tone (usually marked limpness), choking or gagging. In some cases, the observer fears that the infant has died. Previously used terminology such as 'aborted crib death' or 'near-miss SIDS' should be abandoned because it implies a possibly misleading close association between this type of spell and SIDS." In this chapter, referral to either NM or ALTE will reflect the terminology of the original study.

The results of studies of sleep organization in normal infants and high-risk infants are summarized in Table 21–1. In each study, except for that of Haddad and associates,[30] infants were recorded at least for an overnight period. All studies have reported some group differences between high-risk and normal infants and the major claims can be categorized into the two following areas:

A. *"Amount of sleep" measures indicate a maturational delay in high-risk infants.*

Several investigators have concluded, through quantitative analysis of sleep, that a developmental delay exists in infants that are perceived to be at high-risk for SIDS. Haddad and colleagues[30] studied NM and control infants at monthly intervals during the first 4 months of life. Although the infants were exposed to 2% CO_2 for a portion of each 1 to 3 hour daytime nap, the authors state that this hypercapnic gas challenge did not influence the distribution of sleep and arousal. While TST during the nap did not differ between infant groups at any age, the percentages of QS/TST and REM/TST showed significant group differences at 2 to 4 months of age. During the period from 1 to 4 months, QS increased from 35 to 55% in normal infants and from 35 to 44% in NM infants. REM sleep showed opposite changes in this time interval, decreasing from 54 to 30% in controls and from 54 to 40% in NM infants.

Guilleminault and associates[31, 32] have also concluded that NM infants demonstrate a maturational delay in the development of sleep. In these studies, 24-hour sleep patterns were compared in 31 full-term control infants and 29 NM infants during the first 6 months of life. Although TST did not differ between infant groups during the first 5 months of life, other sleep measures showed significant differences. At 3 and 6 weeks of age, NM infants had more REM sleep than controls in the afternoon hours, and at 6 weeks and 3 months of age, NM infants had a significantly larger number of sleep-onset REM periods. At 3 months of age, the amount of stage 2 NREM was about one half of the value in NM compared with control infants (9 vs 19% of TST). At each developmental age, the hourly distribution of NREM and REM did not differ between the two infant groups. It is of interest to note that at each age, NM infants had fewer body movements during sleep.

In contrast, Sterman and colleagues[24, 33] have proposed an "accelerated maturation" hypothesis for SIDS, which states that an increase

Table 21–1. SLEEP PATTERNS IN NORMAL INFANTS, HIGH-RISK INFANTS, AND SIDS VICTIMS

Study	POP	Study Type	Postnatal Age @ Study	Major Claim
Haddad (1981)	C 19 N 13	1–3 hr, daytime nap	1–4 mo	N have a maturational *delay* in sleep distribution: %QS in C > N; %AS in C < N.
Harper (1981)	C 20 S 20	12 hr, overnight	1 wk–6 mo	Analysis of *temporal sequencing* of states is critical. S have an increased tendency to remain asleep, or a relative failure to arouse, compared with C.
Sterman (1982)				EEG power spectral analysis suggests *accelerated* CNS maturation in S compared with C.
Harper (1983)	C 25 S 25	12 hr, overnight	1 wk–6 mo	Differences in sequencing of sleep states between S and C extend until 6 mo of age.
Guilleminault (1983)	C 31 N 29	24 hr	3 wk–6 mo	Sleep patterns in N reflect a maturational *delay* relative to C: N have more REM at 3 and 6 wk; consolidation occurs earlier in C.
Navelet (1984)	C 19 S 24 N 34	8 hr, overnight	1–12 mo	Differences between "at-risk" (S,N) and C greatest at < 12 wks. S,N had shorter AW bout durations, more %AS, and increased QS and AS bout durations compared with C.
Samson-Dollfus (1988)	N 14 S 34	8.3 hr, overnight	6 mo	AW was less in N relative to S; QS stage 3 in N was greater than in S.
Challamel (1988)	C 20 N 31	10.5 hr, overnight	1.5–6 mo	N exhibit a deficiency in arousal mechanisms. TST at 1.5, 4.5 and 6 mo in N > C; AW at 1.5 and 3 mo in N < C. %AS in N at 3 mo > C.
Hoppenbrouwers (1989)	C 25 S 25	12 hr, overnight	1 wk–6 mo	*High variability* found within and between groups for all measures. AS–AW transition patterns were more common in C; in contrast, AS–QS transition patterns tended to occur in S.
Schechtman (1992)	C 66 V 16	12 hr, overnight	2–65 days	SIDS victims showed decreased AW and increased sleep during the early morning hours. At < 1 mo of age, SIDS victims had less REM than control infants.

C, Controls; N, "Near-miss" for SIDS; S, Sibling of SIDS victim; V, SIDS victim; AS, Active sleep; AW, Wakefulness; QS, Quiet sleep; REM, REM sleep; TST, total sleep time.

in metabolic activity (indicated by increases in heart and respiratory rates) facilitates state development via enhanced forebrain modulation of brainstem structures. Support for this hypothesis includes the observations that: (a) elevated thyroid hormone levels, which have been reported in the perinatal period in SIDS victims[34, 35] (but see cautionary remarks regarding interpretation of thyroid hormone level data),[36, 37] could increase the rate of maturation of CNS and sleep mechanisms; and (b) EEG-spindle activity, a hallmark of NREM sleep in adults, occurred earlier in siblings of SIDS than in control infants.[33] Sterman and Hodgman[24] note that in two previous studies[30, 38] where a relative reduction in QS in high-risk infants has been reported, recording periods occurred during daytime naps. A reduction in QS during the day in the high-risk

infants, according to Sterman and Hodgman, is consistent with the "accelerated maturation" hypothesis, since a shift in sleep consolidation towards the nighttime hours would result in less daytime sleep. These authors also point out the necessity to consider environmental factors that could contribute to group differences in maturation, such as the increased attention and stimulation given to siblings of SIDS by caregivers.

B. *The organization of sleep and arousal is disturbed in high-risk infants and in infants who later succumb to SIDS.*

In the early 1980s, Harper and colleagues[39–41] made a key observation that changed the focus of studies of infant sleep: Analysis of the specific order of sleep and AW (temporal sequencing) yields information about the development of sleep that may not be apparent from examination of the total amount or percentages of sleep states alone. Twenty SIBS and 20 matched controls were recorded overnight during the first week of life and subsequently at 1, 2, 3, 4, and 6 months of age, and each minute of the record was scored as AW, AS, or QS. Several features of sleep organization were common to both groups, including (a) an increase in low- (0–0.6 cycles/hr) and mid- (0.6–1.3 cycles/hr) frequency repetition of QS until 3 to 4 months of age and (b) a decrease in low-frequency (0–0.6 cycles/hr) repetition of AS with increases in age. However, differences in sleep organization appeared as early as the first week of life, where SIBS were found to have relatively longer intervals between AS bouts. At 2 and 3 months of age, spectral analysis revealed that some of the SIBS had longer intervals between AW periods compared with controls. These results indicate that SIBS have difficulty in making the transition from sleep to AW and may have a problem arousing from sleep. Furthermore, the finding that differences in sleep organization exist as early as the first week of life suggests that prenatal influences may be important determinants in the development of sleep in these infant groups.

Perhaps a more direct examination of the hypothesis that infants at risk for SIDS have altered sleep architecture derives from studies of state organization in infants who later succumbed to SIDS. Schechtman and colleagues found that infants who later died with a determination of SIDS exhibited much less waking during the end of the sleep period (a time of peak incidence for SIDS) and more waking in the period immediately following sleep onset, thus suggesting an altered circadian pattern of state organization.[42, 43]

A paucity of waking epochs during sleep that appears to characterize state organization in infants at risk has been seen in other laboratories as well. Challamel and colleagues[44] found that NM infants, relative to controls, had (a) more TST at 1.5, 4.5, and 6 months of age, (b) fewer awakenings (> 1 min) at 1.5 and 3 months, (c) an increase in REM at 3 months, and (d) a decrease in stage 2 NREM at 6 months of age. The authors view the increased REM at 3 months in NM infants as secondary to the decrease in awakenings seen at this age. The hypothesis of a long-standing deficit in arousal mechanisms in NM infants is supported by the finding that some NM infants studied at 9 and 12 months of age still had fewer awakenings than controls. In a separate

investigation, NM infants had less AW than SIBS at 6 months of age.[45] Similarly, Navelet and associates[46] studied sleep organization in control and high-risk (NM and SIBS) infants using overnight PSG and found that high-risk infants less than 3 months of age had less AW, which was in agreement with the findings of Harper and associates.[39] Awakenings occurred 3 to 5 times more often (per 100 min of a given sleep state) in AS compared to QS. High-risk infants also had more AS and longer QS and AS bout lengths, resulting in an increase in sleep-cycle duration. These authors concluded that the sleep patterns of high-risk infants indicate a disturbance of sleep-wake organization and that a decrease in AW or an increase in the arousal threshold, independent of homeostatic regulation *during* sleep, may increase the risk for SIDS. The studies suggest a disturbance in state organization and an apparent dampening of arousal mechanisms and provide an important context in which to pursue the hypothesis that a failure of neural mechanisms regulating sleep and arousal is a key factor in SIDS. Diminished myelination has been reported in rostral brain areas of SIDS victims[47] and may underlie some of the state-related findings described here (for review see ref. 5). Other recent neuropathologic and neurochemical findings that suggest disturbances in the regulation of sleep, breathing, and arousal mechanisms in SIDS victims include: (a) decreased striatal dopamine[48]; (b) an immature developmental pattern of increased neurotensin binding sites in the nucleus tractus solitarius (NTS) of the medulla[49]; (c) decreased beta-endorphin levels in the pons and medulla[50]; and (d) hypoplasia of the arcuate nucleus of the ventral medulla.[51] Conflicting results have been reported regarding the size and density of hypoglossal neurons, which play a major role in regulating upper airway tone.[52, 53] It is important to appreciate the technical difficulties in analyzing human tissue, which are complicated by both antemortem and postmortem factors.[54]

It could be argued that an appropriate clinical diagnostic test for risk of SIDS could be the assessment of state organization in infants. However, it is important to note that the preceding findings represent group differences, that not all state measures will differentiate risk groups, and that exceptionally high variability characterizes state measures in individuals.[25] *Intragroup* variability may result from environmental and infant factors or from the instability of recording measures collected on only one night at any given developmental age. *Intergroup* variability may also be influenced by suppositions about the homogeneity of infant groups; for example, SIBS have been considered to be at four- to tenfold higher risk for SIDS than control infants. Even allowing for the high end of this spectrum (i.e., a 2% vs 0.2% incidence of SIDS in SIBS), a practical question is whether (and when) a consistent disorder or abnormality occurs in all SIBS or, considering the other extreme, whether 98% of SIBS do not differ from controls.

Another important point of discussion relates to scoring and classification of infant sleep, since uniform agreement on this issue is lacking. For example, at 3 months of age, infant sleep patterns are routinely scored using adult criteria[23]; prior to this age, an infant scoring manual is available.[55] Techniques that use cardiorespiratory assessment of sleep state,[56] video analysis,[28] and a mattress sensitive to respiration and motion[29] have been implemented and validated. Criteria differ for assessment of "indeterminate sleep," which occupies 10 to 20% of TST. Classification of infant sleep also becomes progressively more difficult at earlier postnatal ages, especially in the preterm infant. An excellent review of technical aspects of sleep scoring in neonates is presented by Scher and associates.[57] It should be stressed that in preterm infants and in term infants during the first postnatal weeks, *two* active sleep periods (low-voltage/continuous EEG activity vs mixed frequency/discontinuous EEG) and *two* quiet sleep periods (high-voltage/continuous EEG vs tracé alternant) exist in each sleep cycle. The differentiation of these subtypes of AS and QS relative to physiologic regulation is an important area for future study.

Respiratory and Cardiac Mechanisms in SIDS

Respiratory Control

Control of respiration during sleep in neonates and adults have been described earlier in this volume, and specific issues related to respiratory pattern and SIDS have been detailed elsewhere (see Chapter 4 and Kryger MH, et al: Principles and Practice of Sleep Medicine, 2nd ed, Chap 15).[58] The most likely fatal scenario in a SIDS event includes *upper airway obstruction*, presumably during sleep. That hypothesis derives from the petechiae found at autopsy in a large proportion (in some structures, such as the lung, up to 85%) of cases.[59] Petechiae are found in a variety of other circumstances; however, the particular distribution within the thorax in SIDS victims argues strongly for substantial negative thoracic pressure generating this sign. Airway obstruction could be generated by a number of mechanisms,[60] including seizure discharge, and may not necessarily be preceded by repetitive occurrences of apnea as is characteristic in the adult OSAS. Examination for repetitive pathologic apnea or other respiratory abnormalities in records of infants at risk for SIDS, or for infants who later succumbed, generally proves negative; however, many of these examinations do not partition the effect of state and thus are limited in evaluating the interaction of respiratory and cardiac rhythms and sleep. Moreover, few studies record upper airway flow and diaphragmatic movements during sleep to detect obstructive events.

Two major characteristics of respiratory control during sleep may contribute to the potential for airway obstruction. First, although respiratory patterning is extremely regular during QS, inspiratory time and negative thoracic pressures are enhanced. Excessive negative pressures accompanied by upper airway obstruction may lead to further airway collapse from the Venturi effect. Second, together with extreme variation in respiratory patterning during REM sleep, a substantial loss of upper airway and thoracic wall muscle tone develops; the decrease in tone is so marked as to cause paradoxical rib cage movement in young infants and a concomitant fall in vital capacity (see Chapter 4).[61] Atonia in upper airway muscles contributes to obstruction by increasing compliance in the pharyngeal airway. Investigations which have partitioned upper air flow and diaphragmatic activity suggest that there may be a propensity for obstructive apnea during AS.[62] SIBS may breathe faster,[63] and infants who later succumb to SIDS have fewer short central apneas (pauses of 4–7 sec) in both QS and REM at ages near the peak incidence of SIDS.[64] These data suggest that respiratory patterning in these infants is less responsive to other physiologic influences (respiratory, baroreceptor, or other somatic input), which normally influences breathing rate. No differences in *overall* respiratory rate or long-term variation has been noted in infants who later die.

A "failure to arouse" (FTA) may play a critical role in SIDS. The ability to make a transition to the waking state after airway obstruction is particularly important. Normally, obstructions of the upper airway are terminated by an arousal, with restoration of upper airway muscle tone by so-called "wakefulness stimuli."[65] It might be argued that the "cause" of the fatal event is initiated by an obstructed upper airway but that the mechanism for failure is an inability to make the transition to the waking state, a transition which a normally adapting infant should accomplish. Within the context of FTA, the relative propensity for arousal from different states is an issue. Responses to nasal obstruction appear to be more frequent in AS compared to QS,[66] but the effectiveness of stimuli to induce arousal may differ by state and age.[19, 67] For example, the percentages of FTA in response to a vibrotactile stimulus remained consistently higher in QS than AS over the first 6 months of life in normal infants,[19] although a significant increase in the percentage of FTA in AS occurred at 3 months of age.

Walker and associates[68] point out that in lambs latencies to arousal in response to acute reductions in blood pressure are longer in REM than in NREM sleep, although arousal is impaired in both sleep states. Yet another perspective is that arousing stimuli in certain infants may *actively inhibit* respiratory and arousal responses by virtue of defective maturation of the neural arousal system.[69]

Recent evidence exists that seizure discharge can lead to prolonged apnea in infants.[70] The propensity for seizure discharge to occur during sleep and the increased disposition for seizures at elevated temperatures hint at a potential mechanism for death in SIDS infants who were excessively warm when found in their cribs. Seizures that originate from subcortical limbic sites may be effective at modifying respiratory patterning,[16] and detection would not be obtained by conventional scalp recording.

Cardiac Patterning

The normal development of heart rate and its variability does not follow simple linear trends from birth; moreover, the trends markedly differ by state.[71] The developmental period near 1 month of age is of particular interest because of a peak in heart rate, a trough in heart rate variation values for QS, and the beginning of disparate trends in variation in other states during that time. The nonuniform overall patterns of heart rate variation direct attention to the different sources of instantaneous variation contributing to moment-to-moment changes in heart rate. It is now apparent that sources of heart rate changes differ radically with sleep state and that different components of the autonomic nervous system are recruited to mediate these changes. Representative patterns of instantaneous heart rate variability as a function of state are shown in Figure 21–1.

Studies of *summary* cardiac rate and variation values have established that infants who later succumb to SIDS have higher heart rates in all states[72, 73] and diminished heart rate variation in waking, particularly by variation induced by breathing; the latter finding required partitioning of sleep state to ascertain the group differences.[73, 74] SIBS also have higher heart rates, especially in QS.[75] There is little evidence to suggest prolonged Q-T intervals are a factor; however, this issue is an area of controversy.[76] Similarly, little evidence exists for clinically significant cardiac arrhythmia in infants who later succumb.[77]

Examination of cardiac interbeat variability provides insights into the nature of physiologic responsivity underlying autonomic control in the developing infant and has the potential for identifying characteristics of infants at risk for SIDS. This utility stems from the exquisite sensitivity of cardiac interval patterning to sympathetic and parasympathetic segments of the autonomic nervous system, and the recognition that components of heart rate variation can be mathematically partitioned to determine the sources of the underlying variation. Summary procedures, such as means, standard deviations, and spectral estimates, are used to describe cardiac variation; dynamic or moment-to-moment interbeat characteristics are often masked by these procedures. Dynamic procedures reveal cardiac interval dispersion differences during sleep states in infants who later succumbed to SIDS; whereas, summary procedures demonstrate differences only in waking.[78] Dynamic procedures have been effective in describing cardiac arrhythmia and interval patterning following acute pharmacologic challenge,[79, 80] cardiac variation in animals subjected to myocardial ischemia,[81] cardiac variation in congenital hypoventilation syndrome ("Ondine's curse"),[82] and in congestive heart failure patients who succumb.[83]

SIDS infants show a distribution of cardiac interbeat dispersion with changing heart rate similar to what is seen in infants with congeni-

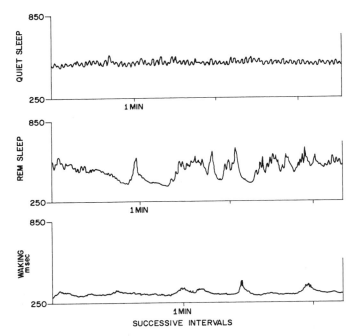

Figure 21–1. The time between cardiac beats (R-R intervals) are successively plotted from one 2-month-old infant during different sleep states; the R-R intervals are plotted on the y axis and successive beats are plotted on the x axis. Note the modulation of intervals at approximately 20 per minute in the QS record. These near-cyclical changes of cardiac intervals result from respiratory-induced influences, the major source of variation in that state. During REM sleep, that modulation is greatly diminished, but influences that modify variation for much longer periods of time appear; these influences exert a much more pronounced effect on overall variability than influences during QS. A similar relative absence of respiratory-related variation as well as a typical increase in heart rate (shorter intervals, lower values on y axis) characterize the waking record. Note that although *overall* variation may be lower in QS, the one interval-next interval changes during the pronounced, sustained accelerations and decelerations of REM and waking may be smaller than the rapid transitions in intervals required for respiratory-related variation in QS (see Fig. 21–2). (From Schechtman VL, et al: Development of heart rate variation over the first 6 months of life in normal infants. Pediatr Res 26:343, 1989.)

tal hypoventilation syndrome[78, 83]; however, the pattern is much less pronounced. Although heart rate showed considerable variation *(and thus was not "fixed")*, one interval-next interval dispersion differed from control infants in that it did not increase as rate decreased (Fig. 21–2). Moreover, cardiac rate appeared to be "clamped" about central values; that is, a change in interval was more frequently followed by a change in the opposite direction in SIDS victims, relative to controls. These findings suggest more rigid control of cardiac variation in SIDS victims, although *overall* variation is only minimally restricted.

The *loss of change* in one interval-next interval variation at different heart rates suggests that the cardiovascular system is less responsive to modulation by other physiologic systems in those infants who succumb. The other physiologic systems may be somatomotor (respiratory influences perhaps being one source), temperature, or even baroreceptor. The interpretation of reduced responsivity is reinforced by examining patterns of heart rate changes: infants who later succumb to SIDS show fewer sustained interbeat changes than controls. Thus, the development of sources contributing to cardiac variability appear to differ in infants at risk.

Other lines of evidence suggest some alteration of the autonomic nervous system in infants who later succumb to SIDS. Both para-

sympathetic and sympathetic components appear to be subtly modified. The evidence for sympathetic activation derives from findings of enhanced sweating in SIDS victims,[84] while the altered variation in heart rate intervals described earlier, including the diminished respiratory influences on heart rate variation, suggests altered vagal outflow.

Thermoregulatory Control

It is well known from numerous studies on adult humans and animals that (a) thermoregulation is influenced both by sleep and circadian factors; (b) body temperature is regulated at a lower level during NREM sleep than during AW; (c) during REM sleep there is a marked inhibition of thermoregulation; and (d) body temperature and the thermal environment are powerful modulators of arousal state distribution. However, there is a paucity of data on the interaction of temperature, thermoregulation, and sleep in infants. A detailed review of the development of thermoregulation in infants is presented elsewhere (see Kryger MH, et al: Principles and Practice of Sleep Medicine, 2nd ed, Chap. 20).

A primary reason for studying the interaction of sleep and temperature in infants is that temperature may play a key role in SIDS mechanisms. Several groups have reported an

Figure 21–2. A useful procedure for evaluating moment-to-moment changes in cardiac intervals is the Poincaré plot. These plots involve displaying each cardiac R-R interval against its predecessor.[120] The resulting plots provide an indication of average rate, dispersion in one interval-next interval values for any observed heart rate, overall heart rate variation, and the trend of dispersion in interbeat interval as rate changes. The plots demonstrate markedly different patterns from SIDS victims and controls during each sleep state. The SIDS plots show a lack of fan-shaped scatter, produced by increased dispersion of points at slower rates, which is apparent in the control plots; instead, these SIDS plots show a uniform dispersion (long, narrow scatter) for all values of interbeat intervals on the x axis. This scatter suggests that particular types of variation are missing in SIDS victims, especially the longer one interval-next interval dispersions at slower rates. The SIDS patterns are similar to patterns observed in infants afflicted with congenital central hypoventilation syndrome ("Ondine's curse").[82] Note that the SIDS infants shown exhibited relatively normal *overall* variation, indicated by the range of intervals on the x axis; thus heart rate is *not* fixed. (From Schechtman VL, et al: Dynamic analysis of cardiac R-R intervals in normal infants and in infants who subsequently succumbed to the sudden infant death syndrome. Pediatr Res 31:606, 1992.)

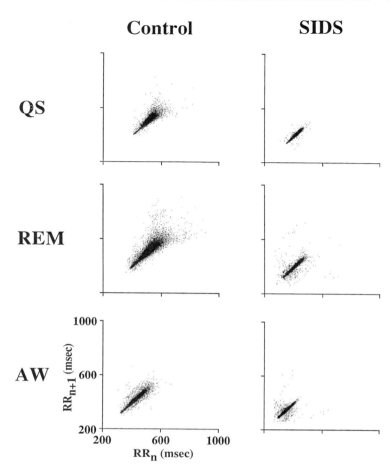

association between cold outdoor temperatures and increased rates of SIDS.[85–87] In some infants, an intrinsic problem of body temperature control may exist. Stanton found higher-than-expected body temperatures in SIDS victims postmortem.[88] Naeye found that some SIDS victims had experienced more bouts of hypothermia and hyperthermia compared with control infants.[89] Kahn and colleagues noted that many infants considered to be at higher risk for SIDS are observed to sweat more than normal infants.[90] Temperature can modulate sleep state distribution with decreased sleep outside of thermoneutrality and a relatively lower percentage of REM sleep as ambient temperature deviates from thermoneutrality.[14] Warm temperatures in the upper thermoneutral zone enhance REM and also result in more apneic periods and reduced upper airway patency.[91–94] Many SIDS victims are reported to have had a mild illness just prior to their death; fever or the sleep disruption resulting from the illness could increase

the number of obstructive apneic events[95] and could result in the depth and duration of recovery sleep with an increased arousal threshold. Thus, temperature could influence SIDS risk by multiple routes via an interaction with sleep, respiratory control, and arousal mechanisms.

In the normal infant, thermoregulatory effector mechanisms (i.e., evaporative water loss; metabolic heat production) are operating soon after birth. Unfortunately, little data are available on the changes in these effector systems during sleep state transitions or how the system response characteristics in REM sleep compare with NREM sleep. An important goal of future research will be to quantify the extent to which thermoregulatory reflexes are inhibited during both REM and NREM sleep states, and also to measure the interaction of thermal and respiratory stimuli on arousal thresholds during sleep stages in the developing infant. Although SIDS victims or infants who were NM for SIDS had been observed to have more frequent episodes of sweating prior to death compared with control infants, it is not possible to relate these findings to sleep-specific disturbances.[62, 90] Since thermoregulatory sweating in adult humans is inhibited in REM,[96, 97] a decrease in evaporative water loss in REM and concomitant increase in core temperature may be precarious for a heavily clothed infant in a warm environment. Finally, temperature may have direct effects on breathing, which may be independent from the influence of temperature on sleep and arousal.[98]

Investigations on the development of sleep in infants have involved solitary sleeping infants. In view of the recent speculation that infant-parent co-sleeping may reduce SIDS risk,[27] it is of interest to consider how the interaction of sleep and temperature might vary with sleeping environment and how this interaction might influence infant development. Although co-sleeping may be associated with potential benefits to the developing infant, it may pose hazards in the case of parental alcohol or substance abuse or if the parents themselves manifest sleep pathology. In terms of thermal modeling, the solitary sleeping environment is a relatively simple system that is characterized by a stable or slowly changing thermal environment with little feedback. In solitary sleepers, however, there is thermal contact during the night when the mother or caregiver feeds the infant. Additionally, Wailoo and associates[99] found that over 75% of infants 3 to 4 months of age aroused the parents at least once during the night. Moreover, the pattern was related to the thermal environment of the infant: the higher the room temperature or the greater the amount of bedclothes, the more often babies aroused their parents and the majority of these infants were found to be sweating. If an infant is unable to arouse in response to a high environmental temperature (or if a parent is unable to respond), then the infant may be at higher risk for SIDS. In contrast, the thermal features of the co-sleeping environment provide more complex interactions with the parents, infant, and surroundings influencing each other, including dynamic thermal stimuli as the position of the parents changes relative to the infant. Parents can also provide immediate protection to the infant in response to inappropriate thermal environments, that is, by regulating room temperature. In some scenarios, however, infants in the co-sleeping environment may have problems keeping cool, and thus it would be of interest to study the

relationship between core body temperature and sleep architecture in co-sleeping infants.

Finally, the prone sleeping position has been associated with increased SIDS risk.[100, 101] Ponsonby and associates[102] concluded that the association between the prone sleeping position and elevated risk of SIDS is increased by four independent factors: the use of natural-fiber mattresses, swaddling, recent illness, and the heat in bedrooms. Guntheroth and Spiers[103] reviewed seven studies on sleeping position and SIDS and calculated that the relative risk for SIDS is increased four- to ninefold in the prone sleeping position; they recommended avoiding placing infants in the prone sleeping position during the first 6 months of life. Similarly, the American Academy of Pediatrics, based on a review of the available literature, recently recommended that healthy infants be positioned on their side or back when being put down for sleep.[104] However, Hunt and Shannon[105] believe that these recommendations are premature, questioning the validity of the relationship reported between sleeping position and SIDS and articulating possible negative effects of the conversion to supine sleeping. They argue that rigorous studies need to be done to test the hypotheses generated by the available epidemiologic data and suggest that any risks associated with the prone sleeping position may be counterbalanced by equivalent risks encountered in the supine sleeping position. Although the effect of prone versus supine sleeping position on sleep architecture and arousal is unclear, some investigators postulated that the mechanisms underlying the association between sleeping position and SIDS involve decreases in heat loss through the face.[106] However, Peterson and associates[107] recently found that the prone sleeping position was associated with only a small decrease in the effectiveness of heat loss. Since core body temperature versus time of night did not differ in infants sleeping prone versus supine, these authors concluded that during the first 6 months of life normal infants can thermoregulate effectively in a variety of thermal environments independent of sleeping position.

A number of recent studies suggest that lethal rebreathing and accidental suffocation may occur in conjunction with the prone sleeping position in specific sleep environments. After examination of the death scene, Kemp and Thach[108] used a rabbit model, in which rabbits breathed into bedding materials through the airway of an infant mannequin to simulate an infant's respiratory microenvironment. They concluded that accidental suffocation by rebreathing was the most likely cause of death in infants who were found face down and certain types of cushions may hamper an infant's ability to turn their head to avoid excessive CO_2 buildup. Therefore, there may be a need to reassess the cause of death in the victims of SIDS who are found with their faces straight down (approximately 25–50%), and the potential for lethal rebreathing needs to be established for conventional infant mattresses, bedding, and sheepskins.[109, 110] Even infants with a head position of 45 degrees relative to the bedding may experience a rapid buildup of CO_2 and depletion of O_2, posing a hazard especially in infants less than 3 months of age whose controlled lifting of the head is still maturing.[111]

Summary

Throughout the fetal, neonatal, and infant developmental period, the maturation of physiologic homeostatic regulatory systems show considerable overlap. Of particular relevance to SIDS are systems controlling arousal states, circadian rhythms, body temperature, breathing, and cardiac control. In the adult, profound interactions occur between these regulatory systems; in the developing infant, dependencies occur between physiologic systems but the description of these interactions is still unfolding. Sleep states, which are also undergoing development, provide overriding switches that change interactions between physiologic systems. At present, it is not possible to conclude which sleep state, AS or QS, represents a more inherently vulnerable period for the infant. AS has been argued to offer protection to the infant by virtue of its phasic stimulation[112]; alternatively, prolonged bouts of AS may result in potentially catastrophic feedback cycles in which homeostasis and arousal are compromised.[14, 91, 113] Higher arousal thresholds have been demonstrated in both AS and QS, indicating that arousal threshold may be species, modality, and age-specific. AS is accompanied by a profound atonia that extends to muscles of the upper airway and may promote airway obstruction. It is quite probable that *each* sleep state may provide periods of varying vulnerability depending on both infant and environmental variables and on sleep history. Most importantly, the nature of sleep states and interactions

with other regulatory systems changes as rostral brain structures mature and modulate more early-developing caudal brain structures.

The available evidence suggests that some infants who succumb to SIDS manifest signs of physiologic and state disturbance from the first week of life. Together with epidemiologic evidence demonstrating that maternal smoking, inadequate prenatal medical care, and maternal anemia are associated with increased risk for SIDS,[114–118] these signs underscore the importance of clarifying the importance of prenatal events in SIDS etiology. The physiologic evidence strongly suggests some alteration in state organization that depresses arousal mechanisms in SIDS victims and some disturbance of autonomic regulation sufficient to impair overall cardiac rate and to modulate influences on heart rate variability. Evidence exists that autonomic influences controlling temperature, or some failure of temperature regulation, may be associated with the fatal event. Additional data point to a disturbance in ongoing respiratory patterning and possibly a failure that includes upper airway obstruction in the terminal event. The event may become catastrophic as a result of the depressed arousal mechanisms described earlier. Since the final event in SIDS appears to be intimately involved with sleep and in the interaction of sleep with other control systems, it is imperative to analyze and understand the role of sleep state effects to clarify mechanisms leading to SIDS.

References

1. Ariagno RL, Glotzbach SF: Sudden infant death syndrome. *In* Rudolph AM (ed): Pediatrics, 19th ed. Norwalk: Appleton and Lange, 1991, pp 850–858.
2. Guntheroth WG: Crib Death: The Sudden Infant Death Syndrome, 2nd ed. Mount Kisco, Futura, 1989, p 324.
3. Schwartz PJ, Southall DP, Valdez-Dapena M: The Sudden Infant Death Syndrome: Cardiac and Respiratory Mechanisms and Interventions. New York, The New York Academy of Sciences, 1988, p 474.
4. Harper RM, Hoffman HJ: Sudden Infant Death Syndrome: Risk Factors and Basic Mechanisms. New York, PMA Publishing Corp, 1988, p 536.
5. Kinney H, Filiano JJ, Harper RM: The neuropathology of the sudden death syndrome. A review. J Neuropath Exp Neurol 51:155, 1992.
6. Steinschneider A: Prolonged apnea and the sudden infant death syndrome: clinical and laboratory observations. Pediatrics 50:646, 1972.
7. Naeye RL: Pulmonary arterial abnormalities in the sudden-infant-death syndrome. N Engl J Med 289:1167, 1973.
8. Naeye RL: Hypoxemia and the sudden infant death syndrome. Science 186:837, 1974.

9. Weese-Mayer DE, Silvestri JM: Documented monitoring: an alarming turn of events. Clin Perinatol 19:891, 1992.
10. Mitchell EA, Ford RP, Stewart AW, et al: Smoking and the sudden infant death syndrome. Pediatrics 91:893, 1993.
11. Schoendorf KC, Kiely JL: Relationship of sudden infant death syndrome to maternal smoking during and after pregnancy. Pediatrics 90:905, 1992.
12. Bentele KH, Albani M: Are there tests predictive for prolonged apnoea and SIDS? A review of epidemiological and functional studies. Acta Paediatr Scand Suppl 342:2, 1988.
13. Harper RM: Physiological mechanisms in SIDS. In Harper RM, Hoffman HJ (eds): Sudden Infant Death Syndrome: Risk Factors and Basic Mechanisms. New York, PMA Publishing Corp, 1988, pp 515–517.
14. Glotzbach SF, Heller HC: Temperature regulation. In Kryger MH, Roth T, Dement WC (eds): Principles and Practice of Sleep Medicine, 2nd ed. Philadelphia, WB Saunders, 1994, pp 260–275.
15. Johnson P: Environmental temperature and the development of breathing. In Harper RM, Hoffman HJ (eds): Sudden Infant Death Syndrome: Risk Factors and Basic Mechanisms. New York, PMA Publishing Corp, 1988, pp 233–248.
16. Harper RM: State-related physiological changes and risk for the sudden infant death syndrome. Aust Paediatr J Suppl:55, 1986.
17. Brady JP, McCann EM: Control of ventilation in subsequent siblings of victims of sudden infant death syndrome. J Pediatr 106:212, 1985.
18. McCulloch K, Brouillette RT, Guzzetta AJ, et al: Arousal responses in near-miss sudden infant death syndrome and in normal infants. J Pediatr 101:911, 1982.
19. Newman NM, Trinder JA, Phillips KA, et al: Arousal deficit: mechanism of the sudden infant death syndrome? Aust Paediatr 25:196, 1989.
20. Davidson-Ward SL, Bautista DB, Sargent CW, et al: Arousal responses to sensory stimuli in infants at increased risk for sudden infant death syndrome. Am Rev Resp Dis 104:A809, 1990.
21. Jouvet-Mounier D, Astic L, Lacote D: Ontogenesis of the states of sleep in rat, cat, and guinea pig during the first postnatal month. Devel Psychobiol 2:216, 1970.
22. Coons S: Development of sleep and wakefulness during the first 6 months of life. In Guilleminault C (ed): Sleep and Its Disorders in Children. New York, Raven Press, 1987, pp 17–27.
23. Hoppenbrouwers T: Sleep in infants. In Guilleminault C (ed): Sleep and Its Disorders in Children. New York, Raven Press, 1987, pp 1–15.
24. Sterman MB, Hodgman J: The role of sleep and arousal in SIDS. In Schwartz PJ, Southall DP, Valdez-Dapena M (eds): The Sudden Infant Death Syndrome: Cardiac and Respiratory Mechanisms and Interventions. New York, The New York Academy of Sciences, 1988, pp 48–61.
25. Hoppenbrouwers T, Hodgman J, Arakawa K, et al: Polysomnographic sleep and waking states are similar in subsequent siblings of SIDS and control infants during the first six months of life. Sleep 12:265, 1989.
26. McKenna JJ: An anthropological perspective on the sudden infant death syndrome (SIDS): the role of parental breathing cues and speech breathing adaptations. Med Anthropol 10:9, 1986.
27. McKenna JJ, Mosko S, Dungy C, et al: Sleep and arousal patterns of co-sleeping human mother/infant pairs: a preliminary physiological study with implications for the study of sudden infant death syndrome. Am J Phys Anthropol 83:331, 1990.
28. Anders TF, Keener M: Developmental course of nighttime sleep-wake patterns in full-term and premature infants during the first year of life. I. Sleep 8:173, 1985.
29. Thoman EB, McDowell K: Sleep cyclicity in infants during the earliest postnatal weeks. Physiol Behav 45:517, 1989.
30. Haddad GG, Walsh EM, Leistner HL, et al: Abnormal maturation of sleep states in infants with aborted sudden infant death syndrome. Pediatr Res 15:1055, 1981.
31. Guilleminault C, Ariagno R, Korobkin R, et al: Sleep parameters and respiratory variables in "near miss" sudden infant death syndrome infants. Pediatrics 68:354, 1981.
32. Guilleminault C, Coons S: Sleep states and maturation of sleep: a comparative study between full-term normal controls and near-miss SIDS infants. In Tildon JT, Roeder LM, Steinschneider A (eds): Sudden Infant Death Syndrome. New York, Academic Press, 1983, pp 401–411.
33. Sterman MB, McGinty DJ, Harper RM, et al: Developmental comparison of sleep EEG power spectral patterns in infants at low and high risk for sudden death. Electroencephalogr Clin Neurophysiol 53:166, 1982.
34. Tildon JT, Chacon MA: Changes in hypothalamic-endocrine function as possible factor(s) in SIDS. In Tildon JT, Roeder LM, Steinschneider A (eds): Sudden Infant Death Syndrome. New York, Academic Press, 1983, pp 211–219.
35. Risse M, Weiler G, Benker G: Comparative histologic and hormonal studies of the thyroid gland with special reference to sudden infant death (SIDS). Z Rechtsmed 96:31, 1986.
36. Schwarz EH, Chasalow FI, Erickson MM, et al: Elevation of postmortem triiodothyronine in sudden infant death syndrome and in infants who died of other causes: a marker of previous health. J Pediatr 102:200, 1983.
37. Wellby ML, Farror CJ, Pannall PR: Importance of postmortem changes in measurements of thyroid function in studies of sudden infant death syndrome. J Clin Pathol 40:631, 1987.
38. Gould JB: SIDS: a sleep hypothesis. In Tildon JT, Roeder LM, Steinschneider A (eds): Sudden Infant Death Syndrome. New York, Academic Press, 1983, pp 443–452.
39. Harper RM, Leake B, Hoffman H, et al: Periodicity of sleep states is altered in infants at risk for the sudden infant death syndrome. Science 213:1030, 1981.
40. Harper RM, Leake B, Miyahara L, et al: Temporal sequencing in sleep and waking states during the first 6 months of life. Exp Neurol 72:294, 1981.
41. Harper RM, Frostig Z, Taube D, et al: Development of sleep-waking temporal sequencing in infants at risk for the sudden infant death syndrome. Exp Neurol 79:821, 1983.
42. Schechtman VL, Harper RM: Time of night effects on heart rate variation in normal neonates. J Develop Physiol 16:349, 1991.
43. Schechtman VL, Harper RM, Wilson AJ, et al: Sleep state organization in normal infants and victims of the sudden infant death syndrome. Pediatrics 89:865, 1992.

44. Challamel MJ, Debilly G, Leszczynski MC, et al: Sleep state development in near-miss sudden infant death infants. *In* Harper RM, Hoffman HJ (eds): Sudden Infant Death Syndrome: Risk Factors and Basic Mechanisms. New York, PMA Publishing Corp, 1988, pp 423–434.

45. Samson-Dollfus D, Delapierre G, Nogues B, et al: Sleep organization in children at risk for sudden infant death syndrome. Sleep 11:277, 1988.

46. Navelet Y, Payan C, Guilhaume A, et al: Nocturnal sleep organization in infants "at risk" for sudden infant death syndrome. Pediatr Res 18:654, 1984.

47. Kinney H, Brody B, Finkelstein D, et al: Delayed central nervous system myelination in the sudden infant death syndrome. J Neuropath Exp Neurol 50:29, 1991.

48. Kalaria RN, Fiedler C, Hunsaker JC, et al: Synaptic neurochemistry of human striatum during development: changes in sudden infant death syndrome. J Neurochem 60:2098, 1993.

49. Chigr F, Denoroy L, Gilly R, et al: Absence of adrenergic neurons in nucleus tractus solitarius in sudden infant death syndrome. Neuropediatrics 24:25, 1993.

50. Pasi A, Mehraein P, Jehle A, et al: Beta-endorphin: regional levels profile in the brain of the human infant. Neurochem Int 20:93, 1992.

51. Filiano JJ, Kinney HC: Arcuate nucleus hypoplasia in the sudden infant death syndrome. J Neuropathol Exp Neurol 51:394, 1992.

52. O'Kusky JR, Norman MG: Sudden infant death syndrome: postnatal changes in the numerical density and total number of neurons in the hypoglossal nucleus. J Neuropathol Exp Neurol 51:577, 1992.

53. Konrat G, Halliday G, Sullivan C, et al: Preliminary evidence suggesting delayed development in the hypoglossal and vagal nuclei of SIDS infants: a necropsy study. J Child Neurol 7:44, 1992.

54. Kopp N, Najimi M, Champier J, et al: Ontogeny of peptides in human hypothalamus in relation to sudden infant death syndrome (SIDS). Prog Brain Res 93:167, 1992.

55. Anders T, Emde R, Parmelee AH: A Manual of Standardized Terminology, Techniques and Criteria for Scoring States of Sleep and Wakefulness in Newborn Infants. Los Angeles, UCLA Brain Information Service, 1971.

56. Harper RM, Schechtman VL, Kluge KA: Machine classification of infant sleep state using cardiorespiratory measures. Electroenceph Clin Neurophysiol 67:379, 1987.

57. Scher MS, Sun M, Hatzilabrou G, et al: Computer analyses of EEG-sleep in the neonate: methodological considerations. J Clin Neurophysiol 7:417, 1990.

58. Glotzbach SF, Ariagno RL: Periodic breathing. *In* Beckerman RC, Brouillette RT, Hunt CE (eds): Respiratory Control Disorders in Infants and Children. Baltimore, Williams and Wilkins, 1992, pp 142–160.

59. Krous HF: The microscopic distribution of intrathoracic petechiae in sudden infant death syndrome. Arch Pathol Lab Med 108:77, 1984.

60. Thach BT, Davies AM, Koenig JS: Pathophysiology of sudden upper airway obstruction in sleeping infants and its relevance for SIDS. *In* Schwartz PJ, Southall DP, Valdes-Dapena M (eds): The Sudden Infant Death Syndrome: Cardiac and Respiratory Mechanisms and Interventions. New York, The New York Academy of Sciences, 1988, pp 314–328.

61. Henderson-Smart DJ, Read DJC: Reduced lung volume during behavioral active sleep in the newborn. J Appl Physiol 46:1081, 1979.

62. Kahn A, Wachholder A, Winkler M, et al: Prospective study on the prevalence of sudden infant death and possible risk factors in Brussels: preliminary results (1987–1988). Eur J Pediatr 149:284, 1990.

63. Hoppenbrouwers T, Hodgman JE, McGinty D, et al: Sudden infant death syndrome: sleep apnea and respiration in subsequent siblings. Pediatrics 66:205, 1980.

64. Schechtman VL, Harper RM, Wilson AJ, et al: Sleep apnea in infants who succumb to the sudden infant death syndrome. Pediatrics 87:841, 1991.

65. Orem J: Neural basis of behavior and state-dependent control of breathing. *In* Lydic R, Biebuyck JF, (eds): Clinical Physiology of Sleep. Bethesda, American Physiological Society, 1988, pp 79–96.

66. Newman NM, Frost JK, Bury L, et al: Responses to partial nasal obstruction in sleeping infants. Aust Paediatr J 22:111, 1986.

67. Igras D, Fewell JE: Arousal response to upper airway obstruction in young lambs: comparison of nasal and tracheal occlusion. J Devel Physiol 15:215, 1991.

68. Walker AM, Horne RS, Bowes G, et al: The circulation in sleep in newborn lambs. Aust Paediatr J Suppl:71, 1986.

69. Morrison AR: Sleep, arousal, and motor control. *In* Harper RM, Hoffman HJ (eds): Sudden Infant Death Syndrome: Risk Factors and Basic Mechanisms. New York, PMA Publishing Corp, 1988, pp 347–359.

70. Southall DP: Role of apnea in the sudden infant death syndrome: a personal view. Pediatrics 81:73, 1988.

71. Harper RM, Hoppenbrouwers T, Sterman MB, et al: Polygraphic studies of normal infants during the first 6 months of life. I. Heart rate and variability as a function of state. Pediatr Res 10:945, 1976.

72. Wilson AJ, Stevens V, Franks CI, et al: Respiratory and heart rate patterns in infants destined to be victims of the sudden infant death syndrome: average rates and their variability measured over 24 hours. Br Med J 290:497, 1985.

73. Schechtman VL, Harper RM, Kluge KA, et al: Cardiac and respiratory patterns in normal infants and victims of the sudden infant death syndrome. Sleep 11:413, 1988.

74. Kluge KA, Harper RM, Schechtman VL, et al: Spectral analysis assessment of respiratory sinus arrhythmia in normal infants and infants who subsequently died of sudden infant death syndrome. Pediatr Res 24:677, 1988.

75. Harper RM, Leake B, Hodgman JE, et al: Developmental patterns of heart rate and heart rate variability during sleep and waking in normal infants and infants at risk for the sudden infant death syndrome. Sleep 5:28, 1982.

76. Schwartz P: The sudden infant death syndrome. *In* Scarpelli EM, Cosui EV (eds): Reviews in Perinatal Medicine. New York, Raven Press, 1981, pp 475–524.

77. Southall DP, Arrowsmith WA, Stebbens V, et al: QT interval measurements before sudden infant death syndrome. Arch Dis Child 61:327, 1986.

78. Schechtman VL, Raetz SL, Harper RK, et al: Dynamic analysis of cardiac R-R intervals in normal infants and infants who subsequently succumbed to the sudden infant death syndrome. Pediatr Res 31:606, 1992.

79. Garfinkel AJ, Walter DO, Trelease RB, et al: Nonlinear dynamics of electrocardiographic waveforms following cocaine administration. Life Sci 48:2189, 1991.

80. Garfinkel A, Raetz SL, Harper RM: Heart rate dy-